Rare Diseases of the Immune System

Series Editors: Lorenzo Emmi, Domenico Prisco

According to the European Parliament, a disease is considered rare when it affects no more than 5 out of 10,000 people. People with rare diseases are not that scarce, however, since we are talking about a phenomenon that affects hundreds of thousands of people in Italy and several millions all over Europe. Many associations, both national and international, have been created in recent years to inform and safeguard patients affected by these syndromes. At the same time, across various disciplines the medical and scientific awareness of the challenges posed by these diseases has risen inexorably. Rare diseases due to alterations in the immune system represent a field of medical science of great interest that is undergoing continuous expansion; these syndromes have a great social and economic impact because they often affect young or very young people at the height of their social activities and relationships. In recent years, much information has been acquired on pathogenesis, diagnosis, and therapy, allowing us to confront these syndromes in a more holistic manner. The series editors are acknowledged experts on immune diseases who have published extensively on various facets of this branch of medicine. This series will be an invaluable resource for immunologists, rheumatologists, hematologists and medical practitioners looking to update their knowledge and a useful educational tool for residents and students.

Indexed in Scopus

Interested authors should contact the corresponding series editor, Lorenzo Emmi at: lorenzoemmi@yahoo.it

Vinod Ravindran • Sham Santhanam
Mohit Goyal
Editors

Rarer Arthropathies

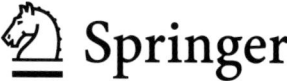 Springer

Editors
Vinod Ravindran
Centre for Rheumatology
Calicut, Kerala, India

Sham Santhanam
Department of Rheumatology
Kauvery Hospitals
Chennai, Tamil Nadu, India

Mohit Goyal
CARE Pain and Arthritis Centre
Goyal Hospital
Udaipur, Rajasthan, India

ISSN 2282-6505 ISSN 2283-6403 (electronic)
Rare Diseases of the Immune System
ISBN 978-3-031-05001-5 ISBN 978-3-031-05002-2 (eBook)
https://doi.org/10.1007/978-3-031-05002-2

This Springer imprint is published by the registered company Springer Nature Switzerland AG
The registered company address is: Gewerbestrasse 11, 6330 Cham, Switzerland

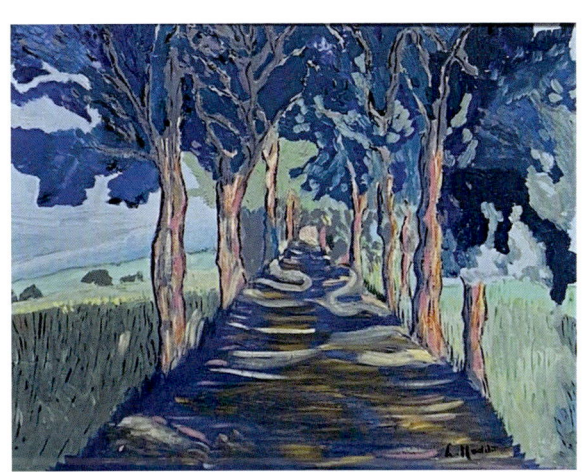

Alberi al mattino
Laura Maddii Emmi
(Private collection)

To my parents.

—Vinod Ravindran

To my parents, wife, and dear daughter and all my teachers.

—Sham Santhanam

To two of my wonderful teachers, Prof. Vijay Goyal, whose teachings helped build my approach to clinical medicine; and Prof. Ashok Kumar, who besides teaching in rheumatology has a great influence on how I strive to work each day.

—Mohit Goyal

Foreword

The diagnosis and management of rarer medical conditions is fascinating for any physician. Like all clinicians, since the time of my training, I get excited when making a diagnosis of a rare rheumatic disease. These cases are the basis of many grand rounds, postgraduate rheumatology meetings, and case reports in medical journals. Their diagnosis requires a high index of suspicion and they are generally challenging to manage. Not only they can masquerade as more common rheumatic conditions, but there are also no guidelines on management to follow. As the literature on these conditions grow, more and more clinicians are likely to diagnose and manage them better.

This book, *Rarer Arthropathies*, provides expert reviews on 19 conditions. There is scant literature on most of these. Conditions such as malignancies, sarcoidosis, tuberculosis, and leprosy can have bothersome musculoskeletal manifestations and timely recognition of these would help clinicians treat these patients better. Ochronosis, basic calcium phosphate-associated arthritis, multicentric reticulohistiocytosis, and RS3PE are though rare conditions but may pose diagnostic and therapeutic challenge. Rarer is an appropriate title for this book since some of the conditions such as palindromic rheumatism and diabetic cheiroarthropathy are not that uncommon. Others such as those associated with treatment by Immune Checkpoint Inhibitors are becoming more common as more patients are treated with these new treatments. Moreover, knowledge of musculoskeletal manifestations of hemochromatosis and fluorosis is important for correct attribution of the manifestations to these causes. On the other hand, recognition of hypertrophic osteoarthropathy is the key to a search for its cause. The volume is further enriched by up-to-date text on SAPHO syndrome and arthritis linked to Chikungunya virus and Brucellosis.

The editors have done a commendable job in bringing together these interesting topics in one volume and engaging authors with tremendous clinical experience and academic repute in the respective fields. Their expertise and knowledge, provides a bird's eye view at the beginning and then take the reader through the details on each topic. The text follows a structure, which remains largely uniform through all the chapters, making it easy to read and also locate the desired detail. Overall, this book provides an invaluable resource for busy practicing clinicians supporting them in the diagnosis and management of these rarer arthropathies.

Professor Ernest Choy
Head of Rheumatology and Translational Research
Institute of Infection and Immunity
Director of Arthritis Research UK CREATE Centre
and Welsh Arthritis Research Network (WARN)
Cardiff University School of Medicine
Cardiff, UK

Preface

Rheumatic diseases are fascinating as well as challenging to diagnose and manage. They can trick even the most experienced of clinicians at times. In general, these diseases often do not exhibit all the characteristics at presentation and evolve over time. Arthritis can be the presenting manifestation of a varied spectrum of autoimmune rheumatic diseases; it can also be seen in the settings of infections, malignancies, and metabolic diseases. Thus, the diagnosis of these rarer arthropathies is a challenge, especially at stages where they do not show features other than that of musculoskeletal system. For a clinician, the diagnosis of a rare disease or the rare presentation of an otherwise common disease brings satisfaction, and the patients get a timely diagnosis and the appropriate treatment. However, in the absence of an awareness of these conditions, one is more likely to miss the diagnosis as these rare arthropathies often mimic the relatively more common entities such as rheumatoid arthritis, spondyloarthritides, or other connective tissue disorders. Missing a malignancy or an infection (considering you may be planning to use immune modulators if you think it is an autoimmune disease) could spell disaster.

The literature available on many of these rare conditions is still extremely limited. In this context, our endeavors of compiling the existing knowledge in this book should hopefully prove useful for clinicians. This volume *Rarer Arthropathies* has 19 well thought out chapters covering a range of topics from rare arthropathies associated with systemic autoimmune diseases, metabolic diseases, and infections to malignancies. The authors, from five different continents, are authorities in their respective fields and have discussed the topics threadbare in an easy-to-understand format. The authors have been researching in these and associated areas and their depth of knowledge and understanding of the topic can be appreciated in this book.

The first five chapters discuss rare arthropathies associated with or variants of systemic autoimmune diseases. Chapter 1 is a review of palindromic rheumatism, a condition often considered related to rheumatoid arthritis. Chapter 2 details the patterns of musculoskeletal involvement in sarcoidosis, the role of imaging and the differentiation of the condition from tuberculosis. Chapter 3 reviews remitting seronegative symmetrical synovitis with pitting edema (RS3PE), a close mimic of many of the common rheumatic diseases and at times the presenting manifestation of an underlying malignancy. Chapter 4 discusses multicentric reticulohistiocytosis, an extremely rare condition with only around 300 cases reported in the literature.

Chapter 5 reviews SAPHO syndrome, sometimes considered a variant of psoriatic arthritis.

Chapter 6 on basic calcium phosphate arthropathies discusses the recognition and management of the Milwaukee shoulder syndrome and calcific periarthritis. Chapter 7 on neuropathic osteoarthropathy discusses this often unrecognized and sub-optimally managed condition and has many excellent clinical images.

The next four chapters cover metabolic diseases presenting as arthropathies. Chapter 8 details musculoskeletal manifestations of diabetes with special focus on cheiroarthropathy. Chapter 9 discusses the features and recognition of arthropathy in hemochromatosis, its genetics and the outcomes with currently available therapy. Chapter 10 on skeletal fluorosis, a condition endemic to the Asian and African countries, discusses the various skeletal manifestations and the preventive strategies. Chapter 11 discusses the pigment deposition disease ochronosis and its differentiation from close mimics such as like ankylosing spondylitis and osteoarthritis.

The next four chapters are on arthritis associated with infections, of which tuberculosis with its myriad osteo-articular manifestations (Chap. 12) and leprosy which is a close mimic of autoimmune inflammatory arthritis (Chap. 13) are more common in tropical and developing countries. Chikungunya (Chap. 14) though also endemic in the tropics has spread globally since the late 2000s, while Brucella arthritis (Chap. 15) is also seen in the Mediterranean region and Middle East. But all of these diseases have increasing global relevance in today's world due to increasing migration and travel.

Chapter 16 details hypertrophic pulmonary osteoarthropathy, a condition that should not be missed as it is usually secondary to an underlying disease which at times can be sinister. Chapter 17 discusses the patterns of carcinomatous arthritis, with useful clinical pointers to underlying malignancy. Chapter 18 covers the identification and tailored management of arthritis associated with immune checkpoint inhibitors. Last but not least, Chap. 19 covers still rarer arthropathies of amyloidosis and sickle cell disease and conditions namely Jaccoud's arthropathy and arthritis robustus, which have a serious dearth of available literature on them.

The book brings together these heterogenous conditions on the accounts of their rarity and their association with arthropathy. The chapters have illustrative tables and flowcharts to emphasize the important take-home messages for the readers. They contain several original clinical, histopathological, and radiographic images.

We hope the book would interest not only the rheumatologists and the physicians managing rheumatic diseases, but all clinicians as patients with these multisystem diseases more often present to other specialists and the primary care physician.

Calicut, Kerala, India   Vinod Ravindran
Chennai, Tamil Nadu, India   Sham Santhanam
Udaipur, Rajasthan, India   Mohit Goyal

Contents

Palindromic Rheumatism

1

Davide Corradini, Kulveer Mankia, and Andrea Di Matteo

1.1 Introduction

Palindromic rheumatism (PR) is an inflammatory condition that is characterized by recurring episodes of pain and swelling in and around the joints (i.e., "flares"), which usually affect either one joint at a time or a few joints together [1].

The word "Palindromic" is derived from the ancient Greek term "Palin dromein," which means "running back again" or "to go backwards". In its current use, a "palindrome" indicates a word or a phrase that is arranged symmetrically around an axis, and consequently it can be spelt the same backward and forward [2]. The term "Palindromic Rheumatism" was used for the first time by Hench and Rosenberg, who described this condition in 1944 [3]. The term "rheumatism" was preferred by the authors to "arthritis" to reflect the typical involvement of peri-articular soft tissues, rather than purely the joints, during the flares [1].

Flares of PR may last from a few hours to several days, but usually less than a week, and do not cause structural joint damage or permanent disability [4]. The intermittent behavior of PR (i.e., the patients are characteristically asymptomatic between the flares) is the key difference that distinguishes this condition from other arthritides, such as rheumatoid arthritis (RA), where joint inflammation becomes persistent if not properly treated [1].

D. Corradini
Rheumatology Unit, University of Cagliari and AOU University Clinic of Cagliari, Monserrato, Italy

K. Mankia
Leeds Institute of Rheumatic and Musculoskeletal Medicine, University of Leeds, Leeds, UK
e-mail: k.s.mankia@leeds.ac.uk

A. Di Matteo (✉)
Rheumatology Unit, Department of Clinical and Molecular Sciences, Polytechnic University of Marche, "Carlo Urbani" Hospital, Ancona, Italy

V. Ravindran et al. (eds.), *Rarer Arthropathies*, Rare Diseases of the Immune System, https://doi.org/10.1007/978-3-031-05002-2_1

Although encountered regularly by most rheumatologists, PR is often regarded as a relatively rare disease. The true incidence is not known. In a retrospective study on around 5000 patients with musculoskeletal symptoms, PR was diagnosed in 2.6% of patients [5]. Similar to RA, women are generally more affected than men (although some studies suggest equal sex distribution) and the average age of disease onset is around 40–45 years [6, 7].

1.2   Pathogenesis

The etiopathogenesis of PR is not completely understood and remains a matter of active debate between experts in the field. PR has been traditionally seen in close connection with RA, with which it shares autoimmune, genetic, and clinical factors [1]. Several studies have demonstrated that around 50% of PR patients will evolve into RA at some point during the disease. The clinical, genetic, and immunological similarities, and the evolution to RA in a considerable proportion of PR patients, suggest that PR may represent a prodromal phase of RA with relapsing-remitting symptoms (a "pre-rheumatoid state"), or an "at-risk" stage of the RA "continuum," rather than a distinct disease entity [6].

Patients with PR have an increased prevalence of HLA-DR shared epitope (SE) alleles compared with controls, which is the strongest genetic risk factor for RA. In patients with PR, homozygosity for SE alleles has been demonstrated to increase the risk of progression to persistent arthritis, and in particular RA [8]. Moreover, RA-related autoantibodies, such as anti-citrullinated protein antibodies (ACPA) and rheumatoid factor (RF), are frequently encountered in patients with PR (from 39 to 68% according to different studies), and often at high titers [5, 9]. Other than ACPA, a recent study also reported on the increased prevalence of anti-carbamylated auto-antibodies (a class of antibodies recently described in RA patients) in patients with PR [10].

While the shared genetic/autoimmune background and some clinical features (i.e., the pattern of joint involvement) advocate a close link between PR and RA, the ultrasound (US) findings detectable in these two conditions are considerably different. The typical US appearance of a RA joint consists of intra-articular synovial hypertrophy, which often exhibits increased vascularization, and bone erosions and/ or cartilage damage as signs of structural damage. Conversely, the US findings of patients with PR show a high prevalence of extracapsular/extra-articular inflammation (Fig. 1.1), such as tenosynovitis, peri-tendonitis of the extensor tendons of fingers, and peri-articular inflammation, but often no synovitis and rarely bone erosions [11].

Another potential mechanism in the etiopathogenesis of PR is auto-inflammation. The relapsing-remitting behavior and clinical presentation of PR flares (i.e., sudden-onset, skin erythema, and intense pain/tenderness) are similar to that seen in patients with microcrystalline arthritis [e.g., gout or calcium pyrophosphate deposition disease (CPPD)] or auto-inflammatory conditions, such as Familial Mediterranean Fever or Whipple's disease [12]. Moreover, the potential

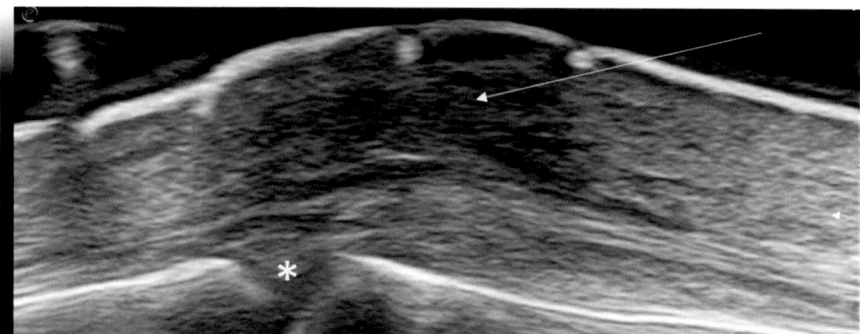

Fig. 1.1 Ultrasound findings of a PR flare. Longitudinal view of the fourth proximal interphalangeal joint in a patient with palindromic rheumatism. The image shows subcutaneous, peri-tendinous edema (arrow) while no synovitis is detected (asterisk). (Courtesy of A. Di Matteo, private collection)

efficacy of colchicine (commonly used in the management of the above conditions) in the prevention of flares in PR represents an additional factor supporting the auto-inflammatory hypothesis for PR [13]. Finally, in a recent Spanish study on 65 PR patients, MEFV mutations in at least one allele were found in more than 10% of patients, and more commonly in those who were ACPA-negative [10]. Mutations of MEFV have also been documented in patients with intermittent hydrarthrosis, a rare condition characterized by transient episodes of joint swelling and effusion mainly involving the knees. Patients with intermittent hydrarthrosis usually do not progress to persistent arthritis and show negative RA-related antibodies [14]. These findings raise the hypotheses that auto-inflammatory genes play a key role in the etiopathogenesis and clinical manifestations of PR and should be investigated, especially in those patients who have negative RA-related antibodies [15].

1.3 Clinical Features

The nature of PR flares is unpredictable. Acute attacks of PR are always of sudden-onset, without any prodrome. Symptoms rapidly escalate, usually reaching their peak within a day. The duration of the flares may range from a few hours to up to a week maximum, generally lasting for 2 or 3 days [1]. The topography of joint involvement in PR is analogous to that observed in patients with RA. The most commonly affected joints are wrists, metacarpophalangeal (MCP) joints, and proximal interphalangeal joints (PIP), while the knees and ankles are less frequently involved [5]. The spine and the sternoclavicular joints are generally spared in both conditions. The knee and ankle are involved in around 30–40% of patients. Less common is the involvement of elbows and hip joints (<20% of cases) [9]. Affected joints present the typical signs of inflammation: tenderness (which may be extremely severe), swelling, and warmth. Erythema of the overlying skin can be observed.

Systemic symptoms, such as fever, are usually absent. At the end of the attack, symptoms remit completely leaving the patient asymptomatic and without residual disability [3].

The natural history of PR follows three main outcomes: clinical remission of the disease (in around 15% of patients); recurrence of flares (without evolution into persistent arthritis) in 40–50% of patients; and evolution into another rheumatic disease, most commonly RA (in around 50% of patients) [4]. Interestingly, progression to RA mostly occurs within the first 2 years of disease onset, and very uncommonly after 10 years [5, 8]. In recent years, several potential risk factors for evolution into RA have been identified in patients with PR. The most studied and well-characterized are ACPA-positivity, homozygosity for SE, female sex, and hand involvement [5]. However, the presence of these predisposing factors is not sufficient to determine progression to RA in PR patients. Indeed, there is a fixed proportion of ACPA-positive PR patients who do not develop RA [9] thus suggesting that other genetic or environmental factors (or a combination of such factors) play a determinant role in the development of chronic arthritis. An important factor to take into account in the interpretation of these data is that most PR patients were on disease-modifying anti-rheumatic drugs, which may potentially have influenced their rate of progression to RA.

1.4   Diagnosis

1.4.1   Differential Diagnosis

In the last 75 years, several classification criteria have been proposed for PR, none of which has been validated or universally adopted [9, 16–18]. As shown in Table 1.1, these criteria share some common features: history of recurring, sudden-onset episodes of arthritis, involvement of at least two different joints during different attacks, and direct observation of the attack by the physician.

Therefore, the diagnosis of PR remains clinical, and it is mainly based on the typical relapsing-remitting presentation of the disease, and on the exclusion of other possible diseases that can cause intermittent arthritis/periarthritis (Table 1.2).

During flares, laboratory tests may show an increase of acute phase reactants, such as C-reactive protein and fibrinogen. Erythrocyte sedimentation rate may be normal or moderately raised. Hemoglobin is usually normal [15]. Positive RA-related antibodies, such as ACPA or RF are frequently identified and can be useful to establish a diagnosis of PR in the context of typical clinical features. However, the detection of ACPA may be a double-edged sword, potentially leading the physician to a wrong diagnosis of RA with a consequent risk of over-treatment; a thorough clinical assessment, including imaging where possible, is therefore essential. For example, the identification of extracapsular inflammation without synovitis with a compatible history and examination would suggest the patient has PR rather than early RA. The duration and persistence of symptoms, as well as the imaging pattern [11], are the most important features to consider in the differential diagnosis between PR and

Table 1.1 Main classification criteria proposed for palindromic rheumatism

Authors (Year)	Criteria
Pasero and Barbieri [16] (1986)	1. History of sudden-onset, recurrent attacks of mono-arthritis 2. Direct observation of an attack by a physician 3. >5 attacks in the last 2 years 4. >2 joints involved (in different attacks) 5. Negativity for X-ray alterations, elevation of acute phase reactants and for rheumatoid factor 6. Exclusion of other recurrent mono-arthritis (e.g., gout, chondrocalcinosis)
Hannonen [9] (1987)	1. Recurrent attacks of sudden-onset mono/polyarthritis and para-articular soft tissue inflammation lasting from a few hours to 1 week 2. Direct observation of an attack by a physician 3. >3 joints involved (in different attacks) 4. Exclusion of other arthritis
Guerne and Weissman [17] (1992)	1. 6-month-history of sudden-onset, recurrent episodes of mono/polyarthritis or soft tissue inflammation 2. Direct observation of an attack by a physician 3. >3 joints involved (in different attacks) 4. No X-ray erosions 5. Exclusion of other arthritis
Gonzalez-Lopez [18] (2000)	Diagnosis of palindromic rheumatism by a rheumatologist and history of brief sudden-onset recurrent episodes of mono/polyarthritis and at least two of the following: – Direct observation of an attack by a physician – >5 attacks in 2 years – >3 joints involved (in different attacks) – No X-ray alterations – Exclusion of other mono-arthritis

RA. Microcrystalline arthropathies, such as gout or CPPD, should also be considered. The clinical presentation of gout, CPPD, and PR is similar (i.e., sudden-onset, painful acute attacks with articular and peri-articular involvement). Different to PR, the first metatarsophalangeal joint is typically involved in gout ("podagra"). Gout should be considered as one of the differential diagnoses in patients with episodic mono or oligoarthritis. It can be confirmed by demonstration of uric acid crystals in the synovial fluid or by typical imaging findings on ultrasonography in the background of elevated uric acid levels. CPPD flares have a predilection for large joints (knee, shoulder, hip) and can last longer than a week.

Predisposing conditions for recurrent episodes of arthritis or tenosynovitis, such as inflammatory bowel diseases, skin psoriasis or recent infections (i.e., gastrointestinal, genitourinary, or respiratory) should also be investigated.

1.4.2 Imaging

Regarding imaging, conventional radiography (CR), magnetic resonance imaging (MRI), and US are helpful in the diagnosis of PR. CR is useful to document the absence of bone erosions. Indeed, all the proposed classification criteria [9, 16–18]

Table 1.2 Differential diagnosis of palindromic rheumatism

Microcrystalline arthropathies
– Gout
– Calcium pyrophosphate deposition disease
– Hydroxyapatite arthritis
Systemic autoinflammatory disorders
– Familial Mediterranean fever
– TRAPS syndrome (Tumour necrosis factor-associated periodic syndrome)
– CAPS syndrome (Cryopyrin-associated periodic syndrome)
– Mevalonate kinase deficiency
Infectious/reactive arthritis
– Septic arthritis
– Reactive arthritis
– Lyme disease
– Whipple's disease
Others
– Rheumatoid arthritis
– Psoriatic arthritis
– Behcet's disease
– Sarcoidosis
– Arthritis associated with inflammatory bowel disease or celiac disease
– RS3PE (Remitting seronegative symmetric synovitis and pitting edema)
– Intermittent hydrarthrosis
– Familial hyperlipoproteinemia
– Hereditary angioedema
– Relapsing polychondritis

for PR include the absence of radiographic damage. If bone erosions are detected, a different diagnosis should be considered, in particular, RA [16]. CR is also useful to detect the presence of calcium pyrophosphate crystal deposits, which should raise the suspicion of CPPD.

On MRI, typical findings consist of extracapsular involvement, such as subcutaneous edema, tenosynovitis (effusion and/or postcontrast enhancement within the tendon sheath), peri-tendinous edema (peri-tendinous effusion and/or postcontrast enhancement outside the tendon sheath), and peri-articular inflammation (extracapsular effusion and/or postcontrast enhancement of the extracapsular tissue) [1]. Synovitis has also been documented but almost always occurs alongside extracapsular inflammation [11]. This is different from RA, where isolated intra-articular inflammation is often seen.

The US is particularly useful for the detection of extracapsular inflammation during flares, such as tenosynovitis, peri-articular soft tissue inflammation, and peri-tendinous edema. Generally, no subclinical inflammation is observed during the asymptomatic phases of the disease [11]. The presence of isolated extracapsular inflammation is an important finding which can help in the differential diagnosis between PR and RA [11, 19]. In the latter, synovitis (with or without joint damage) is the predominant US abnormality [19]. However, peri-articular inflammation on the US has also been observed in other rheumatic conditions, such as psoriatic arthritis [20] and systemic lupus erythematosus [21], and therefore cannot be regarded as a specific feature of PR.

US is also useful for the identifications of crystal deposits, which may indicate the presence of gout or CPPD, the main conditions to consider in the differential diagnosis of PR. Other than the "double contour sign," which is arguably the most representative US finding in patients with gout, articular and tendinous monosodium urate microcrystal deposits of various morphology (i.e., "hard tophi," "soft tophi," "uratic clouds") can be detected in patients with gout [22]. On the other hand, the detection of hyperechoic spots/deposits within the hyaline fibrocartilage (i.e., the femoral condyle hyaline cartilage), or in the fibrocartilaginous structures of the knee (i.e., menisci), wrist (i.e., triangular fibrocartilage), and hip (i.e., acetabulum) suggest the diagnosis of CPPD [23].

1.5 Management

The management of patients with PR is notoriously difficult; because of the absence of clinical trial data and universally agreed guidelines for the treatment of PR, this is largely based on the clinician's personal preferences and experience [24]. Over the last 75 years, several treatments for PR have been described in the literature (Table 1.3).

Table 1.3 Main pharmacological treatments for palindromic rheumatism

Therapeutic goal	Treatment
Treatment of acute attacks	Nonsteroidal anti-inflammatory drugs (NSAIDs) – Acetylsalicylic acid – Indomethacin – Naproxen
	Systemic corticosteroids – Prednisone
	Analgesics – Paracetamol
Prevention of flares	Conventional disease-modifying anti-rheumatic drugs (DMARDs) – **Antimalarials (best evidence)** – Azathioprine – Leflunomide – Methotrexate – Sulphasalazine – D-penicillamine (not used in current rheumatology practice) – Gold (not used in current rheumatology practice)
	Biological DMARDs – Rituximab (promising role)
	Colchicine
	Systemic steroids – Prednisolone
Prevention of rheumatoid arthritis development	Conventional DMARDs – **Antimalarials (promising role)** – Gold (not used in current rheumatology practice)
	Biological DMARDs – Rituximab (promising role)

However, no randomized controlled trials have been carried out to evaluate the efficacy and safety of these treatments, with the majority of the studies addressing these aspects being case reports, case series, or small single-center retrospective studies being published more than 20 years ago. Treatments in PR are usually administered with the following purposes: to reduce the pain and inflammation during flares, to prevent or reduce the incidence of flares or their intensity, and to prevent progression to persistent arthritis. Nonsteroidal anti-inflammatory drugs, or short-term courses of oral corticosteroids, are commonly considered first-line therapy to control symptoms during acute attacks. Interestingly, despite these treatments being widely used in daily clinical practice, data supporting their efficacy for the treatment of PR flares are scarce [1]. The "autoinflammation hypothesis" provides the rationale for the use of colchicine. However, no study has ever evaluated the efficacy of colchicine during flares. Similarly, no studies investigating the potential role of interleukin-1 inhibitors have been carried out.

For the prevention of recurrent attacks, there is some evidence supporting the use of antimalarial drugs (i.e., hydroxychloroquine or chloroquine). In a non-randomized study of 90 patients with PR, hydroxychloroquine resulted in disease remission in half of the patients [8]. Similar results were observed in a more recent study, where clinical records of 92 patients were retrospectively analyzed; antimalarials use resulted in a reduction of the number and intensity of flares in 50% of patients [25]. While minimal evidence supports the use of methotrexate [17] or sulfasalazine [10], good results in preventing the recurrence of flares were observed in studies evaluating the efficacy of gold [9, 26, 27] and D-penicillamine [9]. However, these treatments are not part of the current rheumatology therapeutic armamentarium because of their toxicity.

Only one study has evaluated the value of biologic agents, with rituximab effective in preventing flares in a cohort of 33 patients with refractory PR [28]. Regarding the prevention (or delay) of the development of persistent arthritis, limited data support the promising role of antimalarials [5, 6, 8, 29].

1.6   Conclusion

Palindromic rheumatism is a distinctive clinical condition with a close connection with RA. The current evidence suggests two potentially different mechanistic pathways in the pathogenesis of PR: autoimmunity (that may lead to RA) and acute attacks with features of an auto-inflammatory component.

The diagnosis of PR is clinical and based on the typical behavior of the disease; short-lasting (i.e., less than a week) recurring flares of articular and peri-articular pain and swelling (i.e., "flares"), without residual disability or joint structural damage are characteristic. Imaging can support the diagnosis of PR by the detection of peri-articular, rather than just articular inflammation, and by showing the absence of joint structural damage (i.e., bone erosions).

The optimum treatment strategy for PR, especially for the treatment of acute flares, remains largely undefined. The most robust available evidence supports the use of antimalarials (i.e., hydroxychloroquine) to reduce the recurrence of PR flares and help obtain disease remission.

References

1. Mankia K, Emery P. What can palindromic rheumatism tell us? Best Pract Res Clin Rheumatol. 2017;31:90–8.
2. Silman A, Smolen JS, Weinblatt ME, et al. Rheumatology, vol. 1. 5th ed. Mosby Elsevier; 2010.
3. Hench PS, Rosenberg EF. Palindromic rheumatism: a "new" oft recurring disease of joints (arthritis, periarthritis, para-Arthritis) apparently producing no articular residues. Report of thirty-four cases; its relation to "angio-neural arthrosis", "allergic rheumatism" and rheumatoid arthritis. Arch Intern Med. 1944;73:293–321.
4. Mankia K, Emery P. Palindromic rheumatism as part of the rheumatoid arthritis continuum. Nat Rev Rheumatol. 2019;15:687–95.
5. Gonzalez-Lopez L, Gamez-Nava JI, Jhangri GS, et al. Prognostic factors for the development of rheumatoid arthritis and other connective tissue diseases in patients with palindromic rheumatism. J Rheumatol. 1999;26:540–5.
6. Sanmartí R, Cabrera-Villalba S, Gómez-Puerta JA, et al. Palindromic rheumatism with positive anticitrullinated peptide/protein antibodies is not synonymous with rheumatoid arthritis. A longterm follow-up study. J Rheumatol. 2012;39:1929–33.
7. Emad Y, Anbar A, Abo-Elyoun I, et al. In palindromic rheumatism, hand joint involvement and positive anti-CCP antibodies predict RA development after 1 year of follow-up. Clin Rheumatol. 2014;33:791–7.
8. Maksymowych WP, Suarez-Almazor ME, Buenviaje H, et al. HLA and cytokine gene polymorphisms in relation to occurrence of palindromic rheumatism and its progression to rheumatoid arthritis. J Rheumatol. 2002;29:2319–26.
9. Hannonen P, Müttönen T, Oka M. Palindromic rheumatism: a clinical survey of sixty patients. Scand J Rheumatol. 1987;16:413–20.
10. Castellanos-Moreira R, Rodriguez-Garcia SC, Cabrera-Villalba S, et al. Anti-carbamylated protein antibody isotype pattern differs between palindromic rheumatism and rheumatoid arthritis. Ther Adv Musculoskelet Dis. 2020;12:1759720X20978139.
11. Mankia K, D'Agostino MA, Wakefield RJ, et al. Identification of a distinct imaging phenotype may improve the management of palindromic rheumatism. Ann Rheum Dis. 2019;78:43–50.
12. Cuervo A, Sanmartí R, Ramírez J, et al. Palindromic rheumatism: evidence of four subtypes of palindromic-like arthritis based in either MEFV or rheumatoid factor/ACPA status. Joint Bone Spine. 2021;88:105235.
13. Schwartzberg M. Prophylactic colchicine therapy in palindromic rheumatism. J Rheumatol. 1982;9:341–3.
14. Cañete JD, Aróstegui JI, Queiró R, et al. Association of intermittent hydrarthrosis with MEFV gene mutations. Arthritis Rheum. 2006;54:2334–5.
15. Sanmartí R, Frade-Sosa B, Morlà R, et al. Palindromic rheumatism: just a pre-rheumatoid stage or something else? Front Med (Lausanne). 2021;25(8):657983.
16. Pasero G, Barbieri P. Palindromic rheumatism: you just have to think about it! Clin Exp Rheumatol. 1986;4:197–9.
17. Guerne PA, Weisman MH. Palindromic rheumatism: part of or apart from the spectrum of rheumatoid arthritis. Am J Med. 1992;93:451–60.
18. Gonzalez-Lopez L, Gamez-Nava JI, Jhangri G, et al. Decreased progression to rheumatoid arthritis or other connective tissue diseases in patients with palindromic rheumatism treated with antimalarials. J Rheumatol. 2000;27:41–6.

19. Di Matteo A, Mankia K, Azukizawa M, et al. The role of musculoskeletal ultrasound in the rheumatoid arthritis continuum. Curr Rheumatol Rep. 2020;22:41.
20. Gutierrez M, Filippucci E, Salaffi F, et al. Differential diagnosis between rheumatoid arthritis and psoriatic arthritis: the value of ultrasound findings at metacarpophalangeal joints level. Ann Rheum Dis. 2011;70:1111–4.
21. Di Matteo A, De Angelis R, Cipolletta E, et al. Systemic lupus erythematosus arthropathy: the sonographic perspective. Lupus. 2018;27:794–801.
22. Filippucci E, Di Geso L, Girolimetti R, et al. Ultrasound in crystal-related arthritis. Clin Exp Rheumatol. 2014;32(1 Suppl 80):S42–7.
23. Filippou G, Scirè CA, Damjanov N, et al. Definition and reliability assessment of elementary ultrasonographic findings in calcium pyrophosphate deposition disease: a study by the OMERACT calcium pyrophosphate deposition disease ultrasound subtask force. J Rheumatol. 2017;44:1744–9.
24. Corradini D, Di Matteo A, Emery P, et al. How should we treat palindromic rheumatism? A systematic literature review. Semin Arthritis Rheum. 2021;51:266–77.
25. Khabbazi A, Mirza-Aghazadeh-Attari M, Goli MT, et al. Is palindromic rheumatism a pre-rheumatoid arthritis condition? Low incidence of rheumatoid arthritis in palindromic rheumatism patients treated with tight control strategy. Reumatol Clin (Engl Ed). 2021;17:7–11.
26. Mattingly S. Palindromic rheumatism. Ann Rheum Dis. 1966;25:307–17.
27. Eliakim A, Neumann L, Horowitz J, et al. Palindromic rheumatism in Israel—a disease entity? A survey of 34 patients. Clin Rheumatol. 1989;8:507–11.
28. Raghavan P, Sreenath S, Cherian S, et al. Efficacy of rituximab in resistant palindromic rheumatism: first report in literature. Clin Rheumatol. 2019;38:2399–402.
29. Mankia K, Di Matteo A, Emery P. Prevention and cure: the major unmet needs in the management of rheumatoid arthritis. J Autoimmun. 2020;110:102399.

Sarcoid Arthropathy

2

Edward Alveyn, Rositsa Dacheva, James Galloway, and Marwan Bukhari

2.1 Introduction

Although sarcoidosis was first described in the late nineteeth century, musculoskeletal involvement in sarcoid was not recognized for another 50 years. Davis and Crotty described in 1952 the case of a 24-year-old white female who presented with polyarthritis in the context of granulomatous skin disease and hilar adenopathy. They attributed the symptoms to two distinct diagnoses—sarcoidosis and rheumatoid arthritis—but looking back with our current understanding of the disease it is highly likely they were describing sarcoid arthropathy [1]. Since those early descriptions of musculoskeletal sarcoid, there have been many papers reporting the myriad patterns of joint involvement ranging from monoarthritis and polyarthritis to axial spondyloarthritis. Muscle and skeletal lesions are also well reported.

Epidemiological studies suggest that between 10 and 15% of people with sarcoidosis develop musculoskeletal manifestations [2–4]. This may well be an underestimate since the diagnosis is sometimes challenging in people with articular complaints alone and sarcoid arthropathy is usually only diagnosed when other extra-articular organs are affected (most patients presenting with musculoskeletal involvement do not get a tissue diagnosis). Numerous phenotypes of articular and skeletal sarcoid exist, ranging from the acute presentation of ankle swelling in Löfgren's syndrome to chronic synovitis, tenosynovitis, nonerosive arthropathy, and dactylitis, in addition to isolated bone disease.

E. Alveyn · J. Galloway
Centre for Rheumatic Diseases, Kings College, London, UK
e-mail: edward.alveyn@nhs.net; james.galloway@kcl.ac.uk

R. Dacheva
Diagnostic and Consultation Centre UMHAT "St. Ivan Rilski", Sofia, Bulgaria

M. Bukhari (✉)
University Hospitals of Morecambe Bay NHS foundation Trust, Kendal, UK
e-mail: Marwan.Bukhari@mbht.nhs.uk

© The Author(s), under exclusive license to Springer Nature Switzerland AG 2022
V. Ravindran et al. (eds.), *Rarer Arthropathies*, Rare Diseases of the Immune System, https://doi.org/10.1007/978-3-031-05002-2_2

2.2   Clinical Features

2.2.1   Löfgren's Syndrome

The most classic, easily recognized manifestation of sarcoid is Löfgren's syndrome, characterized by the triad of hilar lymphadenopathy, ankle pain, and erythema nodosum typically in the lower limbs. The clinical presentation is often around spring, and the lymphadenopathy is usually asymptomatic [5, 6]. On careful examination of the joint, the swelling is usually periarticular rather than of true ankle synovitis. Ultrasound or radioisotope imaging demonstrates a pattern of disease affecting subcutaneous tissues and tendon structures rather than the intra-articular space [7]. The erythema nodosum is typically over the anterior shins and is more common in women presenting with Löfgren's rather than men. Löfgren's usually affects the lower limbs and it is less common to see small joint involvement in this syndrome [8].

Laboratory investigations in Löfgren's demonstrate mild elevation of inflammatory markers and in about 15% of people there is an elevated serum angiotensin-converting enzyme (ACE), but the presence of ACE is neither diagnostic nor a predictor of outcome [9, 10]. Genetically, there are associations with polymorphism in the HLA gene (e.g., HLA-DQB1*0201) [11]. The vast majority of patients with Löfgren's recover without any intervention, with symptoms lasting between 3 and 6 months. Treatment is entirely symptomatic; most patients manage with nonsteroidal anti-inflammatory drugs (NSAIDs) alone or with a low dose of corticosteroids for a short period [12].

A closely related clinical syndrome to Löfgren's is Heerfordt's syndrome (uveoparotid fever), characterized by parotid gland enlargement, uveal inflammation, and occasionally cranial nerve palsy [13, 14]. The prognosis of Heerfordt's syndrome is less well-described in the literature, but in many cases follows a pattern of spontaneous resolution. Other patterns of sarcoid involving other tissues such as the lung parenchyma, myocardium, or other visceral organs are not recognized in Löfgren's syndrome. These usually correspond to a higher risk of chronic disease.

2.2.2   Chronic Arthritis

Among patients with long term sarcoidosis, the most frequent manifestations are in the lung parenchyma and the skin; chronic joint inflammation is relatively uncommon, affecting between 1 and 5% of patients. In contrast to the typical presentation of Löfgren's, elevated levels of serum ACE or serum soluble interleukin-2 receptor (sIL2R) are more common in chronic arthritis (in over 50% of patients) reflecting a higher total background burden of granuloma. There are four main patterns of chronic arthritis recognized in sarcoidosis [15]:

1. Nondeforming polyarthritis with granulomatous synovitis
2. Chronic tenosynovitis

3. Nonerosive Jaccoud's pattern deforming arthropathy
4. Dactylitis

2.2.2.1 Granulomatous Synovitis

Chronic arthritis characterized by granulomatous inflammation within the synovium is rare but well-described [16]. Affected joints can include both the lower limb articular structures involved in Löfgren's, but also the small joints of the hands or feet and rarely the sacroiliac joints. Inflammatory back pain in patients with sarcoidosis certainly justifies the use of magnetic resonance imaging for further evaluation. A study performed in Birmingham, UK in which patients with sarcoidosis were systematically evaluated for the presence of sacroiliac disease observed that over 6% of patients had radiographic evidence of spondyloarthropathy [17]. There are certainly some similarities between seronegative spondyloarthritis and sarcoidosis, including the association with inflammatory eye and lung disease and spinal inflammation. It is however important to highlight that although there are some clinical similarities, the diseases are distinct as there is no association of HLA-B27 with the spondyloarthritis seen in sarcoid.

2.2.2.2 Tenosynovitis

Tenosynovitis is well-described in the setting of sarcoid, commonly in the absence of arthritis [18]. Clinically, there is often visible swelling around either the anterior tendon structure of the ankle or the extensor tendon compartments of the wrist. The recognition of tenosynovitis has advanced with the advent of widely available ultrasound imaging, and several studies show that a high proportion of people with sarcoid predominantly have tendon inflammation rather than joint inflammation. Clinically it can be hard to separate the two although, in general, there is less restriction of joint movement with tenosynovitis compared with arthritis. The characteristic ultrasound features of tenosynovitis are demonstrated in Fig. 2.1.

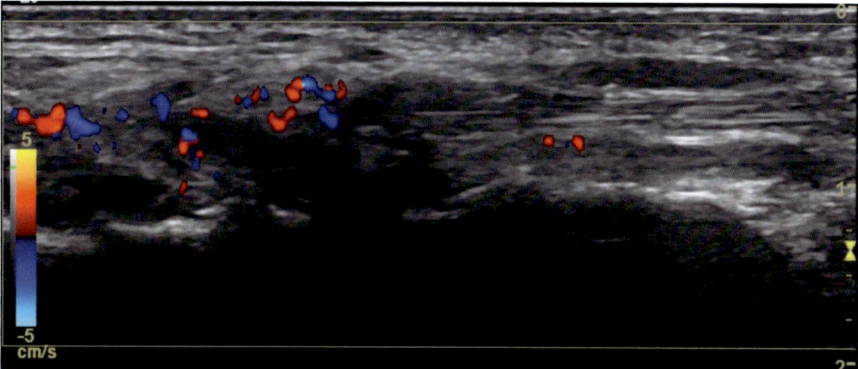

Fig. 2.1 Doppler ultrasound image of the wrist and distal forearm, showing intra-substance tendon heterogeneity, tendon sheath inflammation, and synovial hypertrophy with Doppler signal visible in both tendons and sheath, all suggestive of active soft tissue inflammation

Fig. 2.2 Sarcoid dactylitis of the fingers, causing painless digital swelling

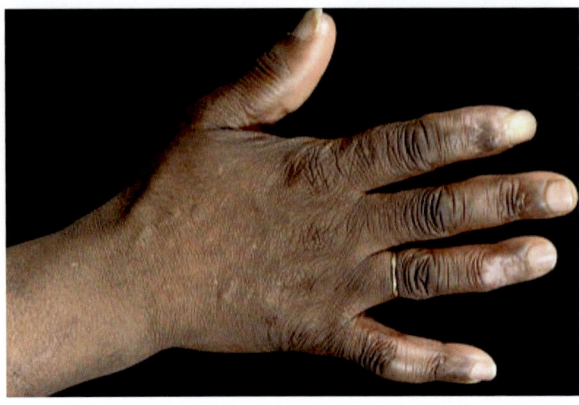

2.2.2.3 Jaccoud's Arthropathy

Jaccoud's arthropathy describes a nonerosive joint deformity with characteristic metacarpophalangeal subluxation and ulnar deviation. The pattern was first described in the context of systemic lupus erythematosus, but is observed in many other diseases including sarcoid and may accompany multisystem involvement [19].

2.2.2.4 Dactylitis

Dactylitis is usually seen as a characteristic feature of seronegative spondyloarthropathies. It is however a very important pattern to recognize in sarcoid and is clinically distinct from the dactylitis observed in, for example, psoriatic arthritis or reactive arthritis. Patients with sarcoid typically describe a painless, progressive, asymmetrical process with an often-deep violaceous discoloration to the overlying skin, and without any nail changes characteristic of psoriatic arthritis (Fig. 2.2). There are almost universal underlying bone changes in patients with sarcoid dactylitis—initially, a lattice-like appearance of the bony architecture is seen—particularly affecting the shafts of the phalanges (in contrast to psoriatic arthritis in which the osseous destruction commences at the articular margin). Over time these changes lead to bone resorption and often shortening of the digits, although again the appearance is quite distinct to that of arthritis mutilans of psoriatic arthritis [20].

2.2.3 Sarcoid Bone Disease

Osseous involvement is a rare form of extrapulmonary sarcoidosis, affecting an estimated 1–13% of people [21]. Bone sarcoidosis is often asymptomatic. The proposed mechanism of its pathogenesis is elevated levels of calcitriol driving increased osteoclastic activity leading to bone resorption. Sarcoid bone lesions are variable in their appearance on imaging and may be visible as lytic lesions (as shown in Fig. 2.3) characterized by cortical defects with preservation of the periosteum (e.g., in the phalanges of hands and feet), permeative "moth-eaten" appearances or destructive, sclerotic lesions [22]. Osseous involvement is often associated with chronic cutaneous

Fig. 2.3 Lytic lesions of the phalanges of the hands in a patient with sarcoidosis, showing lacy or lattice-like appearances, bone resorption and joint destruction, most prominently at the interphalangeal joints of the fifth digits

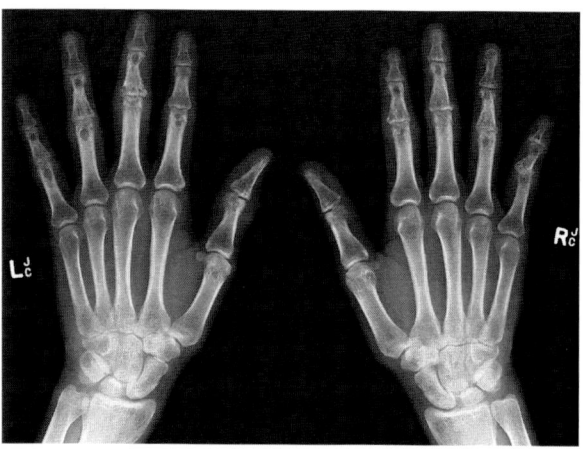

Table 2.1 The typical articular and osseous manifestations of sarcoidosis

Types of involvement	Clinical features	Imaging
Löfgren's syndrome arthropathy	Acute ankle pain and swelling, usually without a clear effusion, in the presence of erythema nodosum and respiratory symptoms	Ultrasound: Periarticular inflammation of the subcutaneous tissues and tendons around the ankle Chest radiography: Hilar lymphadenopathy
Granulomatous synovitis	Synovitis of the hands or feet with or without periarticular inflammation; sacroiliitis	Doppler ultrasound: Synovitis/ tenosynovitis Conventional radiography: sacroiliac joint sclerosis and erosions Magnetic resonance imaging: marrow edema
Tenosynovitis	Anterior ankle or extensor compartment wrist pain and swelling without significant effusion or restriction of movement	Ultrasound: Tendon sheath swelling, increased vascularity, and edema.
Jaccoud's arthropathy	"Correctable" deformity of the metacarpophalangeal joints with subluxation resembling rheumatoid arthritis	Hand radiography: Metacarpophalangeal joint subluxation and ulnar deviation; absence of erosions
Dactylitis	Digital swelling and erythematous/ violaceous discoloration, often asymmetrical and painless	Conventional radiography: Soft tissue swelling; lattice-like bony destruction of the phalangeal shafts with resorption in advanced disease
Sarcoid bone disease	Frequently asymptomatic; may be incidentally discovered. Occasionally there are pathological fractures	Conventional radiography: Variable— lytic, permeative, or sclerotic lesions, commonly of the phalanges, axial skeleton, or long bones

sarcoid including lupus pernio and chronic plaques and rarely affects people with no skin involvement. Axial involvement (particularly of the lumbar spine and pelvis) is common among patients with sarcoid bone disease, as are lesions of the long bones.

The key features of bone disease have been summarized in Table 2.1.

2.3 Diagnosis

2.3.1 Clinical Approach

The first and most valuable aspect of diagnosis in sarcoid arthritis is recognizing organ involvement in other tissue areas. In addition to the classic lung and skin manifestations, clinicians should be vigilant for ocular involvement, typically described as "granulomatous uveitis," an ophthalmological term referring to the characteristic appearance of the anterior chamber of the eye with globules of inflammatory cells adhering to the posterior margin of the cornea. This description does not imply that there has been any histological evidence of a granuloma—an error that is commonly made by other specialists when interpreting the clinical records of colleagues from the ophthalmology department. Care should also be taken to assess for evidence of neurological, cardiac, or hepatic sarcoid.

A crucial point to remember is that even in people with sarcoidosis affecting one organ, other diseases can develop elsewhere concomitantly, potentially confounding accurate diagnosis if the new findings are erroneously attributed to sarcoid. It is therefore imperative to recognize a clinical syndrome compatible with sarcoid and carefully consider alternative causes for any new features identified, including infection and other autoimmune granulomatous processes. A useful rule of thumb is that in most patients who develop multisystem sarcoid, involvement of the affected organs will occur within the first few years of symptom onset. Therefore, if a patient presents with respiratory symptoms and ocular inflammation but without joint inflammation, and 10 years later develops swelling in an ankle, it would be important to consider alternative diagnoses for the cause of ankle swelling (e.g., gout). In contrast, the diagnostic value of a lymph node or skin biopsy would be much greater in a patient presenting with musculoskeletal symptoms contemporaneously to symptoms in the eye, skin, or lung.

The most notable mimic of sarcoid is Mycobacterium tuberculosis infection, another granulomatous disease with acute or chronic onset, prominent pulmonary features, and the potential for musculoskeletal involvement. Particularly in endemic regions, clinicians must be mindful of the similarities and distinguishing features of sarcoid as compared with tuberculosis, some of which are outlined in Table 2.2. The variable presentations of both diseases defy easy categorization, though tuberculosis generally favors an asymmetrical or unilateral distribution more likely to involve the large joints, with histological differences in the appearances of the infection-driven granulomas and characteristic pulmonary features distinct from those of sarcoidosis.

2.3.2 Laboratory Investigations

Given the absence of a highly sensitive and specific biomarker for sarcoidosis, no single laboratory test is sufficient to provide a definite diagnosis. However, elevations in the serum levels of sIL2R and ACE can provide evidence to support a

Table 2.2 Important similarities and differences in the presentations of sarcoidosis and tuberculosis

Clinical characteristics	Sarcoid	Tuberculosis
	Granulomatous diseases, frequently with insidious onset and multiorgan involvement	
Musculoskeletal involvement	Small joints of the hands and feet, ankles, axial skeleton	Spine, large joints (hips, knees, ankles). Osteomyelitis is possible in almost any bone
– Distribution	Commonly bilateral	Frequently unilateral/focal/monoarthritis
Radiological appearance	Variable: sclerotic, lytic, or permeative bony lesions. Characteristic lacy/lattice-like appearances especially in the hands	Phemister's triad: juxta-articular osteopenia, marginal erosions, joint space narrowing + destruction Spine: Anterior vertebral destruction, abscess formation
– Chest imaging	Mediastinal lymphadenopathy—bilateral, symmetrical Cavity formation is uncommon Pulmonary nodules Fibrotic changes: reticular opacities traction bronchiectasis	Diverse radiographic patterns including miliary disease Upper lobe predominance Asymmetrical changes Cavitating lesions
	Tree-in-bud appearances and lymph node calcification seen in both diseases	
Extra-articular manifestations	May be asymptomatic, or with few extra-articular symptoms. Other organ disease—chest, eye, skin, heart, liver, CNS	Pain and constitutional symptoms are more common (fever, night sweats, weight loss), though frequently absent. Occasionally discharging sinuses. Other organ symptoms, e.g., chest
Laboratory findings	↑ soluble IL-2 receptor ↑ angiotensin-converting enzyme ↑ Vitamin D ↑ calcium	↓ Vitamin D – Mantoux – Interferon-gamma release assay – TB culture
Histology	Noncaseating granulomas consisting of epithelioid and multinucleated giant cells Adjacent CD4 + Th cell predominant inflammatory reaction (B cells less prominent) Schaumann and asteroid bodies may be seen	Caseating granulomas with visible acid-fast bacilli and CD4+/CD8+ T cells Prominent inflammatory reaction including B cells

diagnosis of active sarcoid. Derangement of liver enzymes, hypercalcemia and elevated serum immunoglobulins are commonly seen in patients with active disease, while markers of systemic inflammation may only be slightly elevated or even normal.

2.3.3 Biopsy

Apart from typical cases of Löfgren's syndrome, it is crucial when making a diagnosis of a sarcoid to obtain tissue evidence of noncaseating granulomatous disease [5, 23]. Ideally, the tissue would be from the organ being assessed for involvement; however, we know that skin tissue or lymph nodes in the lung are far more accessible sites to biopsy compared to, for example, synovium. For this reason, diagnoses of musculoskeletal sarcoid are frequently made based upon multiple organ involvement and a tissue diagnosis from a remote site.

When there is diagnostic uncertainty, sampling from joint tissue can be very valuable. Although joint effusions can occur in sarcoidosis, they are relatively uncommon and synovial fluid from sarcoid patients is usually nondiagnostic. When evaluated there is usually a relatively mild inflammatory infiltrate which is often a mixture of neutrophils and lymphocytes with a slight mononuclear predominance [24]. In contrast, a synovial biopsy can be very valuable as this may show the presence of noncaseating granulomas. An important caveat concerning synovial biopsies is that in the current era there has been a move towards less invasive synovial sampling using ultrasound combined with automated biopsy needles. There is some evidence to suggest that needle biopsies have a much lower pick-up for granulomatous inflammation, meaning that a negative result from a biopsy sampled in this way should be interpreted with caution. It may be preferable to request semi-open or arthroscopic procedures for the acquisition of these samples.

2.3.4 Imaging

Imaging of sarcoid arthritis can be very informative. Plain radiographs of affected joints may show underlying skeletal abnormalities. Patterns range from the lattice-like appearance seen in the phalanges of the hand, as shown in Fig. 2.3, to large lytic lesions that can occur in long bones adjacent to joints. Most valuable is radioisotope imaging with FDG-PET, which has the ability not only to identify FDG avid lesions (granulomatous sarcoid deposits are highly avid) but also helps to understand the extent of disease in other organs and tissues—which can be diagnostically invaluable [25]. Figure 2.4 demonstrates not only articular and periarticular sarcoid in large and small joints but also extensive lymphadenopathy and muscular sarcoid lesions.

2.4   Management Strategies for Sarcoid Arthritis

2.4.1   Initial Treatment

There is a dearth of evidence from clinical trials to guide the management of musculoskeletal sarcoid. However, strategies can be applied from knowledge of disease response in other organ systems and experience from other patterns of inflammatory arthritis. In general, mild symptoms are managed with NSAIDs. If these are insufficient, oral glucocorticoid (e.g., prednisolone 10–15 mg once daily then tapered to

Fig. 2.4 FDG PET-CT image showing widespread tracer uptake, including in the small joints of the hands, the left elbow, and both knees, where both synovial and periarticular involvement can be seen. Note also the widespread lymph node avidity and nodular foci in the muscles of the upper limbs

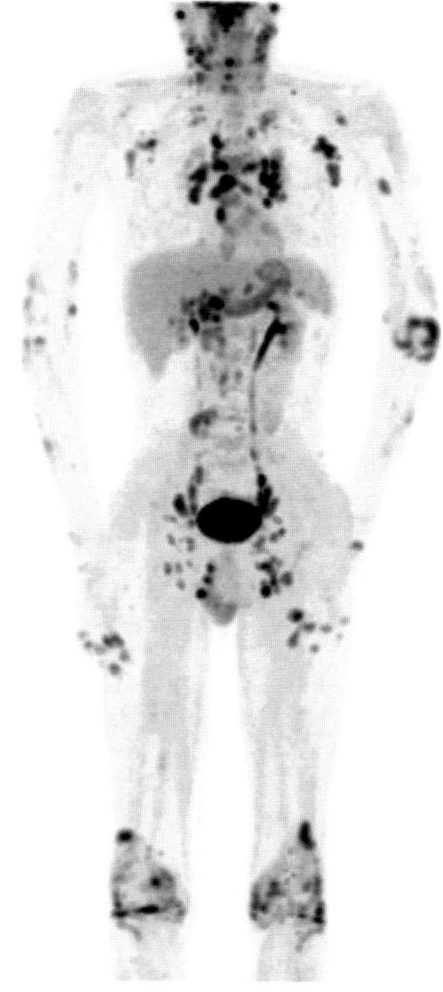

the lowest dose needed to control symptoms) is the next most commonly endorsed treatment. However, there is growing awareness of the risks of chronic exposure to glucocorticoids concerning infection, metabolic bone disturbance, cardiovascular events, and diabetes. A low threshold for offering a second-line agent is therefore likely to reduce the burden of steroid-induced side effects.

2.4.2 Disease-modifying Agents

For mild musculoskeletal symptoms, hydroxychloroquine is the first option, used at a dose of 5 mg/kg per day (based upon actual body weight) providing there is no preexisting retinal disease or renal impairment, based on evidence of the efficacy of antimalarial therapy in pulmonary sarcoidosis [26], and its preferable side effect profile compared to chloroquine. For some patients, symptomatic management without hydroxychloroquine is all that is required, and this may allow the glucocorticoid to be tapered down to a low dose or even stopped.

Some clinicians will also add low dose colchicine (e.g., 500 or 600 micrograms twice daily) in addition to the hydroxychloroquine. There is very little evidence to support this but as a relatively safe approach, it is a reasonable option to trial in patients with mild symptoms, particularly if there is a reluctance to increase immunosuppression.

In patients resistant to these strategies the next line of therapy is methotrexate, typically at a dose of 15–25 mg once weekly accompanied by folic acid supplementation. If there is an inadequate response to oral therapy or if there are side effects, using parenteral (subcutaneous) methotrexate at equivalent doses can be very helpful. Although there is relatively limited data on the use of methotrexate in articular disease, there is a robust evidence base for its effect in other organs affected by sarcoid (e.g., skin and nervous system) [27]. Alternative drugs to methotrexate that have been used in sarcoidosis and for which there are case reports or limited series include leflunomide and sulfasalazine [28].

2.4.3   Biologic Therapy

There is also reasonable literature for the use of certain TNF inhibitors in sarcoidosis [29, 30]. Though there are no head-to-head comparisons of different agents in the class, infliximab arguably has the strongest supporting evidence for the treatment of sarcoid with joint involvement, not only in the form of case reports but also a randomized trial, which primarily looked at respiratory outcomes but did include articular disease as a secondary endpoint [29]. Typically, infliximab is used at a dose of 5 mg/kg intravenously alongside methotrexate in patients with disease resistant to methotrexate monotherapy. TNF alpha is also mechanistically important in granuloma formation and therefore there is a strong rationale for using TNF inhibitors for the treatment of systemic sarcoid, with the possible exception of etanercept, which has failed to show significant benefit for systemic sarcoid [31, 32]. Notably, (like methotrexate) TNF blockade is effective for other manifestations of sarcoid such as in the skin and the brain [33, 34].

In patients who decline intravenous therapy or in whom infliximab is not tolerated, adalimumab is the logical next agent of choice given its similar mechanism of action. There is no evidence for other biologic agents such as rituximab in sarcoid arthropathy. While there is some optimism around the role of JAK inhibition in sarcoid, this is an area that remains to be studied.

In patients who are resistant to therapy, it is always important to revisit the diagnosis and consider alternative explanations for the joint involvement. Sometimes surgical intervention with synovectomy can be an option and this can also help confirm the diagnosis histologically.

2.5 Conclusion

The articular manifestations of sarcoidosis are relatively uncommon but vital to consider in patients with sarcoidosis, as well as in any patient with unexplained persistent bone or joint disease. Prompt and appropriate treatment can effectively reduce symptom burden, prevent irreversible damage, and substantially improve quality of life. Tissue diagnosis and imaging interpreted by clinicians with experience in managing articular sarcoid are invaluable, and advances in minimally invasive biopsy and imaging techniques would likely help improve the speed and accuracy of diagnosis. The patterns and severity of presentations are heterogeneous, meaning therapy tailored to the individual patient is essential and alternative diagnoses should be considered throughout treatment. The paucity of robust clinical trial data for many of the drugs used to treat these manifestations of sarcoid means there is significant opportunity for advancement of care, either through rigorous comparison of the treatments currently in use or via well-conducted trials of more novel targeted immunomodulators such as JAK inhibitors.

References

1. Davis MW, Crotty RQ. Sarcoidosis associated with polyarthritis. Ann Intern Med. 1952;36(4):1098–106.
2. Valeyre D, Prasse A, Nunes H, Uzunhan Y, Brillet PY, Müller-Quernheim J. Sarcoidosis. Lancet. 2014;383(9923):1155–67.
3. Baughman RP, Teirstein AS, Judson MA, Rossman MD, Yeager H Jr, Bresnitz EA, et al. Clinical characteristics of patients in a case control study of sarcoidosis. Am J Respir Crit Care Med. 2001;164(10 Pt 1):1885–9.
4. Hillerdal G, Nöu E, Osterman K, Schmekel B. Sarcoidosis: epidemiology and prognosis. A 15-year European study. Am Rev Respir Dis. 1984;130(1):29–32.
5. Mana J, Gomez-Vaquero C, Montero A, Salazar A, Marcoval J, Valverde J, et al. Lofgren's syndrome revisited: a study of 186 patients. Am J Med. 1999;107(3):240–5.
6. Glennas A, Kvien TK, Melby K, Refvem OK, Andrup O, Karstensen B, et al. Acute sarcoid arthritis: occurrence, seasonal onset, clinical features and outcome. Br J Rheumatol. 1995;34(1):45–50.
7. Le Bras E, Ehrenstein B, Fleck M, Hartung W. Evaluation of ankle swelling due to Lofgren's syndrome: a pilot study using B-mode and power Doppler ultrasonography. Arthritis Care Res (Hoboken). 2014;66(2):318–22.
8. Visser H, Vos K, Zanelli E, Verduyn W, Schreuder GM, Speyer I, et al. Sarcoid arthritis: clinical characteristics, diagnostic aspects, and risk factors. Ann Rheum Dis. 2002;61(6):499–504.
9. Studdy PR, Bird R. Serum angiotensin converting enzyme in sarcoidosis—its value in present clinical practice. Ann Clin Biochem. 1989;26(Pt 1):13–8.
10. Ramos-Casals M, Retamozo S, Sisó-Almirall A, Pérez-Alvarez R, Pallarés L, Brito-Zerón P. Clinically-useful serum biomarkers for diagnosis and prognosis of sarcoidosis. Expert Rev Clin Immunol. 2019;15(4):391–405.
11. Grunewald J, Eklund A. Löfgren's syndrome: human leukocyte antigen strongly influences the disease course. Am J Respir Crit Care Med. 2009;179(4):307–12.
12. Ungprasert P, Crowson CS, Matteson EL. Clinical characteristics of sarcoid arthropathy: a population-based study. Arthritis Care Res. 2016;68(5):695–9.
13. Dua A, Manadan A. Heerfordt's syndrome, or uveoparotid fever. N Engl J Med. 2013;369(5):458.

14. Sharma SK, Soneja M, Sharma A, Sharma MC, Hari S. Rare manifestations of sarcoidosis in modern era of new diagnostic tools. Indian J Med Res. 2012;135(5):621–9.
15. Bechman K, Christidis D, Walsh S, Birring SS, Galloway J. A review of the musculoskeletal manifestations of sarcoidosis. Rheumatology. 2017;57(5):777–83.
16. Thelier N, Assous N, Job-Deslandre C, Meyer O, Bardin T, Orcel P, et al. Osteoarticular involvement in a series of 100 patients with sarcoidosis referred to rheumatology departments. J Rheumatol. 2008;35(8):1622–8.
17. Erb N, Cushley MJ, Kassimos DG, Shave RM, Kitas GD. An assessment of back pain and the prevalence of sacroiliitis in sarcoidosis. Chest. 2005;127(1):192–6.
18. Al-Ani Z, Oh TC, Macphie E, Woodruff MJ. Sarcoid tenosynovitis, rare presentation of a common disease. Case report and literature review. J Radiol Case Rep. 2015;9(8):16–23.
19. Sukenik S, Hendler N, Yerushalmi B, Buskila D, Liberman N. Jaccoud's-type arthropathy: an association with sarcoidosis. J Rheumatol. 1991;18(6):915–7.
20. Olivieri I, Scarano E, Padula A, Giasi V, Priolo F. Dactylitis, a term for different digit diseases. Scand J Rheumatol. 2006;35(5):333–40.
21. Sparks JA, McSparron JI, Shah N, Aliabadi P, Paulson V, Fanta CH, et al. Osseous sarcoidosis: clinical characteristics, treatment, and outcomes—experience from a large, academic hospital. Semin Arthritis Rheum. 2014;44(3):371–9.
22. Wilcox A, Bharadwaj P, Sharma OP. Bone sarcoidosis. Curr Opin Rheumatol. 2000;12(4):321–30.
23. Iannuzzi MC, Rybicki BA, Teirstein AS. Sarcoidosis. N Engl J Med. 2007;357(21):2153–65.
24. Pettersson T. Sarcoid and erythema nodosum arthropathies. Baillieres Best Pract Res Clin Rheumatol. 2000;14(3):461–76.
25. Brandao Guimaraes J, Nico MA, Omond AG, Silva FD, Aivazoglou LU, Carneiro BC, et al. Radiologic manifestations of musculoskeletal sarcoidosis. Curr Rheumatol Rep. 2019;21(3):7.
26. Baltzan M, Mehta S, Kirkham TH, Cosio MG. Randomized trial of prolonged chloroquine therapy in advanced pulmonary sarcoidosis. Am J Respir Crit Care Med. 1999;160(1):192–7.
27. Kaye O, Palazzo E, Grossin M, Bourgeois P, Kahn MF, Malaise MG. Low-dose methotrexate: an effective corticosteroid-sparing agent in the musculoskeletal manifestations of sarcoidosis. Br J Rheumatol. 1995;34(7):642–4.
28. Sahoo DH, Bandyopadhyay D, Xu M, Pearson K, Parambil JG, Lazar CA, et al. Effectiveness and safety of leflunomide for pulmonary and extrapulmonary sarcoidosis. Eur Respir J. 2011;38(5):1145–50.
29. Judson MA, Baughman RP, Costabel U, Flavin S, Lo KH, Kavuru MS, et al. Efficacy of infliximab in extrapulmonary sarcoidosis: results from a randomised trial. Eur Respir J. 2008;31(6):1189–96.
30. Ulbricht KU, Stoll M, Bierwirth J, Witte T, Schmidt RE. Successful tumor necrosis factor alpha blockade treatment in therapy-resistant sarcoidosis. Arthritis Rheum. 2003;48(12):3542–3.
31. Utz JP, Limper AH, Kalra S, Specks U, Scott JP, Vuk-Pavlovic Z, et al. Etanercept for the treatment of stage II and III progressive pulmonary sarcoidosis. Chest. 2003;124(1):177–85.
32. Baughman RP, Lower EE, Bradley DA, Raymond LA, Kaufman A. Etanercept for refractory ocular sarcoidosis: results of a double-blind randomized trial. Chest. 2005;128(2):1062–47.
33. Amber KT, Bloom R, Mrowietz U, Hertl M. TNF-α: a treatment target or cause of sarcoidosis? J Eur Acad Dermatol Venereol. 2015;29(11):2104–11.
34. Baughman RP, Lower EE, du Bois RM. Sarcoidosis. Lancet. 2003;361(9363):1111–8.

Remitting Seronegative Symmetrical Synovitis with Pitting Edema (RS3PE)

3

Christopher J. Edwards and Salvatore Bellinvia

3.1 Introduction

The first description of remitting seronegative symmetrical synovitis with pitting edema (RS3PE) dates back to 1985 when McCarty et al. observed a series of older adults presenting with symmetrical polyarthritis and peculiar pitting edema over the hands, with the original intention of defining a distinct subset of patients with elderly onset rheumatoid arthritis (RA) [1]. In the 1990s, several groups reviewed the clinical and laboratory features as well as outcomes of patients fulfilling the characteristics of RS3PE syndrome first described by McCarthy, to better characterize the real nature of this syndrome as a separate disease entity [2]. Their works emphasized demographic, clinical, and imaging similarities between RS3PE and different rheumatic conditions, in particular its relation with polymyalgia rheumatica (PMR), suggesting that these disorders could be part of the same clinical disease spectrum. A strong association between several solid tumors and hematological diseases was also described. Subsequently, distinctive genetic and pathogenic characteristics have been described and thus the concept that this condition is a distinct clinical entity has become prevalent. RS3PE is now regarded as a well-defined rarer arthropathy that is to be distinguished from other rheumatic diseases which may also present with swelling of distal extremities, biochemical evidence of raised inflammatory markers and negative rheumatoid factor, including seronegative RA, peripheral spondyloarthropathies and PMR.

C. J. Edwards
Department of Rheumatology and NIHR Clinical Research Facility, University Hospital Southampton NHS Foundation Trust, Southampton, UK
e-mail: cedwards@soton.ac.uk

S. Bellinvia (✉)
Department of Internal Medicine, Azienda Sanitaria Provinciale, Messina, Italy
e-mail: salvo.bellinvia@libero.it

© The Author(s), under exclusive license to Springer Nature
Switzerland AG 2022
V. Ravindran et al. (eds.), *Rarer Arthropathies*, Rare Diseases of the Immune System, https://doi.org/10.1007/978-3-031-05002-2_3

23

3.2   Epidemiology

RS3PE appears to be a rare disease for which accurate estimates of incidence and prevalence are lacking. Few studies have attempted to better understand the epidemiological characteristics of the disease, suggesting this may represent ~0.1% of new diagnoses among outpatients aged over 50 years in rheumatology clinics [3]. RS3PE occurs almost exclusively in elderly individuals, with the highest prevalence in the 70–79 age group, and is more common in men than in women (male to female ratio 4:1). The familial aggregation has not been reported but genetic linkage studies have demonstrated human leukocyte antigen (HLA) associations of RS3PE with HLA-B7 and HLA-A2 haplotypes, suggesting an important role for antigen selection and presentation. However, these associations have not been confirmed in various subsequent immunogenetic studies and need further validation in larger patient cohorts. Both RA and PMR are known to be associated with specific alleles of HLA-DR4. Noteworthy in this regard is the lack of association between HLA-DR (DR4) antigens and disease susceptibility in RS3PE, reinforcing again the notion that this disease should be regarded as a different condition from these much more common rheumatic diseases presenting with similar clinical features [4].

3.3   Pathogenesis

The cause of RS3PE is unknown. A role for infectious agents such as *Parvovirus B19*, *Streptobacillus moniliformis*, *Mycoplasma pneumoniae,* and *Helicobacter pylori* or instillation of Bacillus Calmette-Guerin (BCG) has been postulated but a definite infectious trigger or environmental factor has not yet been identified. The specific pathogenic mechanisms are also poorly understood. However, more recent work has revealed vascular endothelial growth factor (VEGF) activity is a key factor in the pathogenesis of RS3PE [5]. As a matter of fact, VEGF is the central signal protein promoting both hypervascularity (synovitis) and increased vascular permeability (subcutaneous edema) which are the clinical hallmarks of the disease. Levels of VEGF in the peripheral blood are notably higher in patients with RS3PE compared to patients with other inflammatory rheumatic disorders including RA or healthy individuals. Moreover, VEGF levels decrease after glucocorticoid treatment, further supporting the view that RS3PE can be classified as a VEGF-associated disorder. Consistent with the extensive inflammation, patients with RS3PE have been found to have a marked increase in IL-6 levels in synovial fluid, suggesting this cytokine might play a major role in the inflammatory disease response. Matrix metalloproteinase-3 (MMP-3) is also elevated in most patients with active RS3PE but serum levels can vary according to whether or not the disorder is associated with malignancies. Of note, MMP-3 is significantly higher in paraneoplastic RS3PE patients than in RS3PE patients without neoplasia and serum levels tend to drastically decrease or normalize after surgical resection of the tumor.

3.4   Pathophysiology

The term remitting seronegative symmetrical synovitis with pitting edema implies a bilateral symmetric acute inflammatory process involving predominantly joints and tendons of the distal extremities accompanied by marked dorsal swelling of the hands or feet with pitting edema, followed by periods of less severe symptoms that do not completely cease without treatment. In fact, distal articular and periarticular structures are both affected in RS3PE patients as has been demonstrated by musculoskeletal ultrasound and MRI findings in several studies [6]. However, articular synovitis seems to be generally mild to moderate in nature, synovial hypertrophy is rare, and bone erosions are virtually absent in RS3PE while extensive carpal (or tarsal) and digital flexor and extensor tendons tenosynovitis appear to be more frequent and severe, accounting for most of the swelling and edema occurring over the hands or feet in patients with RS3PE. Vascularity is also typically very pronounced in joints and tendons of RS3PE patients as confirmed by imaging studies, in keeping with the enhanced VEGF activity which is widely recognized as a key factor in the disease pathogenesis [7].

3.5   Clinical Features

The clinical presentation of RS3PE is characterized by sudden onset of joint pains in the distal upper extremities with puffy edematous hands in a patient over the age of 60. It is typically the abrupt onset of painful swelling of the dorsum of both hands, usually pitting and causing significant limitation of movement and function [8], that prompts the patient with RS3PE to seek medical attention.

Symptoms in RS3PE involve aching with significant swelling which is generally bilateral although a unilateral presentation of RS3PE has been also recognized in a minority of cases [9]. Involvement of the distal extremities occurs most commonly at the dorsal wrists and metacarpophalangeal joints and less frequently at the ankles and feet. Peripheral joints are by far the most affected but the involvement of large joints such as elbows, shoulders, and knees can be occasionally seen. Heat and redness can be prominent features of RS3PE and involved joints and soft tissues are often distinctively warmer on palpation.

Morning stiffness is usually present and lasts for about an hour but this finding is less consistent than other inflammatory arthropathies, reflecting the severity of synovial inflammation in the individual patient. In addition, pain can easily wake patients up during the night as is typical of other inflammatory rheumatic conditions. Joint pain and swelling can result in remarkable difficulties with activities of daily living (ADL). Patients can struggle with simple tasks requiring the use of their hands such as dressing, personal hygiene, or opening jars due to reduced grip strength and loss of movement but they can also experience walking difficulties if distal lower extremities are affected. Rare patients, particularly in the oldest age groups, can also present with constitutional signs and symptoms including fever, weight loss, generalized aching, and fatigue. Reports of weight loss and anorexia should always prompt a search for occult malignancy.

Clinical examination of hands would show soft tissue swelling around the MCP joints which can often be found early in the course of RS3PE but the contribution of both tendon and joint involvement to this finding make this assessment rather non-specific. The clinical hallmark of RS3PE is acute swelling of the whole hand with pitting edema over the dorsum producing the characteristic "boxing glove" sign. Tenosynovitis of the extensor tendons is more likely to cause this clinical finding although involvement of the flexor tendons is also commonly seen. Reduced grip strength can be observed in the early phase of clinical presentation and is a rather sensitive indicator of synovial inflammation. As a result of a restricted range of movement with loss of active flexion, patients are often unable to make a fist. Thickening of the extensor tendons can rarely be detected by palpation of the dorsal aspect of the involved joints.

On the wrists, visible swelling at the dorsum with marked pitting edema is characteristic of the disease and should always be noted on physical examination. Both extensor and flexor tenosynovitides are common findings and major contributors to the development of edema as a result of effusion within tenosynovial sheaths. Loss of extension can be detected early in the clinical course of the disease. Flexion contractures can be seen quite frequently and in some cases can persist for a variable amount of time after the resolution of painful swelling following treatment. Tendon thickening can be observed with a low frequency and similarly tendon rupture at the wrist is very rare.

Lower extremities, particularly rearfoot and ankle, are less often involved in RS3PE and clinical findings show a similar pattern to that occurring in the hands and wrists. Involvement of peroneal tendons, posterior tibial tendon, and tendons of the anterior compartment of the ankle leads to diffuse swelling over the dorsum of the foot with painful inversion and eversion and limited range of movement. Metatarsophalangeal joints are not commonly affected and the Achilles tendon is usually spared.

3.6   Investigations

3.6.1   Laboratory Findings

There are no laboratory tests diagnostic of RS3PE. Acute-phase reactants, including the erythrocyte sedimentation rate (ESR) and C-reactive protein (CRP), are nearly always increased in patients with RS3PE and they could be markedly elevated [10]. Direct comparisons of the diagnostic value of CRP and ESR in RS3PE have not been conclusive but CRP is usually considered a more reliable index of inflammation as ESR levels tend to physiologically rise with age more significantly than does the CRP. Consistent with a systemic inflammatory acute response, normocytic anemia (anemia of chronic inflammation) and thrombocytosis can be observed in some cases together with alpha-1 and -2 fraction elevation on serum protein electrophoresis. Serologic tests, such as rheumatoid factor (RF), cyclic citrullinated peptide (CCP) antibodies, and antinuclear antibodies (ANA), are typically negative and are often useful to exclude other rheumatic conditions. However, results for these serologic studies need to be interpreted in the clinical setting as the prevalence of positive assays also tends to increase with age. MMP-3 and VEGF levels were found to be elevated in research studies of RS3PE and might represent promising diagnostic biomarkers but their use in clinical practice has not yet been validated.

3.6.2 Imaging

In patients with RS3PE, soft tissue swelling as a result of tenosynovial inflammation and articular synovitis are best observed on ultrasonography or magnetic resonance imaging (MRI). Characteristic features of tenosynovitis of flexor and extensor tendons and synovial inflammation can be seen by the use of these modalities but imaging is not a mandatory requirement for the diagnosis of RS3PE. Musculoskeletal ultrasound (MSUS) allows a cost-effective assessment of synovitis, tenosynovitis, and subcutaneous tissue edema of the hands and feet although it is highly operator-dependent [11]. Power Doppler (PD) signal is also very useful to detect increased vascularity in joints and tendons under examination. Tenosynovitis is defined as the presence of anechoic material within the tendon sheaths often associated with PD signal in axial and transverse planes. MRI of the hands and feet can be more sensitive than MSUS in detecting synovial and tenosynovial inflammation but is more costly and not usually required for the diagnosis of RS3PE in clinical practice. Radiographs of the wrists, hands, and feet are typically requested as part of the initial assessment. Conventional radiographs can show soft tissue swelling but joint space narrowing and erosive damage are virtually absent in RS3PE.

3.6.3 Diagnosis

RS3PE is essentially a clinical diagnosis. The diagnosis should be suspected in a patient over the age of 50 years presenting with an acute inflammatory and often symmetric onset of tenosynovitis and arthritis in the distal extremities with puffy edematous hands and/or feet and in whom the findings are not explained by any other condition. Following the first description of RS3PE, classification criteria including the age of onset, pitting edema of hands and seronegativity for rheumatoid factor have been proposed by Olivé et al. in 1997 [12]. Further criteria for classification have been proposed in 2016 by Karmacharya et al. in a systematic review and meta-analysis revisiting RS3PE [13] (Table 3.1).

Despite the clear criteria, correct recognition of RS3PE presents a challenge for several reasons: a considerable degree of expertise is required as the diagnosis relies on clinical features; the differential diagnosis is broad and includes both inflammatory and noninflammatory causes of pitting edema of upper and lower extremities; evaluation and follow-up of these patients may lead to associated neoplastic and rheumatic diseases.

Table 3.1 Features of RS3PE

McCarthy et al. description [1] (1985)
Pitting edema of the dorsum of both hands (and/or feet)
Sudden onset of polyarthritis
Seronegative for RF
No development of radiologically evident erosions
No association with HLA-DRB1 alleles
Excellent response to glucocorticoids and good prognosis
Olivé et al. classification criteria [12] (1997)
1.   Bilateral pitting edema of both hands
2.   Sudden onset of polyarthritis
3.   Age of onset ≥50 years
4.   Seronegative for RF
Karmacharya et al. revisited classification criteria [13] (2016)
1.   Abrupt onset
2.   Marked pitting edema of hands (and/or feet)
3.   Age of onset ≥60 years
4.   Good response to short course of medium dose steroids (10–20 mg)
5.   Seronegativity for RF and ACPA
6.   Absence of radiographic joint erosions

Patients may be diagnosed with RS3PE when they meet all of the criteria proposed by Olive et al. and/or Karmacharya et al.

RF rheumatoid factor, *ACPA* anti-citrullinated protein antibody

3.7   Associated Conditions

3.7.1   RS3PE and Malignancies

The incidence of neoplastic disease is significantly higher in RS3PE patients than in the general elderly population. Both hematological malignancies and solid tumors have been reported in association with RS3PE in multiple studies. Hematological diseases have included non-Hodgkins lymphoma, myelodysplastic syndrome, and leukemia. Solid tumors associated with RS3PE have encompassed adenocarcinoma of the prostate, malignancies of the gastrointestinal tract, lung, breast, ovary, and bladder [14].

Most often RS3PE precedes the discovery of malignancy by a time ranging from several months to a few years. However, signs and symptoms of RS3PE can present concurrently with or occasionally after the associated neoplasia. The term "paraneoplastic RS3PE" has also been used to describe clinical features of RS3PE occurring at the same time or shortly after a diagnosis of malignancy. Paraneoplastic RS3PE is characterized by a less significant response to steroids with a marked improvement after successful medical therapy or surgical treatment of the associated hematological malignancy or solid tumor [15].

Assessment for the presence of underlying malignancy is therefore a key consideration in the evaluation of a patient with diagnosed or suspected RS3PE [16]. Appropriate screening by age and gender should be completed as soon as the diagnosis is considered and patients should be counseled about signs and symptoms and assessed for physical findings attributable to malignancy at presentation and each follow-up visit.

3.7.2 RS3PE and Other Rheumatic Diseases

A definite diagnosis of RS3PE can occasionally overlap with other rheumatic diseases including systemic lupus erythematosus, gout, Sjogren's syndrome, polyarteritis nodosa, ankylosing spondylitis, or systemic conditions such as diabetes mellitus, sarcoidosis, and amyloidosis. Moreover, patients initially diagnosed with RS3PE can also eventually develop clinical features of different rheumatic conditions including RA, PMR, and peripheral spondyloarthritis. However, establishing whether the latter occurrence defines a true association of RS3PE or is more related to the *forme fruste* of subsequent diagnoses can be very challenging in these cases.

3.8 Differential Diagnosis

Various rheumatic and non-rheumatic disorders can present with swelling of the distal extremities and should be differentiated from RS3PE as part of the diagnostic process [17, 18].

3.8.1 Non-rheumatic Disorders

Pitting edema is a common sign in daily clinical practice and a range of etiologies should be considered while examining patients with generalized or localized soft-tissue edema. Bilateral edema can result from cardiovascular (cardiac failure), hepatic (liver failure), or renal disease (renal failure, nephrotic syndrome) while unilateral edema can arise from venous thrombosis or lymphatic obstruction. Other disorders such as complex regional pain syndrome (CRPS) can also have a similar presentation. Painful swelling and biochemical evidence of inflammation are typically absent in noninflammatory systemic causes of pitting edema while bilateral involvement of dorsal hands and feet in RS3PE helps rule out conditions associated with localized unilateral edema.

3.8.2 Rheumatic Disorders

The most challenging considerations in the differential diagnosis of RS3PE are PMR, elderly onset rheumatoid arthritis, and non-psoriatic spondyloarthritides (Table 3.2).

Table 3.2 Differentiating features between RS3PE, PMR, RA, and non-psoriatic SpA

Clinical characteristics and response to treatment	RS3PE	PMR	RA	Non-psoriatic SpA
Gender	Male predominance	Female predominance	F ≈ M	Male predominance
Pitting edema	Prominent	Rare	Infrequent	Rare
Wrist and MCP joints synovitis	Common Mild	Unusual	Common Mild to severe	Uncommon in axial-SpA Often unilateral, asymmetric, and lower limbs are more affected
PIP joints synovitis	Unusual	Rare	Prominent	Uncommon in axial-SpA Often unilateral, asymmetric, and lower limbs are more affected
Pelvic and shoulder girdle pain and stiffness	Rare	Prominent	Unusual	Not prominent Often unilateral, asymmetric
Fever	Infrequent	Infrequent	Rare	Rare
Response to low dose steroids	Excellent[a]	Good	Moderate	Poor
Clinical course	Remission with glucocorticoid treatment	Frequent relapses and recurrences despite glucocorticoid treatment	Remission rare without DMARDs	Remission rare without NSAID or DMARDs
Laboratory and Imaging				
Rheumatoid factor	Negative	Uncommon	Common	Rare
ACPA	Negative	Uncommon	Common	Rare
Radiographic erosion	Absent	Absent	Yes	Yes
Tenosynovitis of extensor and flexor tendons by US or MRI	Marked	Rare	Mild	Uncommon

MCP metacarpophalangeal, *PIP* proximal interphalangeal, *ACPA* anti-citrullinated protein antibody

[a] Poorer response to steroids is observed in paraneoplastic RS3PE compared to idiopathic RS3PE

There is no significant difference with respect to the age of onset and raised inflammatory markers in PMR. RS3PE is much more common in men while PMR is more frequent in women. Distal symptoms and signs are infrequent in PMR and when present are less pronounced than RS3PE. Proximal symptoms with some degree of stiffness and limited range of motion about the shoulders and the hips can be observed on careful musculoskeletal examination in RS3PE but this does not represent a predominant feature. Relapses and recurrences despite steroid treatment are frequent in PMR compared to RS3PE.

In older patients presenting with peripheral symmetric polyarthritis, the possibility of elderly onset RA should be considered. Measurement of rheumatoid factor and antibodies to the cyclic citrullinated peptides (anti-CCP) can help distinguish RS3PE from classic seropositive RA but this can be challenging where RA is seronegative [19]. The age of onset is typically higher in RS3PE than seronegative RA and levels of CRP and ESR are usually higher in RS3PE. A significant number of tender or swollen joints, especially small joints of the hands and feet, is more indicative of seronegative rheumatoid arthritis while ankles appear to be more affected in RS3PE. The correct differentiation of these two forms is also important in terms of outcomes as the malignancy incidence rate is much higher in RS3PE compared to rheumatoid arthritis.

Distal pitting edema can be seen in late-onset spondyloarthritis. However, involvement of distal extremities is usually unilateral or asymmetric in SpA and lower limbs are more commonly affected. The pattern of joint involvement, the presence of extra-articular features of spondyloarthritis such as uveitis, the association with HLA B27, and a good response to NSAIDs help differentiate SpA from RS3PE.

Other diseases such as psoriatic arthritis (PsA), crystal-induced arthritis, amyloid arthropathy, and connective tissue diseases can cause pitting edema over the hands and feet. Typical skin findings and radiographic changes in PsA, the presence of calcium pyrophosphate dihydrate (CPPD) or monosodium urate (MSU) crystals in synovial fluid in CPPD arthropathy and gout respectively, progressive swelling nonresponsive to treatment in amyloid arthropathy, ANA positivity, and clinical signs or symptoms of connective tissue diseases can be useful distinctions to guide clinicians towards the correct diagnosis.

3.9   Management

The main goal of treatment in RS3PE is a relief of symptoms and resolution of pitting edema. Low-dose glucocorticoids (starting dose 10–20 mg/day of prednisone or equivalent) are recommended for all patients diagnosed with RS3PE and response to treatment is typically dramatic within days [20]. The initial dose needs to be tailored to the individual patient taking into account their weight, the severity of symptoms, and comorbidities such as diabetes mellitus, severe hypertension, or heart failure. RS3PE associated with neoplasia is characterized by a poorer response to steroids compared to idiopathic RS3PE while lack of response to glucocorticoids should prompt reconsideration of the diagnosis. There is a limited role for glucocorticoid-sparing agents and current evidence does not support their use in RS3PE. The CRP and to a lesser extent the ESR can serve as useful indicators in monitoring treatment response to steroids and managing dose reduction. Notably, early reduction of CRP to normal levels is a predictive factor associated with suppression of disease activity [21]. The duration of treatment is variable. However, glucocorticoids can be tapered off and discontinued within a few months in most patients. Recurrences and relapses are very infrequent with adequate treatment.

3.10 Conclusion

Remitting seronegative symmetrical synovitis with pitting edema is a rare arthropathy affecting almost exclusively older adults. Sudden onset of polyarthritis and dorsal edema of both hands are the clinical hallmarks of the disease. Response to low-dose glucocorticoids is usually brisk and accompanied by complete resolution of signs and symptoms. A diagnosis of RS3PE entails careful screening for underlying malignancies and differential diagnosis with more common rheumatic diseases sharing similar clinical presentation.

References

1. McCarty DJ, O'Duffy JD, Pearson L, Hunter JB. Remitting seronegative symmetrical synovitis with pitting oedema. RS3PE syndrome. JAMA. 1985;254:2763–7.
2. Schaeverbeke T, Fatout E, Marcé S, Vernhes JP, Hallé O, Antoine JF, Lequen L, Bannwarth B, Dehais J. Remitting seronegative symmetrical synovitis with pitting oedema: disease or syndrome? Ann Rheum Dis. 1995;54:681–4.
3. Okumura T, Tanno S, Ohhira M, Nozu T. The rate of polymyalgia rheumatica (PMR) and remitting seronegative symmetrical synovitis with pitting oedema (RS3PE) syndrome in a clinic where primary care physicians are working in Japan. Rheumatol Int. 2012;32(6):1695–9. Published online 2011 Mar 24. https://doi.org/10.1007/s00296-011-1849-3.
4. Queiro R. RS3PE syndrome: a clinical and immunogenetical study. Rheumatol Int. 2004;24:103–5.
5. Arima K, Origuchi T, Tamai M, Iwanaga N, Izumi Y, Huang M, Tanaka F, Kamachi M, Aratake K, Nakamura H, Ida H, Uetani M, Kawakami A, Eguchi K. RS3PE syndrome presenting as vascular endothelial growth factor associated disorder. Ann Rheum Dis. 2005;64(11):1653–5. https://doi.org/10.1136/ard.2004.032995.
6. Cantini F, Salvarani C, Olivieri I, Barozzi L, Macchioni L, Niccoli L, Padula A, Pavlica P, Boiardi L. Remitting seronegative symmetrical synovitis with pitting oedema (RS3PE) syndrome: a prospective follow up and magnetic resonance imaging study. Ann Rheum Dis. 1999;58(4):230–6.
7. Li H, Altman RD, Yao Q. RS3PE: clinical and research development. Curr Rheumatol Rep. 2015;17(8):49.
8. Eguia HA, Garcia JFP, Diez CR, Edwin A Eguia A. Remitting seronegative symmetrical synovitis with pitting oedema (RS3PE) case presentation and comparison with other polyarthritides affecting older people. Age Ageing. 2017;46(2):333–4.
9. Olivieri I, Salvarani C, Cantini F. RS3PE syndrome: an overview. Clin Exp Rheumatol. 2000;18(4 Suppl 20):S53–5.
10. Salam A, Henry R, Sheeran T. Acute onset polyarthritis in older people: is it RS3PE syndrome? Cases J. 2008;1(1):132.
11. Kawashiri SY, Suzuki T, Okada A, Tsuji S, Takatani A, Shimizu T, Koga T, Iwamoto N, Ichinose K, Nakamura H, Origuchi T, Kawakami A. Differences in musculoskeletal ultrasound

findings between RS3PE syndrome and elderly-onset rheumatoid arthritis. Clin Rheumatol. 2020;39(6):1981–8.

12. Olivé A, del Blanco J, Pons M, Vaquero M, Tena X. The clinical spectrum of remitting seronegative symmetrical synovitis with pitting edema. The Catalán Group for the Study of RS3PE. J Rheumatol. 1997;24(2):333–6.

13. Karmacharya P, Donato AA, Aryal MR, Ghimire S, Pathak R, Shah K, Shrestha P, Poudel D, Wasser T, Subedi A, Giri S, Jalota L, Olivé A. RS3PE revisited: a systematic review and meta-analysis of 331 cases. Clin Exp Rheumatol. 2016;34(3):404–15.

14. Emamifar A, Hess S, Gildberg-Mortensen R, Jensen Hansen IM. Association of remitting seronegative symmetrical synovitis with pitting oedema, polymyalgia rheumatica, and adenocarcinoma of the prostate. Am J Case Rep. 2016;17:60–4.

15. Yajima S, Ooeda T, Inoue M, Suzuki H, Matsumoto S, Masuda H. Paraneoplastic remitting seronegative symmetrical synovitis with pitting oedema (RS3PE), improved following surgical resection of prostatic carcinoma: a case report. Urol Case Rep. 2020;32:101232.

16. Manzo C, Natale M. Polymyalgia rheumatica in association with remitting seronegative sinovitis with pitting oedema: a neoplastic warning. Can Geriatr J. 2017;20(2):94–6.

17. Varshney AN, Singh NK. Syndrome of remitting seronegative symmetrical synovitis with pitting oedema: a case series. J Postgrad Med. 2015;61(1):38–41.

18. Eguia HA, Parodi Garcia JF, Ramas Diez C, Eguia A EA. Remitting seronegative symmetrical synovitis with pitting oedema (RS3PE) case presentation and comparison with other polyarthritides affecting older people. Age Ageing. 2017;46(2):333–4.

19. Higashida-Konishi M, Izumi K, Hama S, Takei H, Oshima H, Okano Y. Comparing the clinical and laboratory features of remitting seronegative symmetrical synovitis with pitting oedema and seronegative rheumatoid arthritis. J Clin Med. 2021;10(5):1116.

20. Nojima Y, Ihara M, Adachi H, Kurimoto T, Nanto S. Impact of low-dose prednisolone on refractory pitting oedema manifesting remitting seronegative symmetrical synovitis with pitting oedema syndrome. J Cardiol Cases. 2016;14(4):119–22.

21. Tani K, Kawaminami S, Okura Y, Tabata R, Yuasa S, Nakanishi Y, Kawahito K, Inaba K, Inaba K, Kondo K, Umetani K, Miyatake A, Suzuki Y, Yamaguchi H. Predictive factors associated with the therapeutic response in patients with polymyalgia rheumatica and remitting seronegative symmetrical synovitis with pitting oedema syndrome. J Med Invest. 2019;66(1.2):112–8.

Multicentric Reticulohistiocytosis

4

Stefano Rodolfi, Adam Greenspan, Michael Klein,
and Carlo Selmi

4.1 Introduction

Multicentric reticulohistiocytosis (MRH) is a rare systemic non-Langerhans cell (LC) histiocytosis. Around 300 cases have currently been reported in the literature, making knowledge about this disease mostly anecdotal, based on isolated case reports or small case series.

Multicentric reticulohistiocytosis is defined as a class C non-LC histiocytosis [1]: a disorder of resident tissue macrophages (i.e., histiocytes) with predominant mucocutaneous involvement and frequent systemic involvement. The first clear description of a case of MRH dates back to 1937, although reports of diseases likely belonging to the MRH spectrum have been reported since 1897. It was only in 1954 that the current name MRH was established by Goltz and Lymon, which took

S. Rodolfi · C. Selmi (✉)
Department of Biomedical Sciences, Humanitas University, Pieve Emanuele, Italy

IRCCS Humanitas Research Hospital, Milan, Italy
e-mail: stefano.rodolfi@humanitas.it; carlo.selmi@hunimed.eu

A. Greenspan
Department of Radiology, University of California, Davis Health, Sacramento, CA, USA
e-mail: agreenspan@ucdavis.edu

M. Klein
Department of Pathology and Laboratory Medicine, Hospital for Special Surgery affiliated with Weill Cornell Medical College, New York, NY, USA
e-mail: KlenM@HSS.edu

© The Author(s), under exclusive license to Springer Nature Switzerland AG 2022
V. Ravindran et al. (eds.), *Rarer Arthropathies*, Rare Diseases of the Immune System, https://doi.org/10.1007/978-3-031-05002-2_4

preference over previously used terms such as lipoid dermo-arthritis, reticulohistio-cytoma, lipid rheumatism, giant cell histiocytomatosis, and giant cell histiocy-tosis [2].

4.2   Clinical Features

Multicentric reticulohistiocytosis more commonly affects Caucasian women with a female to male ratio ranging from 2:1 to 3:1 [3]. Disease onset is usually in the fourth decade of life, although it has been described in children [4] and the elderly [5].

The major clinical manifestations of MRH are destructive polyarthritis and papu-lonodular mucocutaneous rash. Arthritis is usually polyarticular, symmetrical, and erosive. In the majority of patients, articular involvement precedes the onset of skin rash by about 3 years [6]. The most affected joints in order of decreasing frequency are hands, knees, shoulders, hips, ankles, elbows, and feet. In approximately 50% of cases, arthritis appears as spondylitis with axial involvement [7]. If untreated joint involvement progresses in a destructive fashion resulting in severe joint deformity with arthritis mutilans. Nonetheless, the articular involvement usually remits approximately over 10 years [8]. Younger age group has been associated with a more aggressive disease phenotype. The articular phenotype is highly similar to that of rheumatoid arthritis (RA), but unlike RA, MRH frequently involves distal inter-phalangeal joints (DIP).

Cutaneous manifestations are invariably present in MRH. They generally appear after 3 years of articular involvement, although skin lesions as an initial sign have occasionally been reported [6]. The characteristic skin lesion is a red-dish-brown to a flesh-colored papulonodular lesion of variable dimensions (few mm to 1 cm or more) often with a cobblestone appearance. Cutaneous lesions most commonly appear on hands and fingers, in particular on the dorsal aspect of metacarpophalangeal (MCP) joints and proximal (PIP) or distal interphalangeal joints (Fig. 4.1).

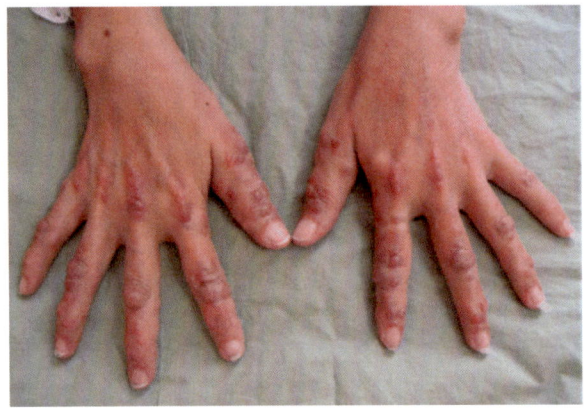

Fig. 4.1 Multiple asymptomatic erythematous nodules on the dorsal aspect of interphalangeal and metacarpophalangeal joints of both hands in a 36-year-old woman with MRH. (Reprinted with permission from [8])

A characteristic finding is the "coral beads sign" represented by periungual papules distributed along the nail folds. Similar to psoriatic arthritis (PsA), inflammation of DIP involves the nail matrix and results in nail changes such as atrophy, longitudinal ridging, and hyperpigmentation. The face is the second most commonly involved region, with papulonodular lesions frequently developing on the forehead, ear, scalp, and nape of the neck [7]. In the worst cases, extensive involvement of the face leads to a permanent disfigurement referred to as "leonine facies." Although hands and face are the most commonly involved sites, nearly all areas can be involved. Cutaneous lesions tend to appear and disappear spontaneously and are usually asymptomatic, though sometimes they can be itchy. Koebner phenomenon and photosensitivity have been described [9, 10]. In addition to the typical papulonodular skin lesion, xanthelasmas can be found in approximately 10% of cases of MRH [7]. Mucosal involvement is also frequent, seen in around one-third of cases, represented by multiple cobblestone-like lesions, usually located on the mucosal surface of the mouth [11].

Multicentric reticulohistiocytosis is considered a systemic disease. Indeed besides articular and cutaneous involvement, which are invariably present, MRH frequently presents with constitutional symptoms such as fever, fatigue, and weight loss [12]. Moreover, MRH can involve several other organs, such as the lung, heart, liver, kidney, urogenital tract, lymph nodes, muscles, eyes, gastrointestinal tract, larynx, and epiglottis [2, 8, 13–16]. Typically organ involvement occurs in the form of nodular infiltrates of histiocytes and/or local inflammation, sometimes evolving to tissue fibrosis. In particular, lung involvement has been reported with either pleural effusion, lung infiltrates, or pulmonary fibrosis [3, 13, 17] while heart involvement can occur in the form of pericardial effusion, myocarditis, or heart failure [18, 19]. Multicentric reticulohistiocytosis is usually a self-remitting disease however the sequelae of the active phases may be permanent and disabling, both physically and psychologically [20]. Arthritis is usually aggressive and frequently results in joint destruction while cutaneous involvement may be particularly disfiguring.

4.3   Diagnosis

4.3.1   Laboratory Investigations

There are no diagnostic laboratory markers for MRH. The inflammatory nature of the disease is sometimes reflected by laboratory tests: C-reactive protein (CRP) and erythrocyte sedimentation (ESR) are elevated in approximately half of the cases [7]; thrombocytosis and mild normocytic anemia have been reported as well. However, in majority, either nonspecific abnormalities or normal laboratory tests are seen. Nevertheless, routine testing with complete blood count, kidney and liver function tests, uric acid, lipid profile, and inflammatory markers should be obtained as they may point to an alternative differential diagnosis. Serum autoantibodies (RF, ACPA, ANA, anti-Ro, and anti-La) are normally negative and when positive may allude to an associated autoimmune condition.

4.3.2   Imaging

Imaging helps characterize the articular involvement as well as in differential diagnosis. Radiographs typically show bone erosions with sclerotic margins, initially located in the para-articular region resembling the erosions of gouty arthritis (Figs. 4.2 and 4.3).

Articular involvement progresses towards joint destruction resulting in arthritis mutilans (Figs. 4.4 and 4.5) and *main-en-lorgnette* (i.e., the typical "opera glass deformity" of the hands). This results in widening of joint spaces, loss of articular cartilage, and subchondral bone resorption.

The absence of periarticular osteopenia is peculiar and may help differentiate MRH from other inflammatory arthritides (most importantly rheumatoid arthritis and psoriatic arthritis). Moreover, the lack of osteophytes and interphalangeal ankylosis is pivotal in distinguishing MRH from erosive osteoarthritis (OA). In case of suspected systemic involvement, a total body contrast-enhanced CT scan may reveal nodular lesions involving target organs. Fluorodeoxyglucose (^{F18} FDG) positron emission tomography (PET) can be employed as well for disease staging and monitoring [24, 25]. MRH lesions, being inflammatory, are characterized by increased uptake of FDG thus enabling FDG-PET to identify the localization of the disease

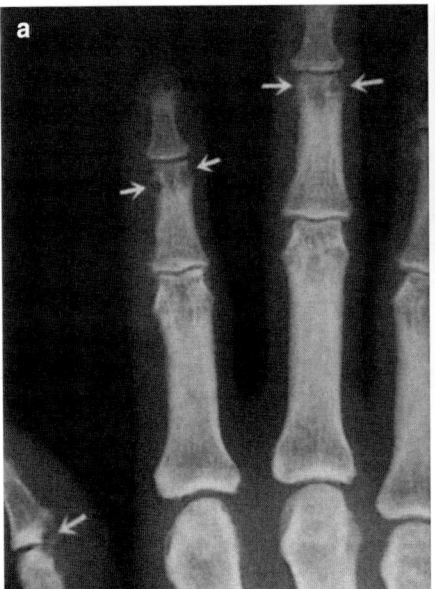
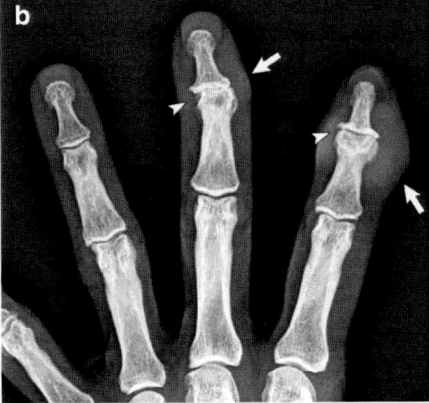

Fig. 4.2 (**a**) A 46-year-old woman presented with distal interphalangeal joints pain and soft tissue swelling. Note erosions with sharp margins at the distal interphalangeal joints (arrows) resembling gout. (**b**) Radiograph of the fingers of the right hand of the 65-year-old woman shows small erosions at the distal interphalangeal joints of the index and middle fingers (arrowheads) associated with soft tissue masses (arrows) resembling gouty tophi. (Reprinted with permission from [21])

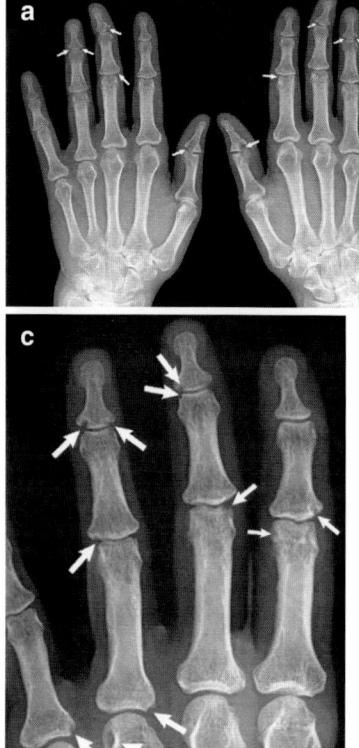

Fig. 4.3 (**a**) Dorsovolar and (**b**) Norgaard views of the hands of a 51-year-old woman who presented with a history of joint pain and swelling, but negative RA factor and normal serum uric acid, show characteristic articular erosions of the proximal and distal interphalangeal joints, as well as the interphalangeal joints of both thumbs *(arrows)*, very similar to erosions of gouty arthritis. (**c**) A coned-down magnified radiograph of the fingers of the right hand shows the erosions *(arrows)* more clearly

(including specific organ involvement), and to screen for the presence of an undetected malignancy (frequently featuring increased FDG uptake).

4.3.3   Histopathology

Synovial fluid analysis is mainly helpful to exclude other causes of arthritis. From the different case series, the only consistent finding has been an increased percentage of multinucleated cells. Nevertheless, exclusion of septic or crystal arthritis is important and easy through arthrocentesis.

Diagnosis of MRH ultimately requires tissue histology. The skin and less frequently the synovial tissue are usually regarded as the primary sites for histologic

Fig. 4.4 Dorsovolar radiograph of both hands of a 57-year-old woman with long-standing polyarthralgia, soft tissue swelling, and deformities of the fingers demonstrates severe destruction of multiple carpometacarpal, metacarpophalangeal, and interphalangeal joints similar to those seen in rheumatoid or psoriatic arthritis. (Reprinted with permission from [22])

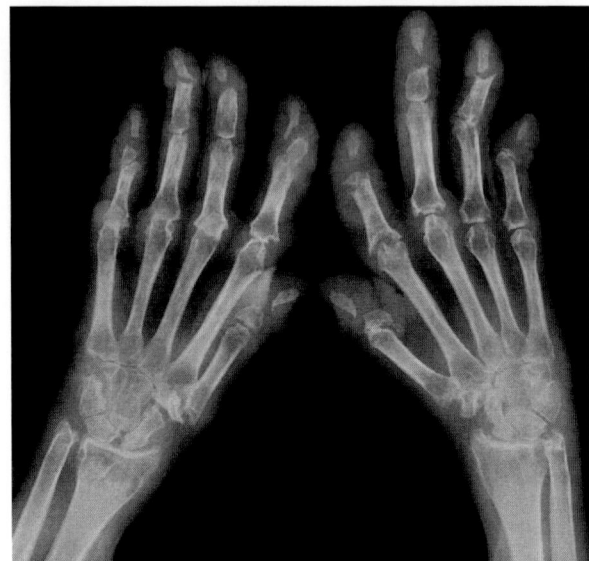

Fig. 4.5 Dorsovolar radiograph of both hands of a 63-year-old man shows arthritis mutilans affecting mainly the distal interphalangeal joints. (Reprinted with permission from [23])

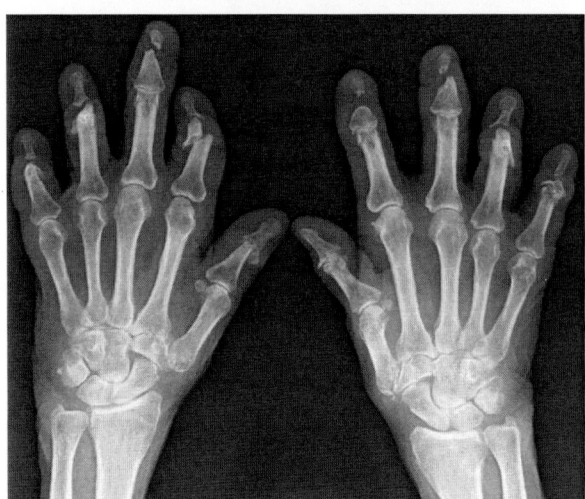

evaluation. Lesions at an early stage show dermal infiltrate of lymphocytes, eosinophils, plasma cells, and sometimes multinucleated histiocytes [26]. These histiocytes are not foamy, which is a characteristic that distinguishes MRH from other histiocytic diseases (e.g., granuloma annulare, sarcoidosis, xanthogranuloma, Erdheim Chester disease, Rosai-Dorfman disease) [8]. During later stages, lesions are characterized by the pathognomonic presence of mononuclear histiocytes with abundant eosinophilic ground glass-like cytoplasm and multinucleated giant cells. Large histiocytes, also called megalocytes, are another typical finding. At this stage foamy histiocytes, along with typical cells, may be detected [27] (Fig. 4.6).

Fig. 4.6 A biopsy specimen of synovium shows foamy histiocytes, multinucleated megalocytes, and typical histiocytes in the fibrous background (H & E, original magnification ×250)

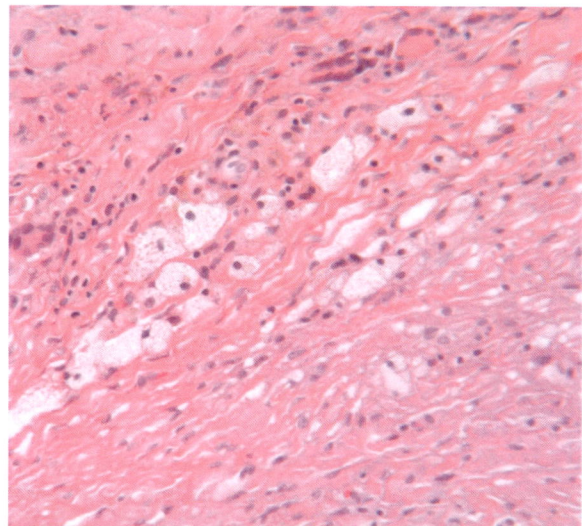

Fig. 4.7 Typical histiocytes, foamy histiocytes, and large histiocytes (so-called "megalocytes") containing PAS-positive material (synovium, PAS stain, original magnification ×400)

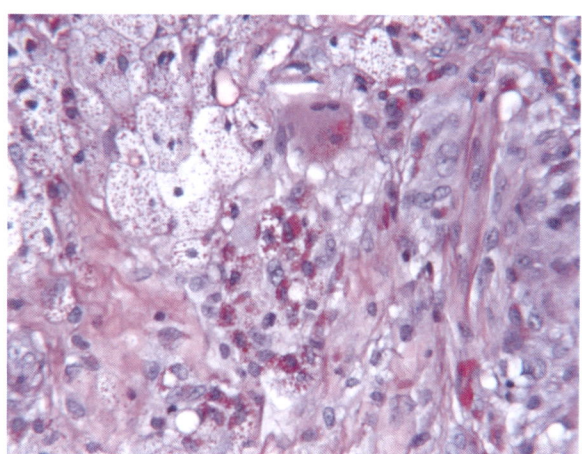

Further staining depicts strong positivity of histiocytes for periodic acid-Schiff (PAS) (Fig. 4.7) and strong expression of macrophage-specific markers such as CD11b, CD14, CD68, CD163, CD206, MAC387, lysozyme, and human alveolar macrophage-56 (HAM-56) [27, 28].

Moreover, MRH histiocytes are positive for vimentin staining and express non-specific esterase and acid phosphatase [28]. The observed strong positivity for CD163 and CD206 together with weak expression of CD86 may reflect a polarization of infiltrating macrophages towards a T2 phenotype, as recently suggested [29]. Importantly, MRH histiocytes stain negative for the Langerhans cell markers CD1a and S100 [28]. Negativity for factor XIIIa is helpful to distinguish MRH from reticulohistiocytoma, a condition also known as solitary cutaneous reticulohistiocytosis, which is characterized by discrete self-limited skin lesions resembling those of MRH [27]. Synovial biopsy is seldom sought due to easier access to skin lesions and shows a similar histological picture with PAS-positive lipid-laden giant cells and histiocytes with eosinophilic ground-glass cytoplasm [30]. Similar findings have been reported in other affected organs, such as the myocardium [19].

At electron microscopy, histiocytes display ultrastructural features of activated mononuclear antigen-processing cells, with prominent nucleoli and numerous Golgi complexes, rough endoplasmic reticulum, lysosomes, mitochondria, and phagosomes [31].

4.4   Pathogenesis

The scarcity of patients' cohorts and the absence of animal models renders the evidence about the pathogenesis of MRH poor. What we know is that inflammation plays a critical role in disease pathogenesis. Analyzed samples of synovial fluid have revealed high amounts of proinflammatory cytokines and inflammatory mediators such as TNFα, IL-1β, IL-6, IL12, prostaglandin E2, and platelet-derived growth factor β [32, 33]. Especially TNFα is a central mediator in MRH, as demonstrated by the reported efficacy of TNFα inhibitors (addressed in detail in the "Treatment" section). Supporting this hypothesis, monocyte chemoattractant protein-1 (MCP-1), a molecule downstream of the TNFα cascade was found elevated in the serum and skin lesion of a patient with MRH, and levels decreased consensually with clinical improvement with anti-TNFα therapy [34]. This inflammatory surge is thought to be generated by the multinucleated giant cells characteristic of MRH: supporting these hypotheses reports have shown cytokine expression by these cells [32], and as mentioned several reports detected macrophage-specific positive staining.

Evidence has pointed out a role for osteoclast activation in the pathogenesis of articular involvement of MRH. Some of the mononuclear cells of MRH infiltrate have been found to express receptor activator of nuclear factor kappa B ligand (RANKL) at immunohistochemical analysis [35]. Stimulation by RANKL positive stromal cells may directly induce differentiation of synovial macrophages into osteoclasts, as demonstrated for rheumatoid arthritis [36, 37]. Supporting this hypothesis, synovial fluid macrophages from an MRH patient were cultured in the presence of macrophage colony-stimulating factor (M-CSF) and RANKL, and they differentiated into osteoclast-like multinucleated giant cells [38]. Moreover, MRH histiocytes were reported to express the osteoclast tissue lytic markers tartrate-resistant acid phosphatase (TRAP) and cathepsin K [39], and thereby further highlighting the central role of osteoclasts in bone resorption in MRH, as in rheumatoid arthritis [40]. Further evidence is provided by the reported clinical efficacy of bisphosphonates in multiple cases of MRH [35, 38, 41].

A clonal origin of MRH cells has been proposed. Recent evidence has demonstrated that Langherans cell histiocytosis and some non-LCH histiocytosis (i.e., Erdheim Chester disease, juvenile xanthogranuloma, Rosai-Dorfman disease) arise from the clonal expansion of a progenitor cell (dendritic cell for LCH, macrophage for non-LCH) harboring mutations in genes involved in tyrosine kinase pathways or intracellular pathways, most commonly the RAS-MAPK pathway [42]. Treatment with BRAF inhibitors or MEK inhibitors has changed the natural course of Erdheim Chester disease [43]. A recent study performed whole-genome sequencing and RNA sequencing in two patients with MRH. One patient presented a novel fusion protein involving kinesin family member 5B and fibroblast growth factor receptor 1 tyrosine kinase (KIF5B-FGFR1), strongly suggesting a gain-of-function tyrosine kinase activity [44]. The other patient presented a driver in-frame deletion of Mitogen-Activated Protein Kinase Kinase 1 (MAP2K1) [44], already reported as a gain-of-function driver mutation in melanoma [45]. The mutational analysis suggested a clonal origin of MRH histiocytes. Finally, the patient with MAP2K1 deletion was successfully treated with chemotherapy [44].

4.5   Association with Other Diseases

Multicentric reticulohistiocytosis is associated with malignancy in about 25% of cases. Association with both solid and hematological cancer has been described. A literature review does not reveal a consistent association with a specific cancer type, indeed almost every type of malignancy has been associated: lung, laryngeal, bronchial, endometrial, ovarian, gastric, liver, sarcoma, leukemia, lymphoma, etc. [46–52]. It is not clear whether MRH should be regarded as a paraneoplastic syndrome in these cases, as treatment of the malignancy did result in disease improvement only on some occasions [53]. Given the extreme rarity of the disease, the association with cancer may be coincidental. Nevertheless, the diagnostic workup of MRH should always include age/gender-specific cancer screening.

The coexistence of MRH with other autoimmune conditions is described in approximately 15% of cases [12]. Several autoimmune diseases have been associated: rheumatoid arthritis [54], systemic lupus erythematosus (SLE) [55], Sjögren syndrome [56], systemic sclerosis [57], and dermatomyositis [58]. Additionally, diseases such as thyroid disease, dyslipidemia, and diabetes mellitus have been associated with MRH [8]; whether this represents a mere coincidence is still under debate. Finally, a significant percentage of patients have been detected with a positive tuberculin test [59]. The conditions associated with MRH have been summarized in Table 4.1.

Table 4.1 Conditions associated with multicentric reticulohistiocytosis

Associated condition	Type
Malignancy	Lung cancer
	Laryngeal cancer
	Bronchial cancer
	Gastric cancer
	Liver cancer
	Endometrial cancer
	Ovarian cancer
	Leukemia
	Lymphoma
	Sarcoma
Autoimmune diseases	Rheumatoid arthritis
	Sjogren syndrome
	Systemic lupus erythematosus
	Systemic sclerosis
	Dermatomyositis
Other diseases	Thyroid disease
	Dyslipidemia
	Diabetes mellitus
	Colitis

4.6 Differential Diagnoses

Sometimes MRH may be misdiagnosed as another autoimmune disease, due to resemblance of clinical presentation. Indeed the differential diagnosis may be challenging, especially when the clinical onset features only articular involvement, as it happens in the majority of cases. The pattern of articular involvement and radiological appearance helps differentiate MRH from other forms of arthritis. Preferential DIP involvement distinguishes it from RA, together with lack of joint narrowing and juxta-articular osteoporosis. The absence of periarticular osteoporosis and periosteal new bone formation distinguishes MRH from PsA, which frequently features DIP arthritis. DIP involvement is typical of erosive osteoarthritis as well, however the absence of marginal osteophytes and joint ankylosis helps in ruling out OA. MRH arthritis can be easily distinguished from crystal arthropathies (i.e., gout and calcium pyrophosphate deposition disease) by demonstrating the absence of urate or calcium pyrophosphate crystals in the synovial fluid examination through polarized light microscopy. Cutaneous manifestations, even though being more specific than articular manifestations, may as well be challenging for the differential diagnosis of MRH, especially when appearing before articular involvement. The main differential diagnosis here is with dermatomyositis (DM): papulonodular lesions typical of MRH when coalescing in the trunk or upper back area may mimic the V-rash or shawl sign of DM, respectively; moreover, hand lesions may be mistaken with Gottron's papules. As mentioned, nail involvement is similar to that of psoriatic arthritis; however, in MRH it is part of a characteristic involvement of the periungual region (i.e., coral beads sign) [60] that makes the disease highly recognizable. Another important differential is with localized granuloma annulare: the disease indeed features cutaneous involvement with erythematous plaques or papules in the dorsal aspect of hands and feet. However, these lesions are highly recognizable due to their annular appearance with circinate borders, and the disease ensues most commonly in young adults, who are rarely affected by MRH. Last, granuloma annulare does not have articular involvement [61]. The differential diagnosis should also include sarcoidosis, xanthoma, fibroblastic rheumatism, lepromatous leprosy, and Farber's disease [62].

4.7 Treatment

Multicentric reticulohistiocytosis is often a self-limited disease, nevertheless early treatment is warranted to prevent the permanent damage of destructive arthritis, dermatitis, or visceral organ involvement. Due to the extreme rarity of the disease, the evidence on treatment efficacy is only limited to case reports and small case series. Nonsteroidal anti-inflammatory drugs (NSAIDs) and steroids are typically used as first-line agents [7]. Generally, patients need to be started on a disease-modifying anti-rheumatic drug (DMARD) to achieve disease remission [7]. The following DMARDs have been employed in the treatment of MRH: methotrexate [63, 64], hydroxychloroquine [63], leflunomide [5], azathioprine [65], cyclosporine A [66] sulfasalazine, mycophenolate [7]. A partial or complete response has been obtained in some cases with alkylating agents such as cyclophosphamide [67, 68], chlorambucil [69], and vincristine sulfate [70]. After the identification of the proinflammatory signature of MRH, selective cytokine inhibition with biologic agents has been employed with promising results. Encouraging data have been reported especially on the efficacy of anti-TNFα, both regarding articular and cutaneous response. Both monoclonal antibodies (infliximab and adalimumab) and recombinant soluble receptor (etanercept) showed clinical efficacy in specific case reports [71–75]. Moreover, in one case clinical improvement was accompanied by a decrease in the serum level of TNFα, further highlighting the critical role of TNFα in MRH pathogenesis [34]. The efficacy of cytokine blockade extends beyond that of anti-TNFα agents. One case of MRH refractory to steroids and methotrexate was successfully treated with IL-6 inhibition through tocilizumab [76]. Furthermore one patient with a strong histological expression of IL-1β and elevated serum IL-1β levels was treated with recombinant IL-1 receptor antagonist (anakinra), achieving both disease remission and normalization of IL-1β levels [77].

Owing to the evidence of osteoclastic activity in MRH, treatment with bisphosphonates has been implemented in some cases. Alendronate, pamidronate, and zoledronic acid have been utilized with beneficial effects both on articular and cutaneous involvement, both as a monotherapy [35] and in combination with steroids and DMARDs [7, 41, 78]. Moreover, the anti-RANKL monoclonal antibody denosumab was used in combination with tacrolimus in the case of MRH [79] and more recent trials suggest that anti-osteoporotic agents targeting cathepsin K may provide new therapeutic options [80].

Finally, the newly introduced concept of multicentric reticulohistiocytosis as a clonal disease [44] opens new frontiers for targeted therapy with tyrosine kinase inhibitors. As for other histiocytosis treatments, inhibitors of the RAS-MAPK-ERK pathway [81] may provide striking clinical benefits. Knowledge is still limited as mutational analysis has recently been performed only on two patients.

Occasionally surgical intervention with arthrodesis or joint replacement may be required in patients with arthritis mutilans.

In summary, treatment of MRH is ought to evolve towards a personalized therapy with biologic agents and tyrosine kinase inhibitors selected upon the immunohistochemical presentation, cytokine profile, and mutational analysis.

4.8   Conclusion

Multicentric reticulohistiocytosis is a systemic non-Langherans histiocytosis with predominant mucocutaneous involvement. It represents a clinical challenge due to the extreme rarity of the disease and its resemblance to other more common inflammatory disorders, especially at the early stages of the disease. Better disease knowledge is required to decrease the rate of underdiagnosis and to start early treatment to prevent the destructive features of MRH. The recently discovered proinflammatory cytokine signature and alteration in tyrosine kinase pathways open up new promising therapeutic options with biologics and antineoplastic drugs.

References

1. Emile JF, Abla O, Fraitag S, Horne A, Haroche J, Donadieu J, et al. Revised classification of histiocytoses and neoplasms of the macrophage-dendritic cell lineages. Blood. 2016;127:2672–81.
2. Barrow MV, Holubar K. Multicentric reticulohistiocytosis. A review of 33 patients. Medicine (Baltimore). 1969;48(4):287–305.
3. Sanchez-Alvarez C, Sandhu AS, Crowson CS, Wetter DA, McKenzie GA, Lehman JS, et al. Multicentric reticulohistiocytosis: the Mayo Clinic experience (1980-2017). Rheumatology (Oxford). 2020;59(8):1898–905.
4. Havill S, Duffill M, Rademaker M. Multicentric reticulohistiocytosis in a child. Australas J Dermatol. 1999;40(1):44–6.
5. Lonsdale-Eccles AA, Haworth AE, McCrae FC, Young-Min SA. Successful treatment of multicentric reticulohistiocytosis with leflunomide. Br J Dermatol. 2009;161(2):470–2.
6. Saba R, Kwatra SG, Upadhyay B, Mirrakhimov AE, Khan FN. Multicentric reticulohistiocytosis presenting with papulonodular skin lesions and arthritis mutilans. Case Rep Rheumatol. 2013;2013:1–4.
7. Tariq S, Hugenberg ST, Hirano-Ali SA, Tariq H. Multicentric reticulohistiocytosis (MRH): case report with review of literature between 1991 and 2014 with in depth analysis of various treatment regimens and outcomes. Springerplus. 2016;5(1, 1):–13.
8. Selmi C, Greenspan A, Huntley A, Gershwin ME. Multicentric reticulohistiocytosis: a critical review. Curr Rheumatol Rep. 2015;17(6):511.
9. Aldridge RD, Main RA, Daly BM. The Koebner's response in multicentric reticulohistiocytosis. Cutis. 1984;34(1):78–80.
10. Taniguchi T, Asano Y, Okada A, Sugaya M, Sato S. Ultraviolet light-induced Köbner phenomenon contributes to the development of skin eruptions in multicentric reticulohistiocytosis. Acta Derm Venereol. 2011;91(2):160–3.

11. Luz FB, Gaspar AP, Kalil-Gaspar N, Ramos-E-Silva M. Multicentric reticulohistiocytosis. J Eur Acad Dermatol Venereol. 2001;15:524–31.
12. Toz B, Büyükbabani N, İnanç M. Multicentric reticulohistiocytosis: rheumatology perspective. Best Pract Res Clin Rheumatol. 2016;30(2):250–60.
13. Yang HJ, Ding YQ, Deng YJ. Multicentric reticulohistiocytosis with lungs and liver involved. Clin Exp Dermatol. 2009;34(2):183–5.
14. Buckley C, Bron A. The ocular and periocular features of multicentric reticulohistiocytosis with paraproteinaemia. A report of two cases. Aust J Ophthalmol. 1981;9(3):207–11.
15. Hotta M, Minamimoto R, Suzuki D, Takahashi A. Multicentric reticulohistiocytosis mimicking malignancy on 18F-FDG PET/CT. Clin Nucl Med. 2017;42(7):567–8.
16. Kocanaogullari H, Ozsan H, Oksel F, Ozturk G, Kandiloglu G, Ustun EE, et al. Multicentric reticulohistiocytosis. Clin Rheumatol. 1996;15(1):62–6.
17. West KL, Sporn T, Puri PK. Multicentric reticulohistiocytosis: a unique case with pulmonary fibrosis. Arch Dermatol. 2012;148(2):228–32.
18. Fast A. Cardiopulmonary complications in multicentric reticulohistiocytosis: report of a case. Arch Dermatol. 1976;112(8):1139–41.
19. Webb-Detiege T, Sasken H, Kaur P. Infiltration of histiocytes and multinucleated giant cells in the myocardium of a patient with multicentric reticulohistiocytosis. J Clin Rheumatol. 2009;15(1):25–6.
20. Trotta F, Castellino G, Lo Monaco A. Multicentric reticulohistiocytosis. Best Pract Res Clin Rheumatol. 2004;18(5):759–72.
21. Greenspan A, Gershwin ME. Imaging in rheumatology—a clinical approach. Philadelphia: Wolters Kluwer; 2018. p. 364, Fig. 10.7
22. Greenspan A, Gershwin ME. Imaging in rheumatology—a clinical approach. Philadelphia: Wolters Kluwer; 2018. p. 363, Fig. 10.5
23. Greenspan A, Gershwin ME. Imaging in rheumatology—a practical approach. Philadelphia: Wolters Kluwer; 2018. p. 363, Fig. 10.6
24. Dietz M, Debarbieux S, Righetti M, Harou O, Tordo J. Paraneoplastic multicentric reticulohistiocytosis on 18F-FDG PET/CT breast carcinoma follow-up. Clin Nucl Med. 2021;46(5):e253–5.
25. Asano T, Suzutani K, Watanabe A, Honda A, Mori N, Yashiro M, et al. The utility of FDG-PET/CT imaging in the evaluation of multicentric reticulohistiocytosis: a case report. Medicine (Baltimore). 2018;97(33):e11449.
26. Heathcote JG, Guenther LC, Wallace AC. Multicentric reticulohistiocytosis: a report of a case and a review of the pathology. Pathology. 1985;17(4):601–8.
27. Zelger B, Cerio R, Soyer HP, Misch K, Orchard G, Wilson-Jones E. Reticulohistiocytoma and multicentric reticulohistiocytosis. Histopathologic and immunophenotypic distinct entities. Am J Dermatopathol. 1994;16(6):577–84.
28. Luz FB, Gaspar AP, Ramos-e-Silva M, Carvalho da Fonseca E, Villar EG, Cordovil Pires AR, et al. Immunohistochemical profile of multicentric reticulohistiocytosis. Skinmed. 2005;4(2):71–7.
29. Kamiya K, Komine M, Murata S, Ohtsuki M. Involvement of M2 macrophages in the pathomechanisms of multicentric reticulohistiocytosis. Int J Dermatol. 2017;56(8):e173–5.
30. Krause ML, Lehman JS, Warrington KJ. Multicentric reticulohistiocytosis can mimic rheumatoid arthritis. J Rheumatol. 2014;41(4):780–1.
31. Caputo R, Gianotti F. Cytoplasmic markers ultrastructural features in histiocytic proliferations of the skin. G Ital di Dermatologia e Venereol. 1980;115:107–10.
32. Bennàssar A, Mas A, Guilabert A, Julià M, Mascaró-Galy JM, Herrero C. Multicentric reticulohistiocytosis with elevated cytokine serum levels. J Dermatol. 2011;38(9):905–10.
33. Nakajima Y, Sato K, Morita H, Torikai S, Hidano A, Nishioka K, et al. Severe progressive erosive arthritis in multicentric reticulohistiocytosis: possible involvement of cytokines in synovial proliferation. J Rheumatol. 1992;19(10):1643–6.

34. Iwata H, Okumura Y, Seishima M, Aoyama Y. Overexpression of monocyte chemoattractant protein-1 in the overlying epidermis of multicentric reticulohistiocytosis lesions: a case report. Int J Dermatol. 2012;51(4):492–4.

35. Goto H, Inaba M, Kobayashi K, Imanishi Y, Kumeda Y, Inui K, et al. Successful treatment of multicentric reticulohistiocytosis with alendronate: evidence for a direct effect of bisphosphonate on histiocytes. Arthritis Rheum. 2003;48(12):3538–41.

36. Cambridge G, Perry HC, Nogueira L, Serre G, Parsons HM, De La Torre I, et al. The effect of B-cell depletion therapy on serological evidence of B-cell and plasmablast activation in patients with rheumatoid arthritis over multiple cycles of rituximab treatment. J Autoimmun. 2014;50:67–76.

37. Clement M, Fornasa G, Loyau S, Morvan M, Andreata F, Guedj K, et al. Upholding the T cell immune-regulatory function of CD31 inhibits the formation of T/B immunological synapses invitro and attenuates the development of experimental autoimmune arthritis in vivo. J Autoimmun. 2015;56:23–33.

38. Adamopoulos IE, Wordsworth PB, Edwards JR, Ferguson DJ, Athanasou NA. Osteoclast differentiation and bone resorption in multicentric reticulohistiocytosis. Hum Pathol. 2006;37(9):1176–85.

39. Codriansky KA, Rünger TM, Bhawan J, Kantarci A, Kissin EY. Multicentric reticulohistiocytosis: a systemic osteoclastic disease? Arthritis Rheum. 2008;59(3):444–8.

40. Gravallese EM, Goldring SR. Cellular mechanisms and the role of cytokines in bone erosions in rheumatoid arthritis. Arthritis Rheum. 2000;43(10):2143–51.

41. Satoh M, Oyama N, Yamada H, Nakamura K, Kaneko F. Treatment trial of multicentric reticulohistiocytosis with a combination of predonisolone, methotrexate and alendronate. J Dermatol. 2008;35(3):168–71.

42. Diamond EL, Durham BH, Haroche J, Yao Z, Ma J, Parikh SA, et al. Diverse and targetable kinase alterations drive histiocytic neoplasms. Cancer Discov. 2016;6(2):154–65.

43. Goyal G, Heaney ML, Collin M, Cohen-Aubart F, Vaglio A, Durham BH, et al. Erdheim-Chester disease: consensus recommendations for evaluation, diagnosis, and treatment in the molecular era. Blood. 2020;135(22):1929–45.

44. Murakami N, Sakai T, Arai E, Muramatsu H, Ichikawa D, Asai S, et al. Targetable driver mutations in multicentric reticulohistiocytosis. Haematologica. 2020;105(2):E61–4.

45. De Unamuno Bustos B, Estal RM, Simó GP, De Juan Jimenez I, Muñoz BE, Serna MR, et al. Towards personalized medicine in melanoma: implementation of a clinical next-generation sequencing panel. Sci Rep. 2017;7(1):495.

46. Hu L, Mei JH, Xia J, Hao QS, Cheng LP, Wu YH. Erythema, papules, and arthralgia associated with liver cancer: report of a rare case of multicentric reticulohistiocytosis. Int J Clin Exp Pathol. 2015;8(3):3304–7.

47. Huang X, Zhang L, Zhang S. Multicentric reticulohistiocytosis with extra-mammillary Paget's disease: a case report. Eur J Med Res. 2013;18(1):38.

48. Tan BH, Barry CI, Wick MR, White KP, Brown JG, Lee A, et al. Multicentric reticulohistiocytosis and urologic carcinomas: a possible paraneoplastic association. J Cutan Pathol. 2011;38(1):43–8.

49. El-Haddad B, Hammoud D, Shaver T, Shahouri S. Malignancy-associated multicentric reticulohistiocytosis. Rheumatol Int. 2011;31(9):1235–8.

50. Hinchman KF, Wu JJ, Soden CE, Waldman J, Dyson SW. Multicentric reticulohistiocytosis associated with Burkitt lymphoma and adenocarcinoma. Cutis. 2008;82(2):113–4.

51. Malik MK, Regan L, Robinson-Bostom L, Pan TD, McDonald CJ. Proliferating multicentric reticulohistiocytosis associated with papillary serous carcinoma of the endometrium. J Am Acad Dermatol. 2005;53(6):1075–9.

52. Nunnink JC, Krusinski PA, Yates JW. Multicentric reticulohistiocytosis and cancer: a case report and review of the literature. Med Pediatr Oncol. 1985;13(5):273–9.

53. Tirumalae R, Rout P, Jayaseelan E, Shet A, Devi S, Kumar K. Paraneoplastic multicentric reticulohistiocytosis: a clinicopathologic challenge. Indian J Dermatol Venereol Leprol. 2011;77(3):318–20.

54. Hoshina D, Shimizu T, Abe R, Murata J, Tanaka K, Shimizu H. Multicentric reticulohistiocytosis associated with rheumatoid arthritis. Rheumatol Int. 2005;25(7):553–4.
55. Saito K, Fujii K, Awazu Y, Nakayamada S, Fujii Y, Ota T, et al. A case of systemic lupus erythematosus complicated with multicentric reticulohistiocytosis (MRH): successful treatment of MRH and lupus nephritis with cyclosporin A. Lupus. 2001;10(2):129–32.
56. Ben Abdelghani K, Mahmoud I, Chatelus E, Sordet C, Gottenberg JE, Sibilia J. Multicentric reticulohistiocytosis: an autoimmune systemic disease? Case report of an association with erosive rheumatoid arthritis and systemic Sjogren syndrome. Joint Bone Spine. 2010;77(3):274–6.
57. Takahashi M, Mizutani H, Nakamura Y, Shimizu M. A case of multicentric reticulohistiocytosis, systemic sclerosis and Sjögren syndrome. J Dermatol. 1997;24(8):530–4.
58. Fett N, Liu RH. Multicentric reticulohistiocytosis with dermatomyositis-like features: a more common disease presentation than previously thought. Dermatology. 2011;222(2):102–8.
59. Gold KD, Sharp JT, Estrada RG, Duffy J, Person DA. Relationship between multicentric reticulohistiocytosis and tuberculosis. JAMA. 1977;237(20):2213–4.
60. Barrow MV. The nails in multicentric reticulohistiocytosis. (Lipoid dermato-arthritis). Arch Dermatol. 1967;95(2):200–1.
61. Piette EW, Rosenbach M. Granuloma annulare: pathogenesis, disease associations and triggers, and therapeutic options. J Am Acad Dermatol. 2016;75:467–79.
62. Lesher JL, Allen BS. Multicentric reticulohistiocytosis. J Am Acad Dermatol. 1984;11(4 Pt 2):713–23.
63. Cash JM, Tyree J, Recht M. Severe multicentric reticulohistiocytosis: disease stabilization achieved with methotrexate and hydroxychloroquine. J Rheumatol. 1997;24(11):2250–3.
64. Gourmelen O, Le Loet X, Fortier-Beaulieu M, Thomine E, Ledan G, Lauret P, et al. Methotrexate treatment of multicentric reticulohistiocytosis. J Rheumatol. 1991;18(4):627–8.
65. Rudd A, Dolianitis C, Varigos G, Howard A. A case of multicentric reticulohistiocytosis responsive to azathioprine in a patient with no underlying malignancy. Australas J Dermatol. 2011;52(4):292–4.
66. Chalom EC, Rosenstein ED, Kramer N. Cyclosporine as a treatment for multicentric reticulohistiocytosis. J Rheumatol. 2000;27(2):556.
67. Ríos Blanco JJ, Barbado Hernández FJ, Gómez Cerezo J, Suárez García I, Contreras Rubio F, Vázquez Rodríguez JJ. Multicentric reticulohistiocytosis. The long course of a rare disease. Scand J Rheumatol. 2002;31(2):107–9.
68. Liang GC, Granston AS. Complete remission of multicentric reticulohistiocytosis with combination therapy of steroid, cyclophosphamide, and low-dose pulse methotrexate. Case report, review of the literature, and proposal for treatment. Arthritis Rheum. 1996;39(1):171–4.
69. Bauer A, Garbe C, Detmar M, Kreuser ED, Gollnick H. [Multicentric reticulohistiocytosis and myelodysplastic syndrome]. Hautarzt. 1994;45(2):91–96.
70. Furey N, Di Mauro J, Eng A, Shaw J. Multicentric reticulohistiocytosis with salivary gland involvement and pericardial effusion. J Am Acad Dermatol. 1983;8(5):679–85.
71. Macía-Villa CC, Zea-Mendoza A. Multicentric reticulohistiocytosis: case report with response to infliximab and review of treatment options. Clin Rheumatol. 2016;35(2):527–34.
72. Kalajian AH, Callen JP. Multicentric reticulohistiocytosis successfully treated with infliximab: an illustrative case and evaluation of cytokine expression supporting anti-tumor necrosis factor therapy. Arch Dermatol. 2008;144(10):1360–6.
73. Kim S, Khatchaturian EM, Dehesa L. Multicentric reticulohistiocytosis: a case report with response to adalimumab. Clin Case Rep. 2020;8(8):1560–3.
74. Motegi SI, Yonemoto Y, Yanagisawa S, Toki S, Uchiyama A, Yamada K, et al. Successful treatment of multicentric reticulohistiocytosis with adalimumab. Acta Derm Venereol. 2016;96(1):124–5.
75. Rodriguez-Cerdeira C, Sanchez-Blanco B, San Millán B, Vilata JJ. Multicentric reticulohistiocytosis treated successfully with etanercept. Open Dermatol J. 2008;2:44–7.

76. Pacheco-Tena C, Reyes-Cordero G, Ochoa-Albíztegui R, Ríos-Barrera V, González-Chávez SA. Treatment of multicentric reticulohistiocytosis with tocilizumab. J Clin Rheumatol. 2013;19(5):272–6.

77. Aouba A, Leclerc-Mercier S, Fraitag S, Martin-Silva N, Bienvenu B, Georgin-Lavialle S. Assessment and effective targeting of interleukin-1 in multicentric reticulohistyocytosis. Joint Bone Spine. 2015;82(4):280–3.

78. Hamamoto K, Goto H, Yamada S, Yoda M, Yoda K, Imanishi Y, et al. THU0386 seven cases of multicentric reticulohistiocytosis treated with intravenous administration of alendronate. Ann Rheum Dis. 2014;73(Suppl 2):315.

79. Mokuda S, Oiwa H. Successful treatment of FKBP51-expressed multicentric reticulohistiocytosis using combination therapy with low-dose denosumab and tacrolimus. Scand J Rheumatol. 2016;45:247–8.

80. Duong LT, Leung AT, Langdahl B. Cathepsin K inhibition: a new mechanism for the treatment of osteoporosis. Calcif Tissue Int. 2016;98(4):381–97.

81. Boonstra J, Rijken P, Humbel B, Cremers F, Verkleij A, van Bergen en Henegouwen P. The epidermal growth factor. Cell Biol Int. 1995;19(5):413–30.

SAPHO Syndrome

5

Steven Truong and Peter Nash

5.1   Introduction

Synovitis, Acne, Pustulosis, Hyperostosis, Osteitis (SAPHO) syndrome involves "osteoarticular" changes of sterile osteitis, sclerotic bony hypertrophy, and synovitis, usually accompanied by pustular skin disease [1].

Diagnosis is challenging due to a highly variable presentation and the absence of validated diagnostic criteria. Diagnosis is made by global impression, relying on the presence of multiple features with moderate or high specificity. Alternate diagnoses including spondyloarthritis, infection, and malignancy must be reasonably excluded by the overall clinical picture, imaging, or bone biopsy.

SAPHO is very rare—prevalence is estimated at less than 1/10,000 in Caucasians and 0.00144/100,000 in Japanese [2, 3]. The actual prevalence may be higher as cases may be diagnosed with the more common, related conditions of spondyloarthritis or pustular skin disease. SAPHO typically onsets at 28–50 years of age and is more common in females [4, 5].

Other adult syndromes of sterile osteitis with multisystem involvement have been described and some meet the definition of SAPHO syndrome. In children, the related syndromes of Chronic Non-bacterial Osteomyelitis (CNO) and Chronic Recurrent Multifocal Osteomyelitis (CRMO) resemble SAPHO but involve less pustulosis and axial disease, and more peripheral osteitis [3].

A multisystem presentation is common, for example, involving Anterior Chest Wall (ACW) synovitis, sacroiliitis, Palmoplantar Pustulosis (PPP), Crohn's disease and axial spondyloarthritis. This suggests shared or overlapping pathophysiology of

S. Truong (✉) · P. Nash
Coast Joint Care, Maroochydore, QLD, Australia

Griffith University School of Medicine and Dentistry, Brisbane, QLD, Australia
e-mail: s.truong@griffith.edu.au

© The Author(s), under exclusive license to Springer Nature Switzerland AG 2022
V. Ravindran et al. (eds.), *Rarer Arthropathies*, Rare Diseases of the Immune System, https://doi.org/10.1007/978-3-031-05002-2_5

these diseases, although a genome-wide study of SAPHO did not find common risk loci. An international survey led by the Group for Research and Assessment of Psoriasis and Psoriatic Arthritis (GRAPPA) reported 49% of SAPHO treating clinicians considered it to be a subtype of spondyloarthritis, 19% a subtype of psoriatic arthritis, 6% reactive arthritis, and 26% a separate entity [6]. Characteristic clinical features shared between SAPHO and psoriatic arthritis include sterile cutaneous microabscesses, sacroiliitis on MRI in 30–40%, and reduced association with HLA-B27. Other specific features of spondyloarthritis are also seen in SAPHO, including enthesitis with bony bridge formation (including vertebral) and peri-entheseal osteitis. Explanations for the infection-like features include the novel concept of "reactive infectious osteitis," a reactive arthritis that can commence and persist without resolution of infection [7]. Resemblance to these conditions and case series guide our choice of treatment.

5.2 Pathophysiology

The pathophysiology of SAPHO is distinct from other arthritides as it has a unique pattern of immune dysfunction and suspected microbial interaction. Clinically it can resemble disseminated bacterial infection or infectious osteitis. Despite the frequent presence of microbes in bone biopsy samples, there is inadequate evidence to confirm causation, suggesting a complex microbial interaction, such as dysbiosis or chronic infection.

Bone marrow biopsies demonstrate sterile osteomyelitis, involving early infiltration with polymorphonuclear neutrophils, followed by a mononuclear cell infiltrate and late-stage sclerosis with osteocytes and marrow fibrosis.

Immune dysregulation of multiple pathways is evident, including elevation of proinflammatory cytokines, low NK cell counts, and increased Th17 cells [8]. Proinflammatory signals of the innate response, including Interleukin (IL)-1, IL-8, IL-17, IL-18, and RANKL are elevated, producing symptoms such as those seen in spondyloarthritis, PAPA (Pyogenic Arthritis, Pyoderma Gangrenosum, and Acne) syndrome and metabolic bone disease [9]. The PAPA syndrome mouse model, PSTPIP2 knockout mice, developed IL-1ß elevation and a SAPHO-like syndrome of synovitis, hyperostosis, and osteitis, multifocal osteomyelitis with macrophage and neutrophil infiltrate of phone, joints, and skin [10].

Cutibacterium acnes (formerly *Propionibacterium acnes*) is a strong stimulator of the NLR/NLRP-inflammasome which produces IL-1ß [11]. *C. acnes* is therefore a species of flora that can trigger innate autoimmunity. *Staphylococcus aureus* and *Streptococcus pyogenes* are believed to play a similar triggering role in psoriasis vulgaris. Supporting this link, *C. acnes* has been isolated in 42–67% of bone biopsy samples and can cause joint erosions in rat models [7, 12]. The reported sensitivity of *C. acnes* culture may be falsely low, reduced by a culture duration of less than 10 days. Other SAPHO associated pathogens include *S. aureus*, *Haemophilus parainfluenzae*, Actinomycetes, syphilis, Veillonella, and Eikenella.

5.3 Clinical Features

Osteoarticular symptoms occur from osteitis, synovitis, and enthesitis. These processes usually occur adjacent to one another but can occur independently and can induce local soft tissue swelling.

The cardinal feature of SAPHO is ACW pain, present in 63–90% with imaging signs in more than 90%. Other common sites include the spine (74–60%), sacroiliac joints (24–39%), peripheral joints (31–83%), mandible (11–13%), and pelvis (4%) [4, 13, 14].

Commonly involved ACW joints are the first sternocostal joints (54%), sternoclavicular joints (SCJ) (38%), sternal angle (37%), the 2–6th sternocostal joints (16%), and adjacent manubrium (85%) [4, 15]. Spinal and peripheral enthesitis is common, especially in the patellar or Achilles tendons. Most individuals experience back pain, involving the thoracic spine (65%), lumbar spine (50%), or cervical spine (50%) and 65% describe inflammatory back pain.

Lifetime skin involvement occurs in most individuals (71–85%) and can commence before, with or after osteoarticular manifestations [5, 16]. A minority (<30%) experience skin lesions that commence more than 2 years after osteoarticular manifestations [17]. The recognized skin manifestations are all neutrophilic pustular dermatoses—PPP, severe acne, and psoriasis vulgaris. Other neutrophilic pustular dermatoses such as hidradenitis suppurativa and pyoderma gangrenosum have been reported as part of SAPHO but are not included in commonly used diagnostic criteria.

Palmoplantar Pustulosis is a subtype of psoriasis involving recurrent sterile pustules and vesicles which is histologically indistinguishable from pustular psoriasis. It is the most common skin manifestation in Caucasians (52–67%) and East Asians (71–92%) [4]. Severe acne is more common in Caucasians with SAPHO (14–40%) than in East Asians (10–16%) and is more common in males [18]. Psoriasis vulgaris is the least common skin manifestation (15–25%), while comorbid PPP and severe acne is uncommon (2–8%).

The natural history of SAPHO is variable, and when symptomatic it has a high impact on quality of life. Disease activity fluctuates with an overall good prognosis of self-limited disease, uncommonly progressing to deformity or permanent loss of function [17]. Single episodes lasting less than 6 months are uncommon (13%). Most cases experience at least one episode lasting more than 6 months (52%), while many suffer a relapsing and remitting disease course (35%) often, with only a few severe episodes in a lifetime [5]. Recurrent episodes move to new sites in most individuals observed over 12 years.

5.4 Diagnosis

Diagnosis of SAPHO is challenging due to its heterogeneous presentation and the lack of validated diagnostic criteria. Infective osteomyelitis can be excluded when typical clinical and imaging features of SAPHO are present or by bone biopsy.

Table 5.1 Commonly used diagnostic criteria for SAPHO syndrome

Benhamou (1988) [19]	Kahn and Khan (1994) [20]	Khan (2003) [21]
At least 1 of the following 4 conditions: 1. Osteoarticular manifestations of acne conglobate, acne fulminans, or hidradenitis suppurativa 2. Osteoarticular manifestation of PPP 3. Hyperostosis (of the ACW, limbs, or spine) with or without dermatosis 4. CRMO involving the axial or peripheral skeleton with or without dermatosis	At least 1 of the following 3 conditions: 1. Chronic recurrent multifocal sterile and axial osteomyelitis, with or without dermatosis 2. Acute, subacute, or chronic arthritis associated with PPP, pustular psoriasis, or severe acne 3. Any sterile osteitis associated with PPP, pustular psoriasis, or severe acne	At least 1 of the following 5 conditions: 1. Bone–joint involvement associated with PPP and psoriasis vulgaris 2. Bone–joint involvement associated with severe acne 3. Isolated sterile hyperostosis/osteitis 4. CRMO (children) 5. Bone–joint involvement associated with chronic bowel diseases. Exclusion: Infectious osteitis, tumoral conditions of bone, noninflammatory condensing lesions of bone

Three preliminary diagnostic criteria are commonly used (Table 5.1) [19–21]. All rely on the identification of sterile osteitis or characteristic imaging features and all include criteria that overlap with related diseases, e.g., pustular psoriasis with arthritis. Therefore, these diagnostic criteria should be used as a guide for experienced clinicians who can recognize or exclude common presentations of SAPHO and related conditions. Most clinicians surveyed reported that the Kahn and Khan criteria are reflective of SAPHO seen in clinical practice but want it updated [6].

A diagnosis can be made when imaging demonstrates the characteristic osteoarticular lesions and distribution of arthritis or presence of skin manifestations. If imaging finds unifocal osteomyelitis or the overall picture is inconclusive for SAPHO, CNO, or CRMO, a bone biopsy should be performed to exclude malignancy or infection [22]. Other mimics on imaging include mixed lytic and sclerotic lesions from lymphoma or multiple myeloma (Table 5.2). Spondyloarthritis and SAPHO can cause enthesitis, spondylodiscitis, and paravertebral ossification, although SAPHO does not produce the delicate marginal syndesmophytes seen in spondyloarthritis [23].

Similarly, the histological findings of sterile osteomyelitis with chronic inflammatory infiltrate are not diagnostic and can be caused by chronic infection, so microbial culture, rRNA amplification, and Mycobacterial polymerase chain reaction testing should be performed. In the GRAPPA survey, a bone biopsy was considered as "not required" in the appropriate clinical circumstances by 55% of clinicians, was "supported" as necessary by 10%, while 35% were uncertain [6].

Table 5.2 Differential diagnosis of SAPHO syndrome

Feature	Differential diagnosis
Synovitis	Rheumatoid arthritis, Spondyloarthritis, Psoriatic arthritis
Acne	PAPA (Pyogenic arthritis, Pyoderma Gangrenosum, and acne) syndrome, Behçet's PASH syndrome (Pyoderma gangrenosum, acne, Suppurative hidradenitis)
	Arthritis associated with hidradenitis suppurativa
Pustulosis	Isolated PPP or pustular psoriasis
	Sonozaki syndrome (pustulotic arthro-osteitis)
	Infiltrative neutrophilic dermatoses, e.g., Sweet's syndrome, Sneddon-Wilkinson disease
	Pyoderma gangrenosum
Hyperostosis	Diffuse idiopathic skeletal hyperostosis
Osteitis	Chronic bacterial osteomyelitis, tuberculosis, secondary syphilis
	Ewing sarcoma, osteosarcoma, metastatic tumors, lymphoma
	Paget's disease
	Eosinophilic granuloma
	Vasculitis affecting bone

5.5 Differential Diagnoses

Assessment for other causes of osteitis must be performed before a diagnosis of SAPHO is made (Table 5.2). This includes other sterile osteomyelitis syndromes which share clinical features with SAPHO and may exist on the same disease spectrum. CNO and its severe form CRMO affect children and young adults, most frequently in the metaphyses of long bones of the lower limbs or the shoulder girdle. Features of spondyloarthritis are absent and only 20% have PPP, severe acne, or psoriasis vulgaris. Axial predominant disease in children with pustulosis is rare so can be diagnosed as SAPHO. Similar to SAPHO, immune dysregulation involves IL-1β, IL-18, and the NLRP3 inflammasome, causing osteolysis and in some cases hyperostosis and bone sclerosis.

Sternocostoclavicular hyperostosis (SCCH) produces ACW osteoarticular disease resembling SAPHO, usually without skin lesions, elevated erythrocyte sedimentation rate (ESR), or C-reactive protein (CRP) or Bone Marrow Edema (BME). SCCH can have enthesitis, axial inflammation or peripheral arthritis, progressive erosions, hyperostosis, or fusion of the sternoclavicular joints. Isolated sterile mandibular osteomyelitis without skin manifestations has been described as mandibular sclerosing osteomyelitis or diffuse sclerotic osteomyelitis.

Acute or chronic osteomyelitis from a low virulence organism can produce non-specific inflammatory changes on imaging or biopsy, which can cause erosions and joint space widening without elevated inflammatory markers. Septic arthritis affecting the SCJ is uncommon to rare, accounting for 1% of all septic arthritis [24]. Pathogens known to infect the SCJ include *S. aureus*, Brucella, *Escherichia coli*, Pseudomonas, TB, and Syphilis. Joint aspiration and culture are moderately sensitive for SCJ septic arthritis (50–77%) while MRI or bone scan have sensitivity approaching 100%.

Several common arthritides can affect the ACW. Moderate to severe SCJ degeneration on imaging is common, reported in 50–100% of people over 60 years of age [25]. It is usually bilateral and may have characteristic degenerative features such as joint space loss, subchondral cysts, osteophytes, and sclerosis. SCJ or manubriosternal arthritis has been reported in spondyloarthritis (39%), psoriatic arthritis (50%), and ankylosing spondylitis (4%). Asymptomatic SCJ chondrocalcinosis occurs in 17% of adults.

5.6   Investigations

The characteristic imaging features of SAPHO are osteitis and hyperostosis. Hyperostosis involves cortical hypertrophy with diffuse osteosclerosis and can narrow the medullary canal. Osteitis involves acute inflammation of medullary bone which often causes medullary sclerosis and less commonly osteolysis.

5.6.1   Imaging

Early imaging changes include osteitis, osteosclerosis with cortical erosions, and soft tissue edema. Inflammation is initially seen in the costoclavicular ligaments, SCJ, and adjacent structures (manubrium, medial clavicles, costal cartilage, first ribs). Late changes include synovitis, marked hyperostosis (especially of the medial clavicle), osteosclerosis, costal cartilage sclerosis, and SCJ or first sternocostal ankylosis.

5.6.1.1 Conventional Radiography
Plain radiography may identify diffuse osteitis, cortical hypertrophy, or osteolysis after more than 3 months of disease. Sclerosis of medullary bone and cortical hypertrophy then occurs, finally producing mixed osteosclerotic and lytic lesions in the late stage. Enthesophytes, sclerosis, erosions, periosteal reactions, joint space loss, or articular osteolysis may occur.

5.6.1.2 Computed Tomography
Computer Tomography (CT) is more sensitive than conventional radiography and can detect early changes including sclerosis and costoclavicular ligament enthesophytes. Spinal lesions evident on CT are present in >90% of SAPHO, involving ≥2 vertebral levels in the vast majority (89%), usually with little or no change in intervertebral disc space [26]. Features include vertebral corner cortical erosions and reactive osteosclerosis of nearby cancellous bone, and asymmetrical syndesmophytes or bony bridges from vertebral corners with or without adjacent endplate ossification [15, 20, 26]. These changes do not resemble the delicate syndesmophytes of spondyloarthritis, and sacroiliac joint sclerosis caused by SAPHO is typically far more extensive than that in spondyloarthritis, especially on the iliac side [15, 23]. CT can also identify features of suppurative

osteomyelitis such as continuous osteolytic lesions (and at times perforating lesions) with even slight sclerosis.

5.6.1.3 Magnetic Resonance Imaging

Magnetic resonance imaging provides high sensitivity imaging of characteristic features including hyperostosis, enthesitis, osteitis, and peri-entheseal and peri-articular inflammation [4, 26]. In addition to diagnostic information, it assesses disease activity and peri-osteitis soft tissue masses and is the preferred imaging modality for imaging suspected SAPHO [6]. The pattern of acute inflammatory change is often sufficient to differentiate SAPHO from acute infection or metastasis and can assess SAPHO disease activity. BME has been reported in up to 89% of cases, including 87% in the sternocostal joints and 38% in the sternoclavicular joints [4]. This study found most to all cases had extensive inflammation, producing BME of the joint capsule, ligaments and surrounding soft tissue, joint effusions, and most had an inflammatory retrosternal soft tissue mass. BME was present in most individuals with spinal bony bridges, and fatty spinal deposits indicative of past inflammation were common (39%). Costoclavicular enthesitis and local hyperostotic foci are considered early diagnostic features. Spondylodiscitis is common in SAPHO, observed in 32–47%; however, its acute and chronic features are also seen in spondyloarthritis and infection. Multiple vertebral corner lesions affecting contiguous vertebrae, and lesions involving the adjacent vertebral endplate or anterior cortex favor SAPHO over other conditions such as metastases, spondyloarthritis, or infection [16].

5.6.1.4 Bone Scintigraphy

Bone scintigraphy is a sensitive test for SAPHO that can characterize bone or articular pain and identify asymptomatic lesions across the body. It can reveal characteristic patterns of osteitis including the "bulls head sign" or multifocal osteitis, which usually involves 3–4 sites [4, 27]. Three common patterns have been described—focused on the SCJ, spine, or costal joints [28]. The absence of SCJ uptake and unifocal SAPHO are uncommon [2]. The utility of bone scintigraphy for the assessment of disease activity is unclear.

5.6.1.5 Positron Emission Tomography

Positron Emission Tomography (PET) typically shows multiple lesions in the ACW and spine with low-moderate fluoro-deoxy glucose (FDG) uptake and concurrent osteolysis and osteosclerosis [29]. PET can often differentiate metastases from SAPHO by interpreting specific articular findings but has an unclear role in disease activity monitoring as it has only a fair-moderate agreement with symptoms [29].

5.6.2 Laboratory Investigations

Serum inflammatory markers ESR and CRP may be raised during acute SAPHO activity, while white cell count is not. ESR elevation has been observed in 57–89%,

CRP elevation in 50–72%, and either in 63% [4, 14, 16, 26]. Inflammatory markers may have a role in monitoring disease activity if elevated at baseline. Other potential markers of disease activity include amyloid A, IgG4, and bone turnover markers [9]. Reported rates of HLA-B27 in SAPHO cohorts are similar to or lower than the general population, perhaps because individuals with a positive HLA-B27 are more likely to be diagnosed with axial spondyloarthritis [4, 5, 18, 26].

5.7   Management

Interventions for SAPHO have been chosen based on our limited understanding of its pathogenesis, effective treatments of similar conditions, and limited evidence from case series.

Non-Steroidal Anti-Inflammatories (NSAIDs) are used to treat osteoarticular pain, with improvement reported in 65–86% and complete response in 34% [14, 30].

Pamidronate is reported as improving osteoarticular pain in 82% with complete remission in 49%, and some reports describe improvement in bone scan uptake and BMO [30]. Skin manifestations improve at rates higher than spontaneous remission. In addition to anti-resorptive actions, pamidronate is believed to have anti-inflammatory actions including inhibition of IL-1β.

Case series of corticosteroids (0.5 mg/kg of prednisolone) describes a temporary response in 81%, with an observed rebound of skin disease worse than baseline when used at high doses [14]. Intra-articular injections have been used for brief relief of arthritis but have minimal to no benefit for osteitis.

Case reports of conventional immunosuppressants suggest limited efficacy. Reports of methotrexate use describe an improvement in pain in half the cases, while enthesitis and skin do not appear to respond. Leflunomide improved pain in all three reported cases while sulfasalazine did not.

Antibiotics including tetracyclines, clindamycin, and azithromycin reportedly improve acne but not PPP and do not provide a lasting effect [12]. A recent pooled analysis of antibiotic case reports ($n = 107$) found about 1/3 of patients had complete resolution of symptoms, 1/3 had a partial response, and 1/3 had no response [30].

Biologic medications have reported efficacy but are associated with paradoxical skin reactions in almost half and flares of preexisting skin manifestations. These events may all be flares of the disease. Tumour necrosis factor (TNF) inhibitor use has been reported in a large case series, which describe complete remission in 3/4, mostly sustained over 17 months and no response in <5% [30]. Osteoarticular pain more frequently responds to TNF inhibition than skin manifestations.

Case series describe nonresponders to pamidronate and TNF inhibitors responding to other biologics including IL-1, IL-6, and IL-17 inhibitors. IL-17 inhibitors appear to have a similar response rate to TNF inhibitors with improvement in pain, BMO, CRP, and skin manifestations. Their rationale for use is that IL-17 inhibition is highly effective for PPP and IL-17 is implicated in the pathogenesis of all clinical components of SAPHO syndrome. Despite their effectiveness against PPP, IL-17 inhibitors have been associated with severe pustular skin reactions. Anakinra

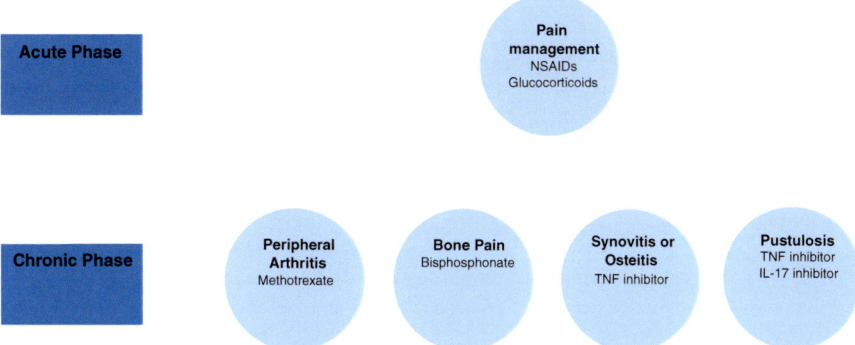

Fig. 5.1 Treatment options in SAPHO

(anti-IL-1) also appears to provide a similar improvement in osteoarticular symptoms to TNF inhibitors but rates of skin response are much lower. Ustekinumab (anti-IL-23) has been used in a limited number of cases with a mixture of complete, partial, and nonresponse, and has successfully been used to treat paradoxical skin reactions. Tocilizumab (anti-IL-6) use has been described in very few cases with inconsistent results. Tofacitinib use has been reported in a few cases with a good response in osteoarticular symptoms.

From limited data and understanding of pathophysiology, treatment choice for this heterogenous syndrome is challenging. Following diagnosis, acute therapy using NSAIDs or corticosteroids is often adequate for pain relief. If a relapsing disease course occurs, long-term treatment can be chosen based on the major disease manifestation, related preexisting diseases, or comorbidities. Bisphosphonates target bone pain, while methotrexate may be preferred in individuals with psoriasis or peripheral arthritis. Severe arthritis or osteoarticular pain favors the use of TNF inhibitors, while arthritis with pustular skin disease or enthesitis may respond best to IL-17 or IL-23 inhibition based on their use in spondyloarthritis and psoriasis. These treatment options have been summarized in Fig. 5.1.

5.8   Conclusion

SAPHO presents a challenge to diagnosis and treatment even for experienced clinicians. It frequently resembles or coexists with other conditions, including life and limb-threatening causes of osteitis. Identification requires careful assessment of clinical manifestations, pathology, and imaging. Its pathophysiology is poorly understood but involves dysregulated innate immune pathways, probably as an aberrant response to skin flora, producing a spondyloarthritis-like syndrome. These findings have prompted the use of broad and targeted immunomodulatory therapies, which are adequate to suppress the relapsing/remitting disease manifestations in most people. Further description of its pathology should inform prognosis and improve diagnosis and treatment.

References

1. Chamot AM, Benhamou CL, Kahn MF, Beraneck L, Kaplan G, Prost A. [Acne-pustulosis-hyperostosis-osteitis syndrome. Results of a national survey. 85 cases]. Rev Rhum Mal Osteoartic. 1987;54(3):187–96.
2. Przepiera-Będzak H, Brzosko M. Clinical symptoms, imaging, and treatment of SAPHO syndrome: a single-center study of 52 cases. Pol Arch Intern Med. 2018;128(6):396–9.
3. Takigawa T, Tanaka M, Nakanishi K, Misawa H, Sugimoto Y, Takahata T, et al. SAPHO syndrome associated spondylitis. Eur Spine J. 2008;17(10):1391–7.
4. Yu M, Cao Y, Li J, Zhang Y, Ye Y, Wang L, et al. Anterior chest wall in SAPHO syndrome: magnetic resonance imaging findings. Arthritis Res Ther. 2020;22(1):216.
5. Colina M, Govoni M, Orzincolo C, Trotta F. Clinical and radiologic evolution of synovitis, acne, pustulosis, hyperostosis, and osteitis syndrome: a single center study of a cohort of 71 subjects. Arthritis Rheum. 2009;61(6):813–21.
6. Furer V, Kishimoto M, Tsuji S, Taniguchi Y, Ishihara Y, Tomita T, et al. The diagnosis and treatment of adult patients with SAPHO syndrome: controversies revealed in a multidisciplinary international survey of physicians. Rheumatol Ther. 2020;7(4):883–91.
7. Rozin AP. SAPHO syndrome: is a range of pathogen-associated rheumatic diseases extended? Arthritis Res Ther. 2009;11(6):131.
8. Xu D, Liu X, Lu C, Luo J, Wang C, Gao C, et al. Reduction of peripheral natural killer cells in patients with SAPHO syndrome. Clin Exp Rheumatol. 2019;37(1):12–8.
9. Zhang S, Li C, Zhang S, Li L, Zhang W, Dong Z, et al. Serum levels of proinflammatory, anti-inflammatory cytokines, and RANKL/OPG in synovitis, acne, pustulosis, hyperostosis, and osteitis (SAPHO) syndrome. Mod Rheumatol. 2019;29(3):523–30.
10. Liao H-J, Chyuan I-T, Wu C-S, Lin S-W, Chen K-H, Tsai H-F, et al. Increased neutrophil infiltration, IL-1 production and a SAPHO syndrome-like phenotype in PSTPIP2-deficient mice. Rheumatol Oxf Engl. 2015;54(7):1317–26.
11. Sahdo B, Särndahl E, Elgh F, Söderquist B. Propionibacterium acnes activates caspase-1 in human neutrophils. APMIS Acta Pathol Microbiol Immunol Scand. 2013;121(7):652–63.
12. Assmann G, Kueck O, Kirchhoff T, Rosenthal H, Voswinkel J, Pfreundschuh M, et al. Efficacy of antibiotic therapy for SAPHO syndrome is lost after its discontinuation: an interventional study. Arthritis Res Ther. 2009;11(5):R140.
13. Li C, Ye Y, Cao Y, Zhang W, Xu W, Wu N, et al. Axial skeletal lesions and disease duration in SAPHO syndrome: a retrospective review of computed tomography findings in 81 patients. Int J Rheum Dis. 2020;23(9):1152–8.
14. Li C, Zuo Y, Wu N, Li L, Li F, Zhang W, et al. Synovitis, acne, pustulosis, hyperostosis and osteitis syndrome: a single centre study of a cohort of 164 patients. Rheumatol Oxf Engl. 2016;55(6):1023–30.
15. Earwaker JWS, Cotten A. SAPHO: syndrome or concept? Imaging findings. Skeletal Radiol. 2003;32(6):311–27.
16. Gao S, Deng X, Zhang L, Song L. The comparison analysis of clinical and radiological features in SAPHO syndrome. Clin Rheumatol. 2021;40(1):349–57.
17. Hayem G, Bouchaud-Chabot A, Benali K, Roux S, Palazzo E, Silbermann-Hoffman O, et al. SAPHO syndrome: a long-term follow-up study of 120 cases. Semin Arthritis Rheum. 1999;29(3):159–71.
18. Li C, Cao Y, Zhang W. Clinical heterogeneity of SAPHO syndrome: challenge of diagnosis. Mod Rheumatol. 2018;28(3):432–4.
19. Benhamou CL, Chamot AM, Kahn MF. Synovitis-acne-pustulosis hyperostosis-osteomyelitis syndrome (SAPHO). A new syndrome among the spondyloarthropathies? Clin Exp Rheumatol. 1988;6(2):109–12.
20. Kahn MF, Khan MA. The SAPHO syndrome. Baillieres Clin Rheumatol. 1994;8(2):333–62.
21. Kahn MF. Proposed classification criteria of SAPHO syndrome. In: Proceedings of the annual meeting of the American College of Radiology, Orlando, Florida. October 23–28, 2003.

22. Hedrich CM, Morbach H, Reiscr C, Girschick HJ. New insights into adult and paediatric chronic non-bacterial osteomyelitis CNO. Curr Rheumatol Rep. 2020;22(9):52.
23. Colina M. Comment on "SAPHO syndrome: imaging findings of vertebral involvement". AJNR Am J Neuroradiol. 2016;37(10):E65–6.
24. Ross JJ, Shamsuddin H. Sternoclavicular septic arthritis: review of 180 cases. Medicine (Baltimore). 2004;83(3):139–48.
25. Edwin J, Ahmed S, Verma S, Tytherleigh-Strong G, Karuppaiah K, Sinha J. Swellings of the sternoclavicular joint: review of traumatic and non-traumatic pathologies. EFORT Open Rev. 2018;3(8):471–84.
26. Xu W, Li C, Zhao X, Lu J, Li L, Wu N, et al. Whole-spine computed tomography findings in SAPHO syndrome. J Rheumatol. 2017;44(5):648–54.
27. Skrabl-Baumgartner A, Singer P, Greimel T, Gorkiewicz G, Hermann J. Chronic non-bacterial osteomyelitis: a comparative study between children and adults. Pediatr Rheumatol Online J. 2019;17(1):49.
28. Cao Y, Li C, Yang Q, Wu N, Xu P, Li Y, et al. Three patterns of osteoarticular involvement in SAPHO syndrome: a cluster analysis based on whole body bone scintigraphy of 157 patients. Rheumatol Oxf Engl. 2019;58(6):1047–55.
29. Sun X, Li C, Cao Y, Shi X, Li L, Zhang W, et al. F-18 FDG PET/CT in 26 patients with SAPHO syndrome: a new vision of clinical and bone scintigraphy correlation. J Orthop Surg. 2018;13(1):120.
30. Huang H, Zhang Z, Zhao J, Hao Y, Zhou W. The effectiveness of treatments for patients with SAPHO syndrome: a follow-up study of 24 cases from a single center and review of literature. Clin Rheumatol. 2021;40(3):1131–9.

Basic Calcium Phosphate-Associated Arthritis

6

Ann K. Rosenthal and Keith Baynes

6.1   Introduction

Basic calcium phosphate (BCP) is a term used to refer to a trio of calcium phosphate crystals including tricalcium phosphate, octacalcium phosphate, and carbonate-substituted hydroxyapatite. These tiny crystals are similar in composition to the normal mineral that is present in the bone matrix and are involved in many forms of pathologic calcification. For example, they are present in breast and prostate cancers, atherosclerotic blood vessels, calciphylaxis seen in end-stage renal disease, and dystrophic calcification seen at sites of tissue injury. BCP crystal deposits can be relatively inert, or aggressively inflammatory, and much about the factors contributing to their formation as well as their interactions with surrounding tissues remains unclear.

In the musculoskeletal system, BCP crystals are present in a variety of settings. They are found in almost all tissue samples from patients with late-stage osteoarthritis (OA) of the hip or knee [1, 2], and are also common components of the synovial fluid in OA [3, 4]. Their presence in OA correlates with disease severity, and a significant body of evidence supports their ability to contribute to joint damage in this setting [5]. BCP crystals can induce inflammatory cytokines [6], contribute to osteoclast formation [7], and alter tissue biomechanics. BCP crystals are also involved in calcific tendinitis, which is a common cause of acute shoulder or hip pain associated with large radiographic crystal deposits.

A. K. Rosenthal (✉)
Division of Rheumatology, Department of Medicine, Medical College of Wisconsin and the Zablocki VA Medical Center, Milwaukee, WI, USA
e-mail: arosenthal@mcw.edu

K. Baynes
Department of Radiology, Medical College of Wisconsin, Milwaukee, WI, USA
e-mail: kbaynes@mcw.edu

© The Author(s), under exclusive license to Springer Nature Switzerland AG 2022
V. Ravindran et al. (eds.), *Rarer Arthropathies*, Rare Diseases of the Immune System, https://doi.org/10.1007/978-3-031-05002-2_6

Two rare forms of arthritis are believed to be caused by BCP crystals. These are Milwaukee Shoulder Syndrome (MSS) and Calcific Periarthritis (CP). These two conditions will be the focus of this review.

6.2   Milwaukee Shoulder Syndrome

6.2.1   Historical Perspective

Milwaukee Shoulder Syndrome was initially described in 1981 by McCarty et al. [8]. Although similar descriptions of elderly patients with large shoulder effusions had been described over 100 years prior [9], McCarty was the first to identify "microspheroid structures" containing hydroxyapatite crystals in these patients. Before his description, this syndrome was known as rotator cuff tear arthropathy, a reference to the severe destruction of the rotator cuff. The largest data collectiion from patients with MSS was published many years ago and described 72 patients in total [10]. Because of the rarity of this condition as well as the challenges involved in conclusively identifying the presence of BCP crystals (described below), MSS is frequently misdiagnosed.

6.2.2   Clinical Features

Milwaukee Shoulder Syndrome currently lacks any validated diagnostic or classification criteria. Based on case collections largely from a single center (Milwaukee), we know that this disease often occurs in elderly women [9]. They present with chronic shoulder swelling associated with a wide range of symptoms. Some affected individuals have severe pain which can be exacerbated at night, and others have very little discomfort [10]. Up to 50% of the patients in some case series also have knee involvement [10], characterized by exuberant effusions with little evidence of inflammation. While BCP crystals have also been implicated in some forms of destructive hand arthritis, this has not been confirmed.

Bilateral shoulder arthritis occurs in 64% of the patients [11]. In some cases, shoulder capsules can rupture resulting in large ecchymoses on the chest wall and upper arm. Rarely, sinus tracks can develop [9].

The knee involvement may be lateral compartment-predominant, which is not typical for most knee OA, but the overlap with calcium pyrophosphate deposition disease (CPPD) in this case series makes it difficult to attribute this to BCP-associated pathology alone [10]. Hip involvement has also been described, as has elbow involvement.

Examination typically shows significant shoulder effusions. Warmth and erythema are not commonly seen. Affected shoulder joints often have clinical evidence of rotator cuff destruction manifest by diminished strength of the arm and impaired active range of motion of the shoulder. In contrast, passive range of motion may be well-preserved. The shoulder joint often feels unstable to the examiner and may easily dislocate.

6.2.3   Epidemiology

The incidence and prevalence of MSS are not known and to our knowledge have never been studied. The literature currently consists of case collections of patients [10, 11]. The age range in existing case collections is 50–90 years. MSS is more common in women. Some risk factors have been proposed, including overuse of the shoulder, use of crutches, and prior shoulder injury. While trends in prevalence are not easily tracked, our center has anecdotally noted a seeming decrease in the prevalence of MSS over the last 20 years.

6.2.4   Diagnosis

Accurate diagnosis remains a major hurdle in MSS. Currently, the diagnosis is made based on clinical features but can be strongly supported by synovial fluid findings and typical changes on radiographs.

6.2.4.1 Synovial Fluid Analysis

Individuals with MSS typically have large glenohumeral joint effusions which can readily be aspirated. If these rupture into the subacromial bursa, aspiration can be performed with a subacromial approach. The fluid can be blood-tinged [12]. White blood cell counts in synovial fluid from MSS patients are typically below 1000 cells/mm^3 and are often extremely low.

6.2.4.2 BCP Crystal Analysis

BCP crystals cannot be readily detected by typical bedside methods used for other types of arthritogenic crystals. BCP crystals are much smaller than monosodium urate (MSU) or calcium pyrophosphate (CPP) crystals and single BCP crystals are below the detection limit for light microscopes. These crystals also lack the characteristic birefringence helpful in differentiating crystals from debris under polarizing light microscopy. Currently, the only widely available method to detect BCP crystals in the clinic is to use Alizarin Red S staining [13]. This test involves 2% Alizarin Red S stain which should be filtered before each use. Typically, a drop of synovial fluid is mixed with a drop of stain on a microscope slide and the slide is examined under plain light microscopy. Aggregated crystals appear as clusters or coins of shiny red staining (Fig. 6.1). This test has been validated for accuracy in two studies using transmission electron microscopy as a gold standard [13, 14]. Its accuracy was about 90% for strongly positive samples. It is important to remember that these observers had significant experience with this stain. In real-world use, the synovial fluid structures stained with Alizarin Red S can be quite difficult to differentiate from debris [15]. Furthermore, Alizarin Red S is not specific for BCP crystals and also stains CPP crystals. This is a particular problem with MSS effusions, as in some case series, up to 40% of patients diagnosed as MSS also had CPP crystals in their synovial fluid [8].

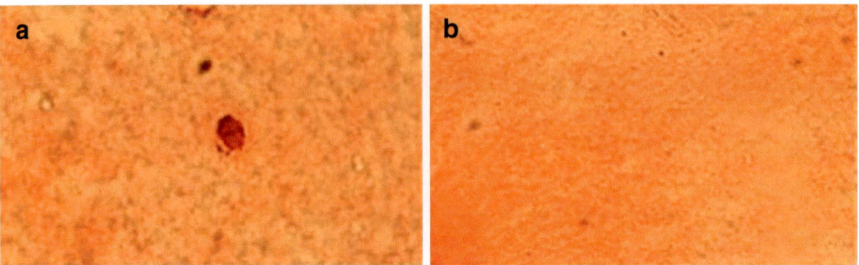

Fig. 6.1 Alizarin Red S staining of synovial fluid BCP crystals. (**a**) Synovial fluid stained with Alizarin Red S shows the typical appearance of a single cluster of BCP crystals under light microscopy (600×). (**b**) Stained synovial fluid sample with no BCP crystals

Fig. 6.2 Radiographic appearance of Milwaukee Shoulder Syndrome (MSS). Shoulder with severe bone and joint destruction as is typically seen in MSS

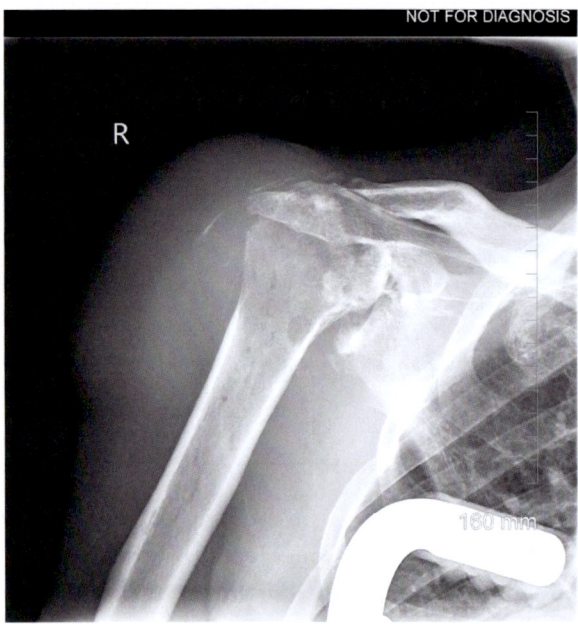

There are several other more accurate ways of identifying BCP crystals. These include techniques such as Fourier transform infrared spectroscopy and transmission electron microscopy with energy dispersive analysis. X-ray diffraction and atomic force microscopy have also been used to identify BCP crystals. These methods are highly accurate for detecting BCP crystals but are not widely available to the clinical community [16].

6.2.4.3 Imaging

Conventional radiography is useful in supporting a diagnosis of MSS (Fig. 6.2). X-rays show evidence of rotator cuff destruction as seen by a "high-riding" glenohumeral head. This is accompanied by considerable bony destruction. Soft tissue calcification may be observed in as many as 55% of cases. There is also evidence of cartilage loss demonstrated by glenohumeral joint space narrowing. There is little information regarding advanced imaging in MSS, although MRI-based imaging may facilitate better characterization of the extent of soft tissue involvement [17].

6.2.5 Pathophysiology

BCP crystal formation is not well understood, but likely involves complex multistep processes [18]. In general, pathologic calcification often occurs at sites of ischemia or tissue damage. Cell death or injury releases many factors which can contribute to calcium phosphate mineralization. In many tissues, small extracellular vesicles participate in pathologic calcification [19]. Changes in extracellular matrix composition [20], and altered circulating levels of mineralization regulators such as FGF23 and fetuin may affect these processes.

Once BCP crystals form, they cause inflammation in some settings, but there is remarkably little inflammation in joints affected by MSS. BCP crystals can induce fibroblast proliferation [21] which can increase the secretion of destructive enzymes and cytokines from the synovium. One theory of MSS pathogenesis that the tissue damage results from increased collagenase activity induced by BCP crystals [22]. Collagenases destroy tendons, ligaments, and joint capsules as well as bone. In vitro, BCP crystals can induce the production of several forms of collagenase from fibroblasts [22] and have similar actions on chondrocytes in synergy with cytokines seen commonly in OA and after injury [23].

6.2.6 Differential Diagnosis

The differential diagnosis for MSS is broad. Other competing diagnoses include posttraumatic OA of the glenohumeral joint, CPPD, amyloid arthropathy, hemochromatosis arthritis, tenosynovial giant cell tumor, neuropathic joint disease (Charcot arthropathy), and the poorly defined syndrome known as rotator cuff arthropathy. Differentiating MSS from these conditions can be difficult. OA of the glenohumeral joint is unusual without a preceding injury. CPPD can be very difficult to distinguish but should be accompanied by radiographic chondrocalcinosis, CPP crystals in synovial fluid, and evidence of additional joint involvement. Amyloid deposition causes large anterior shoulder "pads," and fluid or tissue from these joints should contain Congo Red positive debris. Giant cell tumors should show proliferative synovitis on MRI, and a diagnosis of Charcot arthropathy requires proof of sensory deficits in the affected shoulder. There is significant clinical overlap with rotator cuff arthropathy and without documenting BCP crystals on synovial fluid analysis, these conditions would be difficult to distinguish from one another.

6.2.7 Management

There is little consensus regarding how best MSS should be treated, and various interventions have not been studied or compared [9]. Physical therapy to maintain existing shoulder motion and function is important. Pain management with acetaminophen or NSAIDs can be used in patients with mild symptoms. Colchicine has been utilized, but there are no data to support its efficacy. With more severe symptoms, the approach typically includes shoulder aspiration and injection with corticosteroids. Tidal irrigation has been reported to be successful in several patients and has been used in conjunction with tranexamic acid injections [24]. If patients have no contraindications, shoulder replacement has also been undertaken successfully [25].

6.3   Calcific Periarthritis

Calcific periarthritis (CP) is defined by the presence of radiographic or histopathologic evidence of calcific deposits at or near the symptomatic joint. This syndrome typically presents with acute monoarticular pain with inflammatory features. It classically occurs around the small joints of the hands and feet. In the great toe, CP has been nicknamed "pseudopodagra" [26]. The overlap between CP and calcific tendinitis is substantial. They likely share common pathophysiology, and periarticular BCP crystals in a small joint may be in or near a tendon. Current knowledge of CP is based on case reports and small case series.

6.3.1   Clinical Features

Calcific periarthritis is a typically monoarticular inflammatory syndrome of acute onset. In a recent study of 15 patients with biopsy-proven CP, 5 cases involved the hands; 7 involved the toes, and 3 were adjacent to the humeral head [27]. These episodes are typically self-limited and most resolve within 3–4 weeks. Although this is usually the case, some patients may have persistent symptoms lasting up to 6 months [28]. The associated pain is often described as throbbing and can be significantly worse at night. Pain can be quite severe in CP and symptoms often precipitate an ER or urgent care visit. While typically monoarticular, in one series, 5 patients had more than one hand joint involved [28]. The pattern of hand involvement is not particularly well studied, but CP may be more common in MCP and PIP joints compared to DIP joints [28]. Elbows can also be involved. The recurrence rate is not known, but in one study of 17 patients, there was no recurrence during the following 12 months after the initial presentation [29].

On physical examination, there is considerable inflammation with redness, warmth, and swelling involving a single joint of the hand or foot. Fever has been described but is unusual. The joint does not typically demonstrate a fluid collection and this is an important factor in differentiating CP from actual inflammatory arthritis. In the foot, CP can affect any joint but is best characterized in the MTPs [26].

6.3.2   Epidemiology

CP is rare, but lacks any validated prevalence or incidence data. The numbers of publications describing CP suggest that it is considerably more common than MSS. The average age in one study of 10 patients with hand involvement was 36 years [30], and there are also a handful of case reports in children [31]. One large case series showed an age range of 31–86 years but also included calcific deposits in the shoulders [27]. Risk factors for CP are not well understood. In most series, about one-third of affected patients describe an antecedent injury [27]. The predominance of women is not fully understood. However, foot involvement has been associated with pregnancy [26], and the constrictive footwear often worn by women has also been postulated to contribute to this pattern.

6.3.3   Diagnosis

The clinical diagnosis of CP is supported by radiographic evidence of periarticular calcification and in rare cases, requires histologic studies.

6.3.3.1 Imaging
The diagnosis of CP is typically made by a careful history and physical examination supported by the presence of periarticular calcific deposits on radiographs. In some cases, the lesions are biopsied to rule out infection or tumors [27]. Conventional radiographs frequently show dense periarticular calcific deposits (Fig. 6.3). When these deposits are very close to the bone, they can produce cortical erosions and can rarely erode into the marrow space [27]. They are typically described as round or oval and may appear cloud-like, dense, amorphous, or homogeneous [32]. In the foot, these deposits can be confused with accessory bones or pieces of bone from prior fractures. While the appearance of CP on conventional radiographs tends to support the diagnosis, newer imaging modalities such as dual-energy computed tomography can differentiate BCP crystal deposits from those of CPP [33].

6.3.3.2 Histology
A recent case series summarized histopathology in 15 biopsies of CP lesions [27]. They found minerals in a basophilic amorphous background with or without an inflammatory infiltrate consisting of histiocytes. Neutrophils were typically absent in this series, but it is noteworthy that some of these lesions had been present for many weeks.

Fig. 6.3 Radiographic appearance of calcific periarthritis. In this radiograph, the fourth MCP joint (circled area) contains a periarticular calcification on the radial aspect of the joint typical of those seen with calcific periarthritis

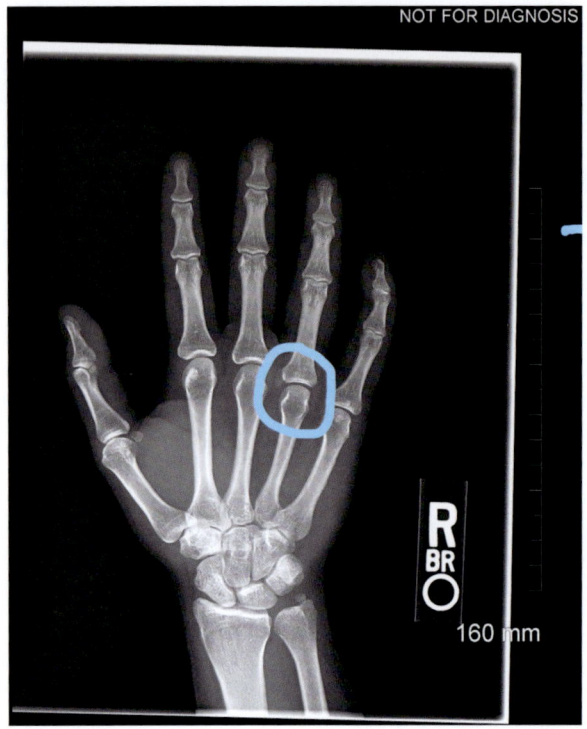

6.3.4 Pathogenesis

The pathogenesis of CP is not understood. Like other syndromes involving pathologic calcific deposits, there may be some element of tissue injury that triggers the formation of calcium phosphate deposits. As mentioned previously in regards to MSS, there are many theories of BCP crystal formation postulated but none have been conclusively proven.

6.3.4.1 Genetic Causes

Unlike MSS, there are genetic causes of CP which may provide some clues as to its pathogenesis. A positive family history of CP or recurrent attacks in multiple joints warrants evaluation for a genetic cause. CD73 deficiency results in recurrent arthritis with CPP and BCP crystals. CD73 is an enzyme that removes the terminal phosphate from ATP and other nucleotides. It is postulated that lack of CD73 alters the ratio of pyrophosphate to phosphate and promotes pathologic mineralization. Recent work by Cudrici et al. in a cohort of patients with CD73 deficiency [34] confirmed that the periarticular calcific deposits were composed of BCP crystals and did not contain CPP crystals. Hypophosphatasia can also cause recurrent episodes of CP. Hypophosphatasia results from deficient levels of alkaline phosphatase. Alkaline phosphatase breaks down pyrophosphate, and can also alter the pyrophosphate to phosphate ratio. Like CD73 deficiency, it is associated with CPP crystal formation inside synovial joints and periarticular BCP crystal formation [35].

6.3.4.2 Idiopathic Causes

Unlike MSS, CP is an inflammatory syndrome. Some have postulated that BCP deposits are likely longstanding but asymptomatic and the symptoms are initiated by a resorptive process [36]. This hypothesis is supported by observations that calcific deposits in calcific tendinitis become less sharp-edged and cloudier-appearing on radiographs when they become symptomatic. Although what triggers BCP crystals to become inflammatory in any setting remains unclear, it is well known that other types of arthritogenic crystals can be dormant in some settings. For example, MSU crystals are often found in uninflamed joints in patients with poorly controlled gout [37]. Once triggered, the inflammatory pathways through which BCP crystals induce inflammation are fairly well studied. Like MSU and CPP crystals, BCP crystals act to induce inflammation through the NLPR3 inflammasome [38]. They can also affect macrophage phenotype and can activate macrophages [39] and dendritic cells through pathways involving Syk and PI3K resulting in induction of damage-associated molecular patterns such as S100A8 and MMP1 [40].

6.3.5   Differential Diagnosis

The differential diagnosis of CP is broad. It includes joint or soft tissue infection, as well as gout, CPPD, and joint injury. Larger calcifications can mimic malignancy if they erode into the adjacent cortical bone. In many of the larger series [41], CP was not considered initially as a diagnosis and this can result in unnecessary invasive testing or aggressive therapies.

6.3.6   Management

No randomized controlled trials of therapy in CP have been reported. The case series describe the use of NSAIDs, local corticosteroids, or anesthetic injections into the lesion. There are case reports of successful use of the bisphosphonate, clodronate, in CP [42]. Iontophoresis with a calcium chelator has been used for large calcific deposits in patients with calcific tendinitis but lacks support in the CP literature. Similarly, platelet-rich plasma therapy has been used in calcific tendinitis of the shoulder [43], but not in CP involving small joints. Typically, the duration of treatment is short, resulting in rapid resolution of symptoms. However, in one retrospective study of 10 patients with CP of the hand, conservative treatment was continued for an average of 11 months [28]. Surgery is rarely used in this setting, but as mentioned above, excisional biopsies may be performed for diagnostic purposes.

6.4 Conclusion

In summary, BCP crystals are associated with the rare arthropathies of MSS and CP. Much about the etiology and management of these types of arthritis remains understudied. Hopefully, future progress in these areas based on clear diagnostic criteria and better methods of BCP crystal detection will lead to improved management strategies for these syndromes.

References

1. Fuerst M, Bertrand J, Lammers L, Dreier R, Echtermeyer F, Nitschke Y, et al. Calcification of articular cartilage in human osteoarthritis. Arthritis Rheum. 2009;60(9):2694–703.
2. Fuerst M, Niggemeyer O, Lammers L, Schafer F, Lohmann C, Ruther W. Articular cartilage mineralization in osteoarthritis of the hip. BMC Musculoskelet Disord. 2009;10:166.
3. Derfus BA, Kurian JB, Butler JJ, Daft LJ, Carrera GF, Ryan LM, et al. The high prevalence of pathologic calcium crystals in pre-operative knees. J Rheumatol. 2002;29(3):570–4.
4. Nalbant S, Martinez JAM, Kitumnuaypong T, Clayburne G, Sieck M, Schumacher HR. Synovial fluid features and their relations to osteoarthritis severity: new findings from sequential studies. Osteoarthr Cartil. 2003;11(1):50–4.
5. Stack J, McCarthy G. Basic calcium phosphate crystals and osteoarthritis pathogenesis: novel pathways and potential targets. Curr Opin Rheumatol. 2016;28(2):122–6.
6. Ea HK, Chobaz V, Nguyen C, Nasi S, van Lent P, Daudon M, et al. Pathogenic role of basic calcium phosphate crystals in destructive arthropathies. PLoS One. 2013;8(2):e57352.
7. Cunningham CC, Corr EM, McCarthy GM, Dunne A. Intra-articular basic calcium phosphate and monosodium urate crystals inhibit anti-osteoclastogenic cytokine signalling. Osteoarthr Cartil. 2016;24(12):2141–52.
8. McCarty DJ, Halverson PB, Carrera GF, Brewer BJ, Kozin F. "Milwaukee shoulder"—association of microspheroids containing hydroxyapatite crystals, active collagenase, and neutral protease with rotator cuff defects. I. Clinical aspects. Arthritis Rheum. 1981;24(3):464–73.
9. Halverson P. Basic calcium phosphate (apatite, octacalcium phosphate, tricalcium phosphate) crystal deposition diseases and calcinosis. In: Koopman W, editor. Arthritis and allied conditions. Philadelphia: Lippincott Williams & Wilkins; 2001. p. 2372–91.
10. Halverson PB, Carrera GF, McCarty DJ. Milwaukee shoulder syndrome. Fifteen additional cases and a description of contributing factors. Arch Intern Med. 1990;150(3):677–82.
11. Halverson PB, McCarty DJ, Cheung HS, Ryan LM. Milwaukee shoulder syndrome: eleven additional cases with involvement of the knee in seven (basic calcium phosphate crystal deposition disease). Semin Arthritis Rheum. 1984;14(1):36–44.
12. Santiago T, Coutinho M, Malcata A, da Silva JA. Milwaukee shoulder (and knee) syndrome. BMJ Case Rep. 2014;2014:bcr2013202183.
13. Paul H, Reginato AJ, Schumacher HR. Alizarin red S staining as a screening test to detect calcium compounds in synovial fluid. Arthritis Rheum. 1983;26(2):191–200.
14. Eggelmeijer F, Dijkmans BA, Macfarlane JD, Cats A. Alizarin red S staining of synovial fluid in inflammatory joint disorders. Clin Exp Rheumatol. 1991;9(1):11–6.
15. Gordon C, Swan A, Dieppe P. Detection of crystals in synovial fluids by light microscopy: sensitivity and reliability. Ann Rheum Dis. 1989;48(9):737–42.
16. Rosenthal AK, Mandel N. Identification of crystals in synovial fluids and joint tissues. Curr Rheumatol Rep. 2001;3(1):11–6.
17. Dewachter L, Aerts P, Crevits I, De Man R. Milwaukee shoulder syndrome. JBR-BTR. 2012;95(4):243–4.
18. Demer LL, Tintut Y. Inflammatory, metabolic, and genetic mechanisms of vascular calcification. Arterioscler Thromb Vasc Biol. 2014;34(4):715–23.

19. Dcrfus B, Kranendonk S, Mandel N, Lynch K, Kushnaryov V, Ryan L. Human osteoarthritic matrix vesicles generate apatite and calcium pyrophosphate dihydrate in vitro. J Bone Jt Surg. 1994;18:502–3.

20. Jubeck B, Gohr C, Fahey M, Muth E, Matthews M, Mattson E, et al. Promotion of articular cartilage matrix vesicle mineralization by type I collagen. Arthritis Rheum. 2008;58(9): 2809–17.

21. Cheung HS, Story MT, McCarty DJ. Mitogenic effects of hydroxyapatite and calcium pyrophosphate dihydrate crystals on cultured mammalian cells. Arthritis Rheum. 1984;27(6):668–74.

22. Cheung HS, Halverson PB, McCarty DJ. Release of collagenase, neutral protease, and prostaglandins from cultured mammalian synovial cells by hydroxyapatite and calcium pyrophosphate dihydrate crystals. Arthritis Rheum. 1981;24(11):1338–44.

23. McCarthy GM, Westfall PR, Masuda I, Christopherson PA, Cheung HS, Mitchell PG. Basic calcium phosphate crystals activate human osteoarthritic synovial fibroblasts and induce matrix metalloproteinase-13 (collagenase-3) in adult porcine articular chondrocytes. Ann Rheum Dis. 2001;60(4):399–406.

24. Epis O, Caporali R, Scire CA, Bruschi E, Bonacci E, Montecucco C. Efficacy of tidal irrigation in Milwaukee shoulder syndrome. J Rheumatol. 2007;34(7):1545–50.

25. Epis O, Viola E, Bruschi E, Benazzo F, Montecucco C. [Milwaukee shoulder syndrome (apatite associated destructive arthritis): therapeutic aspects]. Reumatismo. 2005;57(2): 69–77.

26. Fam AG, Rubenstein J. Hydroxyapatite pseudopodagra. A syndrome of young women. Arthritis Rheum. 1989;32(6):741–7.

27. Lehmer LM, Ragsdale BD. Calcific periarthritis: more than a shoulder problem: a series of fifteen cases. J Bone Joint Surg Am. 2012;94(21):e157.

28. Kim J, Bae KJ, Lee DW, Lee YH, Gong HS, Baek GH. Effective period of conservative treatment in patients with acute calcific periarthritis of the hand. J Orthop Surg Res. 2018;13(1):287.

29. Kim JK, Park ES. Acute calcium deposits in the hand and wrist; comparison of acute calcium peritendinitis and acute calcium periarthritis. J Hand Surg Eur Vol. 2014;39(4):436–9.

30. Yosipovitch G, Yosipovitch Z. Acute calcific periarthritis of the hand and elbows in women. A study and review of the literature. J Rheumatol. 1993;20(9):1533–8.

31. Budnick I, Horasek S, Aboulafia A. Idiopathic chronic calcific periarthritis in a child. Am J Orthop (Belle Mead NJ). 2011;40(11):576–8.

32. Vinson EN, Desai SV, Reddy S, Goldner RD. AJR teaching file: periarticular calcifications in two patients with acute hand pain. AJR Am J Roentgenol. 2010;195(6 Suppl):S76–9.

33. Pascart T, Falgayrac G, Norberciak L, Lalanne C, Legrand J, Houvenagel E, et al. Dual-energy computed-tomography-based discrimination between basic calcium phosphate and calcium pyrophosphate crystal deposition in vivo. Ther Adv Musculoskelet Dis. 2020;12:1759720x20936060.

34. Cudrici CD, Newman KA, Ferrante EA, Huffstutler R, Carney K, Betancourt B, et al. Multifocal calcific periarthritis with distinctive clinical and radiological features in patients with CD73 deficiency. Rheumatology (Oxford). 2021;61(1):163–73.

35. Guanabens N, Mumm S, Moller I, Gonzalez-Roca E, Peris P, Demertzis JL, et al. Calcific periarthritis as the only clinical manifestation of hypophosphatasia in middle-aged sisters. J Bone Miner Res. 2014;29(4):929–34.

36. Uhthoff HK, Loehr JW. Calcific tendinopathy of the rotator cuff: pathogenesis, diagnosis, and management. J Am Acad Orthop Surg. 1997;5(4):183–91.

37. Bomalaski JS, Lluberas G, Schumacher HR Jr. Monosodium urate crystals in the knee joints of patients with asymptomatic nontophaceous gout. Arthritis Rheum. 1986;29(12):1480–4.

38. Pazár B, Ea HK, Narayan S, Kolly L, Bagnoud N, Chobaz V, et al. Basic calcium phosphate crystals induce monocyte/macrophage IL-1β secretion through the NLRP3 inflammasome in vitro. J Immunol. 2011;186(4):2495–502.

39. Mahon OR, Kelly DJ, McCarthy GM, Dunne A. Osteoarthritis-associated basic calcium phosphate crystals alter immune cell metabolism and promote M1 macrophage polarization. Osteoarthritis Cartilage. 2020;28(5):603–12.

40. Corr EM, Cunningham CC, Helbert L, McCarthy GM, Dunne A. Osteoarthritis-associated basic calcium phosphate crystals activate membrane proximal kinases in human innate immune cells. Arthritis Res Ther. 2017;19(1):23.
41. Doumas C, Vazirani RM, Clifford PD, Owens P. Acute calcific periarthritis of the hand and wrist: a series and review of the literature. Emerg Radiol. 2007;14(4):199–203.
42. Monteforte P, Molfetta L, Grillo G, Brignone A, Rovetta G. Disodium clodronate in painful nonresponsive periarthropathy of the hip. Int J Tissue React. 2000;22(4):111–5.
43. Seijas R, Ares O, Alvarez P, Cusco X, Garcia-Balletbo M, Cugat R. Platelet-rich plasma for calcific tendinitis of the shoulder: a case report. J Orthop Surg (Hong Kong). 2012;20(1):126–30.

Neuropathic Osteoarthropathy

7

Parthajit Das, Srijita Ghosh Sen, and Sumit Datta

7.1   Introduction

Neuropathic osteoarthropathy or neurogenic osteoarthropathy (NOA) represents a spectrum of chronic, progressive, noninfectious, and destructive musculoskeletal conditions associated with a neurosensory deficit. Common associations are diabetes mellitus, syringomyelia, syphilis, and other neuropathies. The clinical manifestations may range from joint effusion, mild cartilaginous fragmentation, preserved or increased bone density at an early stage to progressive bone loss or hypertrophy, bony or joint disorganization and/or dislocation due to laxity of periarticular soft tissue structures including ligaments, tendons, etc. There are ambiguities about the exact pathogenesis of NOA. Early diagnosis and institution of effective therapeutic measures remain challenges because of a lack of awareness and paucity of pathognomonic clinical signs to distinguish from other foot-related ailments such as osteoarthritis, soft tissue or joint infections, inflammatory joint disorders, and foot/ankle sprain or fracture.

It is believed that "neuropathic arthritis" was first described by Sir William Musgrave as a complication of venereal disease in 1703. In 1831, John Kearsley Mitchell, an American physician, reported a case of "Tuberculosis of the spine" with neuropathic arthropathy. It was subsequently elucidated by Jean-Martin Charcot in 1868, a French pathologist and neurologist, in his "Neurotrophic theory" recognizing a causative relationship between neuropathic arthropathy and tabes dorsalis. At the seventh International Medical Congress (1881), "Charcot's disease" was established as a distinct pathological entity. In 1936, W.R. Jordan established the association between neurogenic arthropathy of the foot/ankle and diabetes mellitus.

P. Das (✉)
Department of Rheumatology, Apollo Multispeciality Hospital, Kolkata, West Bengal, India

S. G. Sen · S. Datta
Department of Radiology, Apollo Multispeciality Hospital, Kolkata, West Bengal, India

This chapter shall discuss the demography, pathogenesis, clinical manifestations, imaging, and treatment options for neuropathic osteoarthropathy.

7.2   Epidemiology

Epidemiologic data about neuropathic osteoarthropathy is sparse. The estimated prevalence of NOA is between 0.1 and 0.9% among people with diabetes [1], and the average duration of diabetes to develop NOA is 10 years [2]. The risk of acquiring a Charcot foot is unrelated to the type of diabetes mellitus (Type 1 or Type 2). McEwen et al. found a significant association between elevated body mass index and NOA [3].

7.3   Clinical Features

A high index of clinical suspicion is essential for the accurate diagnosis of NOA because of its variable presentation. Neuropathic arthropathy commonly manifests as a slowly progressing arthropathy over months or years, accompanied by recurrent acute attacks. The natural history of clinical and radiological progression has been described by the modified Eichenholtz classification through the following stages; Stage 0—prodromal/inflammatory, Stage 1—development, Stage 2—coalescence, and Stage 3—consolidation (Table 7.1) [4]. The demographics and the predilection of joint involvement may be suggestive of different etiologies of NOA (Table 7.2).

Table 7.1 Eichenholtz classification of clinical and radiological progression of neuropathic arthropathy [4]

Stage	Clinical findings	Radiological findings
Stage 0 (Prodromal/ Inflammatory)	Red, hot, swollen foot No deformity	No changes yet are seen. Normal radiograph
Stage I (Development)	Erythema, foot edema, elevated temperature, no pain	Bony debris at joints, fragmentation of subchondral bone, joint subluxation, and/or fracture-dislocation
Stage II (Coalescence)	Decreased signs of inflammation	Worsening of stage 1 features. Absorption of bony debris with new bone formation. Coalescence of large fragments with sclerosis of bone ends. Mild increase in stability
Stage III (Consolidation)	Resolution of inflammation. Changes in overall foot architecture due to underlying final bony remodeling can lead to new pressure points which are at risk of ulceration	Remodelling of affected bones and joints

Table 7.2 Common sites of involvement and various etiologies of neuropathic arthropathy

Disease	Area of involvement
Peripheral neuropathy (Diabetes, Leprosy, Alcohol, Charcot-Marie -tooth disease)	Predominantly foot and ankle
Syringomyelia	Shoulder, elbow, wrist
Spinal cord injury	Spine, knees
Tabes dorsalis	Knee, hip
Congenital insensitivity to pain	Multiple joints may be involved

Fig. 7.1 A typical Charcot foot in acute active phase: red, hot, and swollen right foot

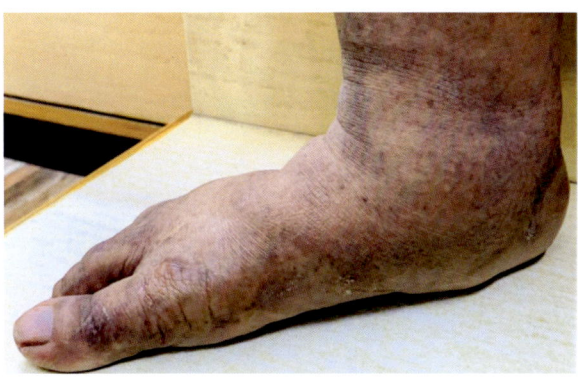

Table 7.3 Mimickers of acute neuropathic arthropathy

1. Osteomyelitis
2. Infection-related arthritis such as tuberculosis and septic arthritis
3. Soft tissue infections—cellulitis
4. Inflammatory arthritis such as rheumatoid arthritis, psoriatic arthritis, and crystal arthropathies
5. Foot/ankle sprain or fracture
6. Deep vein thrombosis

Diabetes primarily affects lower limb joints such as foot, ankle, and knees; syringo-myelia usually affects the shoulder or elbow; and tabes dorsalis (rare these days) is known to affect the knees, hips, and ankles. Although unusual, involvement of upper limb joints can also occur in patients with diabetes.

Patients with acute NOA usually present with sudden onset unilateral redness, warmth, and swelling of the joint (Fig. 7.1), often painless due to underlying poly-neuropathy and may be accompanied by a history of minor trauma. Infection, cel-lulitis, deep venous thrombosis, and inflammatory arthropathies should be considered as important differentials (Table 7.3). Radiological and laboratory results are often normal at this stage.

The clinical features specific to individual joints in NOA have been discussed in Table 7.4. Without early recognition and treatment, progression can be rapid, and irreversible joint damage can occur within 6 months (Fig. 7.2). Prudent use of

Table 7.4 Clinical features of Neuropathic arthropathy

Joints involved	Causes	Clinical features	Treatment
Upper extremity			
Shoulder	Syringomyelia (80% of cases) Diabetes, Cervical spondylosis, Arnold-Chiari malformation	Painless swelling due to distension of the glenohumeral joint and subacromial-subdeltoid bursa In advanced cases, the entire humeral head and neck can be reabsorbed	Protective immobilization of the shoulder joint Limited role of surgical intervention
Elbow	Syringomyelia, Diabetes mellitus, Syphilis, Congenital insensitivity to pain	Joint swelling with instability or dislocation Compression of the ulnar nerve and posterior interosseous nerve are known complications	Dynamic functional bracing aiming to neutralize varus and valgus stresses
Wrist	Diabetes mellitus, Syringomyelia, Leprosy, Syphilis, Congenital insensitivity to pain	Painless swelling of the wrist joint and/or loss of strength, and paresthesia of the hand	Immobilization of the wrist joint, using casts until swelling and redness are settled
Spine			
	Traumatic spinal cord injury (Dorso lumbar spine), Congenital insensitivity to pain, Diabetes mellitus, Tabes dorsalis (rare)	Spinal pain and deformity, low impact fractures, and in advanced cases compressive myelopathy	Treatment is initially conservative Circumferential arthrodesis may be performed in case of significant instability
Lower extremity			
Foot and ankle	Diabetes Mellitus, Other neuropathies, Leprosy, Congenital insensitivity to pain Myelomeningocele	Acute NOA usually presents with red, hot swollen joint, which often goes unrecognized Common foot deformities seen are the bony prominences at unusual places, "rocker bottom foot" etc At a later stage, joint damage can be severe and irreversible Skin is mostly preserved, but NOA can coexist with foot pressure ulceration	Discussed in the treatment section

Table 7.4 (continued)

Joints involved	Causes	Clinical features	Treatment
Knee	Traumatic spinal cord injury, Congenital insensitivity to pain, Diabetes mellitus, Tabes dorsalis	Common presentations are joint swelling and crepitus, which may cause significant joint instability	Management is usually conservative with offloading in a total contact cast and/or knee bracing and non-weight-bearing In advanced cases, arthrodesis or total knee arthroplasty may be considered
Hip	Idiopathic, Tabes dorsalis	Painless, or minimal pain disproportionate to the degree of arthropathy Joint space narrowing and subchondral sclerosis are usual features Intra-articular debris is common in the hypertrophic type and intra-articular fracture is often noted Disproportionate destruction of the femoral head, with relative sparing of the acetabulum, may be present	Internal fixation is performed for a femoral neck fracture Treatment is initially conservative for resorptive hip, as surgery is usually unsuccessful Arthrodesis, bone graft, or total hip arthroplasty may be considered for advanced cases

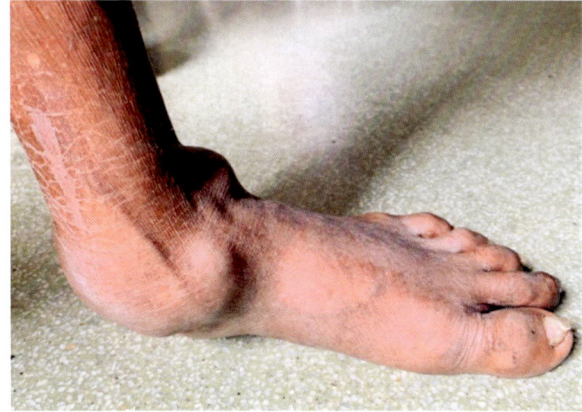

Fig. 7.2 Chronic deforming arthropathy

imaging modalities such as plain radiography, bone scintigraphy, magnetic resonance imaging (MRI), or 18F-fluorodeoxyglucose positron-emission tomography (PET) may aid the early diagnosis of NOA.

7.4　Pathogenesis

The underlying pathogenesis of NOA remains poorly understood. Initially, there were two accepted theories for the pathogenesis of NOA. The "neurotraumatic theory" emphasized that repetitive microtrauma with the loss of proprioception may lead to progressive joint destruction [5] while the "neurovascular theory," stated that the excess blood flow and demineralized bony state may accompany neuropathic arthropathy [6]. Other possible pathogenetic mechanisms are discussed below.

7.4.1　Proinflammatory State

The "inflammatory theory" stresses the pathogenic role of local joint inflammation and the increased expression of proinflammatory cytokines, including IL-1 β, IL-6, and TNF-α [7]. Serum concentrations of TNF-α and IL-6 are elevated at the onset of acute Charcot foot, which are significantly reduced following resolution. The proinflammatory state is related to the bone turnover observed in NOA [7].

7.4.2　Role of the Osteoprotegerin-RANKL-RANK Axis

Proinflammatory cytokines have a positive influence on the activity of the metabolic pathway consisting of Osteoprotegerin (OPG), receptor activator of nuclear factor kappa-B (RANK), and receptor activator of nuclear factor kappa-B ligand (RANKL) axis. RANKL is responsible for the differentiation of osteoclast precursor cells to mature osteoclasts. RANKL binds with the RANK receptor (located on the surface of preosteoclasts, mature osteoclasts), which in turn leads to the differentiation of preosteoclasts into mature osteoclasts. OPG acts as the soluble decoy receptor for RANKL, preventing its binding with RANK. This relationship between RANKL and OPG is disrupted in patients with NOA, and an unregulated synthesis of RANKL results in excessive bony turnover and bony accumulation [8]. Regardless of the initiating mechanism, an initial resorptive phase may occur in the development of a neuropathic joint, which is then followed by a hypertrophic repair phase.

7.4.3　Other Factors

There are other factors such as advanced glycation end products (AGE) and reactive oxygen species (ROS) which may contribute to the development of NOA in diabetes. Excess accumulation of AGE in tissues such as tendons, bone, or cartilage may activate AGE-RAGE (receptor for advanced glycation end products) pathway, leading to increased osteoclastogenesis through enhanced RANKL activation and higher predisposition to low impact fracture [9]. Moreover, associated autonomic neuropathy may result in vasomotor changes resulting in reduced skin and bone blood flow, leading to ischemia and skin ulcerations.

7.5   Genetics

Previous studies have suggested the involvement of genetic factors associated with OPG and RANKL variants in the development of NOA. A positive association with G alleles for OPG variants (245T>G, 1181G>C, and 1217C>T) was found with NOA when compared to patients with diabetic neuropathy and healthy controls [10]. The allele and genotype frequencies of RANKL variants (290C>T, 643C>T, and 693G>C) have been found to occur more frequently in patients with NOA and neuropathy [11].

The osteoclasts differentiate from monocytes. It is believed that gene methylation in monocytes, monocyte-derived microparticles, or miRNAs can influence monocyte-to-osteoclast differentiation, and may have a permissive role in the development of NOA [12]. A few differentially methylated genes including HMGA1, MAPK11, and PPP2R5D were expressed in monocytes from patients with NOA.

These genetic markers could become a useful and convenient screening tool to predict the development of NOA in high-risk patients. However, more robust studies are necessary to confirm their usefulness as a diagnostic tool.

7.6   Diagnostic Approach

A strong clinical suspicion is needed to diagnose NOA because of its multifaceted presentation and several mimickers. Therefore, thorough history taking and clinical examination (Table 7.4), appropriate laboratory and radiological investigations, and exclusion of NOA mimickers are the key considerations toward making the diagnosis of NOA. Figure 7.3 depicts the diagnostic approach to Neuropathic Osteoarthropathy.

7.6.1 Laboratory Investigations

The complete hemogram (hemoglobin, white cell, and platelet count) may be within normal limits and acute phase reactants may be appropriate for the patient's age, sex, and body weight in NOA uncomplicated by infection. Synovial fluid analysis may be sterile, with no organisms on microscopy or no crystals. Elevated acute phase reactants such as erythrocyte sedimentation rate (ESR) and C-reactive protein (CRP) should raise the possibility of infection, e.g., cellulitis,

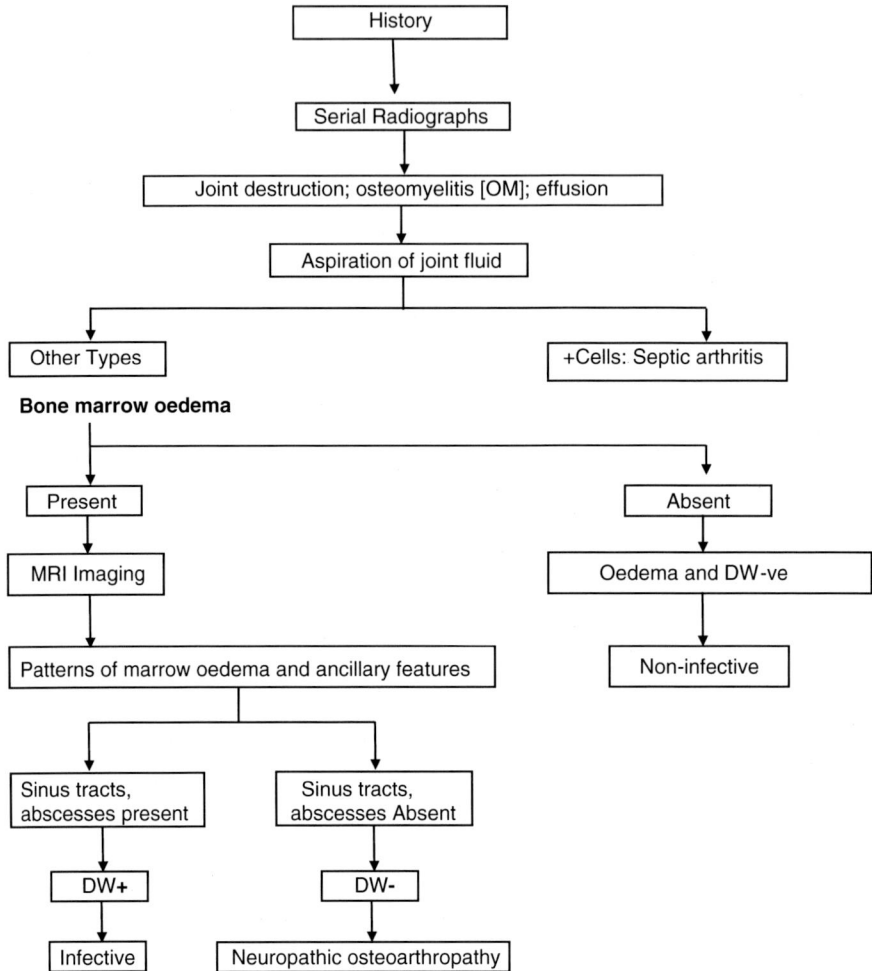

Fig. 7.3 Diagnostic approach to neuropathic osteoarthropathy. *DW* Diffusion Weighted sequence [B value: 800–1000 s/mm²]

osteomyelitis, septic arthritis, inflammatory arthropathies, or gout. The synovial fluid study may be useful if a differential diagnosis of septic arthritis or gout is considered. The immunological assays may aid the diagnosis of inflammatory arthropathies.

7.6.2 Nerve Conduction Study

Manifestations of diabetic neuropathy may range from small fiber-predominant neuropathy as an early manifestation to distal symmetric polyneuropathy as the disease progresses. Nerve conduction study findings of Syringomyelia include low amplitude compound muscle action potential, low amplitude F response with delayed latency, or loss of F response with normal sensory nerve action potentials (SNAPs). In Leprosy, it is the sensory velocity that is impaired suggesting a diffuse neuropathy, amplitude, and the duration of action potential remaining within normal range. Congenital insensitivity to pain will demonstrate normal motor nerve conduction parameters, with reduced response amplitude or evoked response on nerve stimulation.

7.6.3 Imaging

7.6.3.1 Radiography
Diagnosis is primarily reliant on typical appearances on radiographs, or by monitoring progressive changes on serial radiography. Radiography assesses the extent of joint destruction and reduction, bony erosion, and calcification with fragmentation. All three types of Neuropathic osteoarthropathy—hypertrophic, atrophic, and mixed are seen differentiated on radiography [13]. The hypertrophic form presents with joint destruction and fragmentation resulting in debris. Bone sclerosis and osteophytes are also seen. The distribution of exuberant osteophytes may mimic advanced osteoarthritis [14] and often differentiation between the two becomes challenging. The atrophic form presents with features of bone resorption, akin to septic arthritis. Mixed form characterizes the combination of hypertrophic and atrophic forms and is common in occurrence. Sites of individual joints and the manifestations of various types of neuropathic osteoarthropathy are discussed in Table 7.5. The radiography findings in individual joints are discussed below.

Spine
Radiography plays a defining role in depicting the involvement of one or more vertebrae of the thoracolumbar spine; traumatic spinal cord injury being the commonest etiology. Diabetes mellitus and congenital insensitivity to pain constitute other causes. Vertebral lysis or sclerosis, loss of normal curvature, narrowing of disc space, and subluxation are the dominant features. With the ongoing process, end-plate osteophytes and calcification of para-spinal soft tissue may be seen. Neuropathic changes develop typically in the first mobile spinal segment, below the caudal end of the fusion, in paraplegics with spinal fusion procedures [15].

Table 7.5 Types of Neuropathic osteoarthropathy (Radiological)

Types	Sites
Atrophic	• Shoulder—In the non-weight-bearing joint of the upper limb. Syringomyelia and peripheral nerve lesions are usually present • Forefoot
Hypertrophic	• Lower limb—large joints (as in knee joint) • Spine
Mixed	Combination of hypertrophic and atrophic forms

Table 7.6 Differential features of neuropathic osteoarthropathy, osteomyelitis, and metastasis

Imaging features	Neuropathic osteoarthropathy	Osteomyelitis	Metastasis
Osseous fragments	Para-vertebral extension and into the spinal canal [16]	Usually involvement of one vertebral body with adjoining discs	No extensive involvement
Vertebral column involvement	All three vertebral columns may be involved	Single vertebral column [17]	All three may be involved
Facet joint	Involvement with fragmentation	No involvement	Mainly pedicular involvement

Differential diagnoses of similar spine involvement with contrasting features and involvement have been mentioned in Table 7.6.

Hip Joint

Neuropathic osteoarthropathy is a relatively rare entity in the hip joint. Septic arthritis and rapidly destructive osteoarthritis are close mimickers of this disease.

Femoral head destruction with acetabular sparing are the characteristic features of NOA; while joint space narrowing, subchondral sclerosis involving both acetabular and femoral head identify rapidly destructive osteoarthritis [18] of the hip. NOA of the hip joint is primarily idiopathic. The radiographic changes range from extensive joint destruction and resorption of the head and neck of the femur to fracture of the head and neck of the femur resulting from a trivial injury [19].

Shoulder

The neuropathic shoulder is relatively uncommon compared to the lower extremity and the commonest cause is syringomyelia (syrinx). Suspicion of neuropathic involvement of the upper extremity should mandate imaging of the cervical cord [20] as shown in Fig. 7.4a and b. This prompts assessment of less common causes such as Arnold-Chiari Malformation and cervical spondylosis including post-traumatic syringomyelia. The clinical manifestations are claw hand and sensory neuropathic changes affecting lateral spinothalamic tracts. Pain and temperature are therefore affected. Eventually, there is a painless effusion of the glenohumeral and subacromial-subdeltoid bursa. Imaging findings include periarticular soft tissue calcification, amputated appearance of proximal humerus, large joint effusion [13], glenoid sclerosis, humeral head flattening [21], and in severe cases, resorption of humeral head and neck simulating amputation. Osseous fragments and debris are seen in fluid distended bursa.

Elbow Joint and Wrist Joint

Neuropathic arthropathy of the elbow joint is quite uncommon, and that of the wrist is even rarer. Even though, syrinx is the commonest cause in elbow joints; diabetes, leprosy, and syphilis also involve these joints. On radiography, mixed atrophic types are commonly encountered, along with joint debris [22].

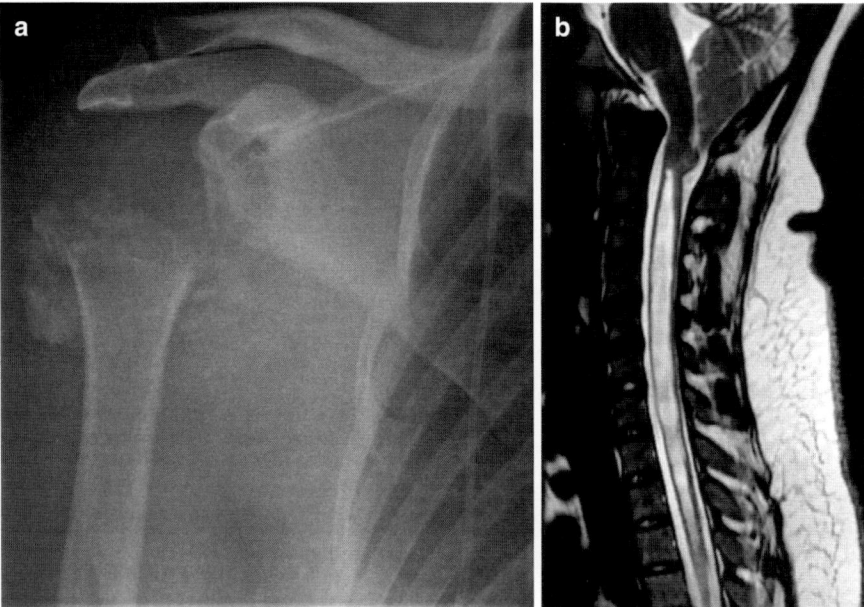

Fig. 7.4 (**a**) Radiograph of right shoulder joint destruction of head of the humerus with disorganization and joint debris. The deformity is also evident. (**b**) MR T2 weighted Image of the cervical spine of the same patient shows a long segment syrinx

In leprosy, claw hand is often seen; with bone resorption in both width and length yielding a tapered appearance at the end of the bone (licked candy stick appearance).

Knee Joint
The knee is the most commonly involved site in syphilis. Diabetes and congenital insensitivity to pain are other etiologies. Syphillis is a forgotten entity and has slipped into history. There is a paradigm shift in site involvement with diabetes, with foot and ankle joints being the most affected sites. CT and MRI images of knee NOA are shown in Figs. 7.5a, b, and 7.6a, b.

Ankle and the Foot Joint
Diabetes mellitus is the commonest cause [23] of NOA in these joints, often precipitated by minor trauma. With disease progression, multiple joints are involved and a vicious cycle sets in, altering the osteo-arthro-kinetics of the joints. The disease process in this severely destructive arthropathy starts in the midfoot region, with subluxation at the second tarsometatarsal joint and progresses laterally [24]. Charcot foot essentially involves inflammation, fragmentation, coalescence, and remodelling (consolidation); and in 23% of the cases recurs with an inflammatory phase, with a mean interval of 27 months [25]. The natural course usually goes through an

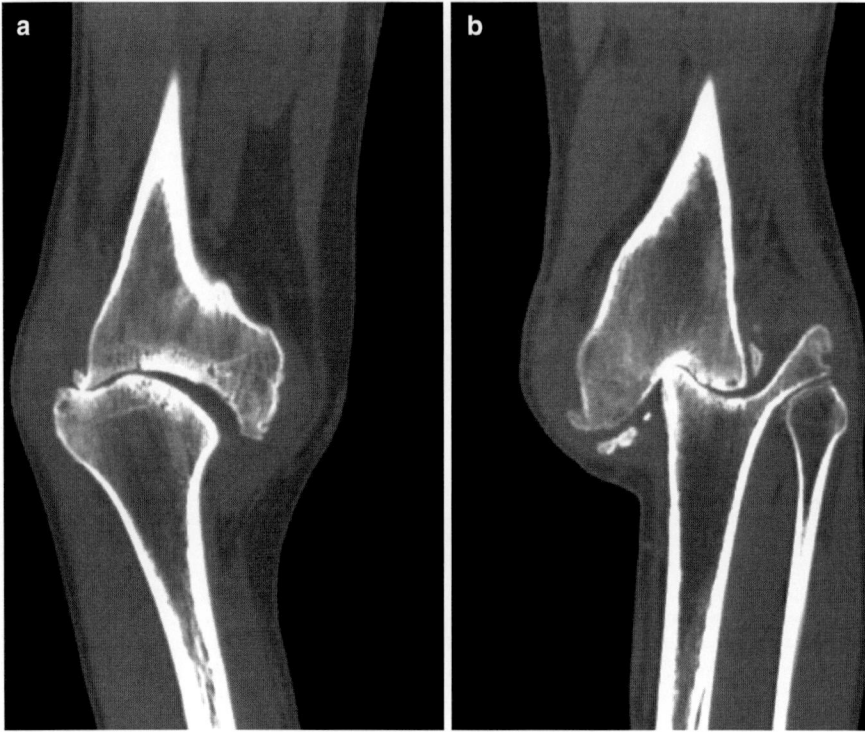

Fig. 7.5 CT scan of the right knee joint: multi-reformatted planar reconstruction in sagittal (**a**) and coronal plane (**b**) shows radio-dense joint debris with subluxation, joint deformity and accompanying subcutaneous edema. (Image courtesy: Dr. Neeti Gupta, Tata Memorial Hospital, Mumbai)

active phase (swollen and warm ankle with foot) and the inactive phase (wherein the foot is no longer warm and hot, but may have residual edema which may be noted occasionally). The result is joint and bone destruction, proliferation, and Rocker-bottom deformity [26] as shown in Fig. 7.7a and b. Imaging of the foot and ankle is classified/categorized based on Brodzky class, which is based on the pattern of joint involvement. Sanders and Frykberg classification [2] concerns the zonal distribution of the disease, and the tarsometatarsal joint involvement [Zone II] is the commonest. The role of imaging [Radiography, MRI with Scintigraphy] is not only to diagnose and stage; but also for monitoring and recognition of complications [27]. This entire gamut aids in planning the management.

The following radiographic measurements are helpful in determining the severity of deformation in a neuropathic joint.

1. **Cuboid height:** To measure this, a horizontal line is drawn from the plantar aspect of calcaneal tuberosity to the plantar surface of the fifth metatarsal head. A perpendicular line is drawn from the plantar surface of the cuboid to the abovementioned horizontal line. The normal limit is about 1.2 cm above that line (Fig. 7.8).

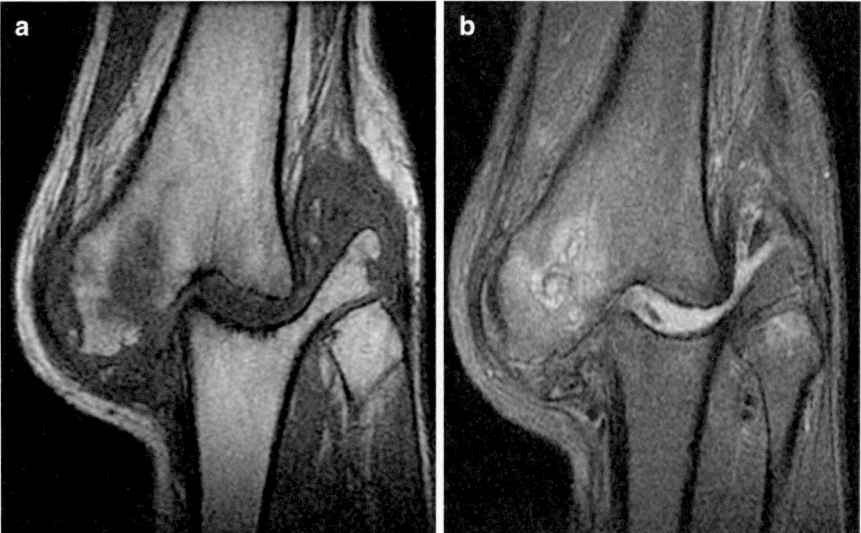

Fig. 7.6 MRI scan of the right knee joint (**a**) T2 Weighted Sequence and (**b**) STIR Sequence reveals disorganization, deformity, and marrow edema of the medial femoral condyle. Subluxation of femorotibial joint

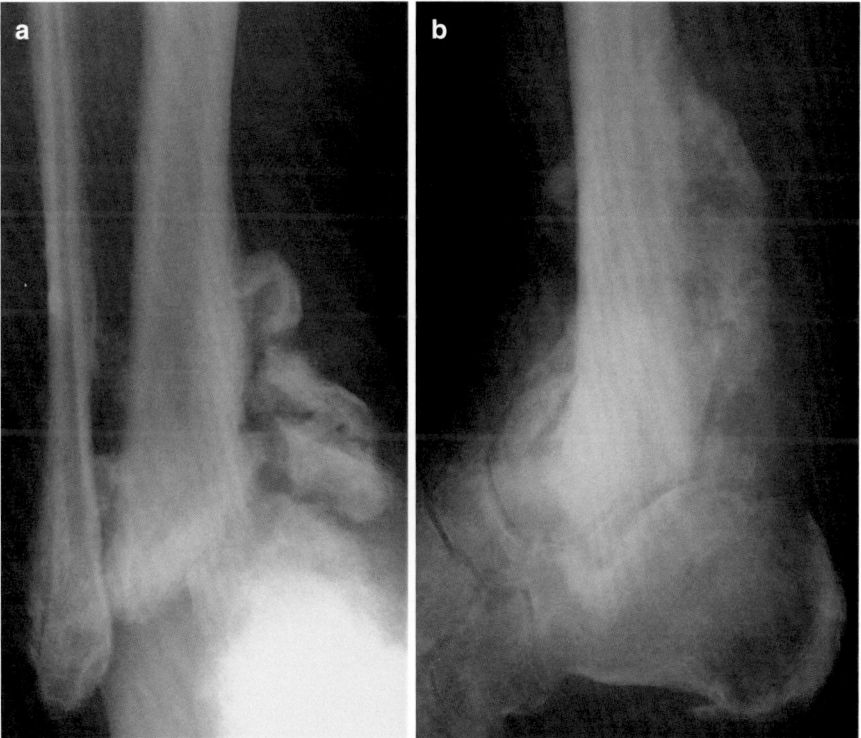

Fig. 7.7 (**a**) Antero-posterior and (**b**) lateral radiograph B of right ankle joint shows destruction, dislocation, and deformity with increased bone density noted

Fig. 7.8 Radiograph of
the left foot shows
diminution of cuboid
height, as delineated by
perpendicular (bold
yellow) line, below the
horizontal (thin
yellow) line

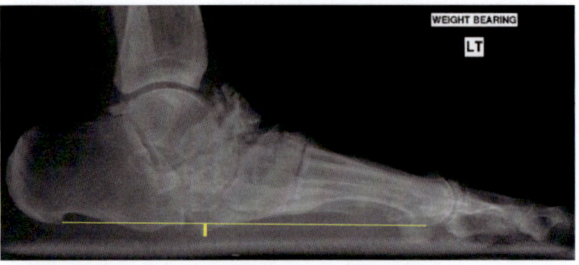

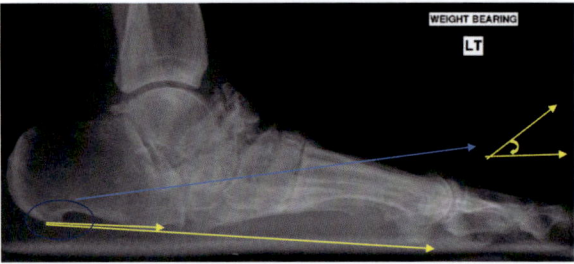

Fig. 7.9 Diminution of the angle subtended between the lines connecting the most plantar aspect of calcaneal tuberosity with the most anterior portion of anterior calcaneum (smaller yellow arrow) and the line connecting the plantar surface of the calcaneum and the fifth metatarsal head (longer yellow arrow). The blue circle and the blue straight line defines the "Calcaneal pitch," in magnification

2. **Calcaneal pitch:** It is defined as an angle between two subtended lines. The first line connects the plantar surfaces of the calcaneum and fifth metatarsal head, while the other connects the most plantar aspect of calcaneal tuberosity and the most anterior portion of anterior calcaneum [28]. The normal value ranges between 20° and 30°. Radiographs may be normal in the early stage of neuropathic osteoarthropathy. In advanced cases, a decrease in the subtended angle is observed (Fig. 7.9).

In the ankle and foot joint NOA, MRI shows synovial cysts, ligamentous disruption, capsular abnormalities (distension and rupture), intra-articular debris, and joint effusion. The changes are grouped into early and late changes.

In the early stage, marrow and soft tissue edema, joint effusion, and subchondral micro-fractures [29] are seen.

In the late stage, there is the presence of marrow edema depending upon the disease activity. Subchondral cysts, bony proliferation with sclerosis, debris, and joint effusion are the mainstay [23]. Dislocations may involve Lisfranc's joint or talar head, with the collapse of the longitudinal arch [29] (Figs. 7.10 and 7.11).

Fig. 7.10 T2 Weighted Sequence: Coronal view of right ankle joint shows destruction, synovial proliferation, and subluxation with deformity

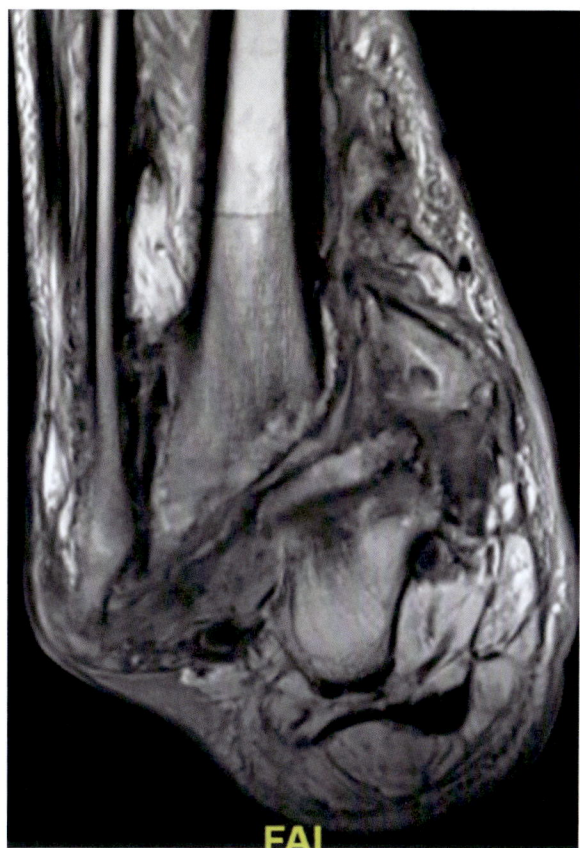

7.7   Treatment

A comprehensive management plan should emphasize prompt clinical diagnosis, early recognition of micro or macro-vascular complications, good quality pre and postoperative care, and optimum control of other comorbidities such as diabetes, cardiovascular disease, morbid obesity, and nephropathy. An experienced team of healthcare professionals including a rheumatologist, endocrinologist, orthopedic surgeon, rehabilitation personnel, occupational therapist, podiatrist, etc., should work cohesively to deliver the optimum care. Fracture prevention liaison service should be encouraged to optimize bone health, minimize the risk of falls and prevent fractures.

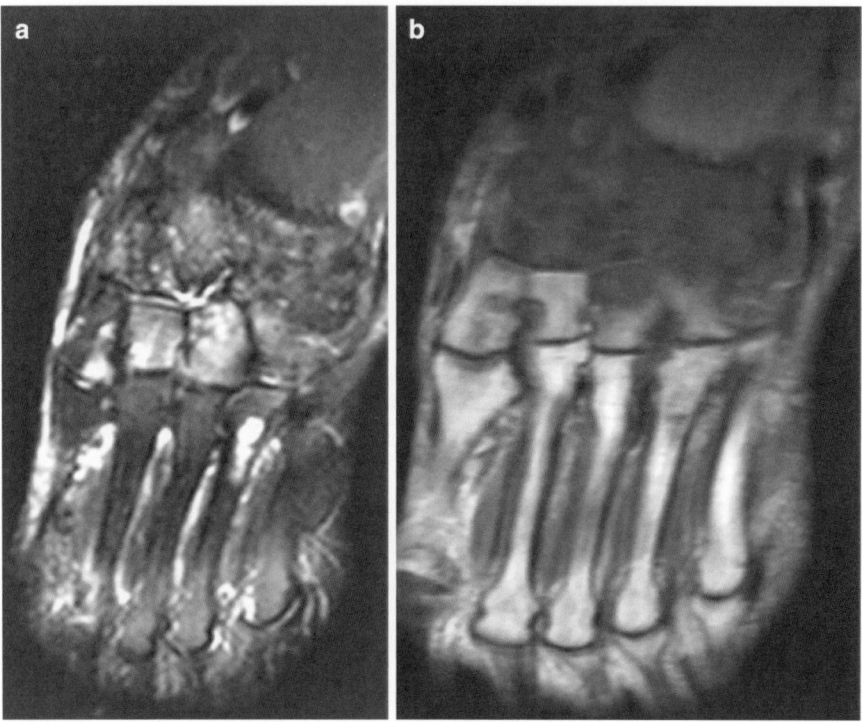

Fig. 7.11 Coronal STIR (**a**) and coronal T2 (**b**) weighted images show hypointensity in the fore-foot region with intermediate intensity on T2 Weighted image reflecting secondary changes, along with joint destruction and deformity

7.7.1 General Measures

Rest and non-steroidal anti-inflammatory drugs (NSAIDs) are often used for optimum pain relief. Immobilization of the affected joint with a sling or specialized cast and restriction of activity is generally recommended for the neuropathic joints. Treatment of underlying disease remains the mainstay of therapy.

7.7.2 Specific Measures

(a) **Upper Limb NOA**

Shoulder, elbow, and wrist NOA are rare diseases and are often preceded by misdiagnosis and unsuccessful treatment. Conservative treatment is usually preferred in these patients, as surgical management can be challenging. Protected immobilization of the upper limb with a sling is recommended for joint stabilization. Supervised intra-articular corticosteroid injection (e.g., glenohumeral joint) may be used at an early stage where indicated.

(b) **Lower Limb NOA**

Conservative management is advocated to prevent further injury to the affected joint. At the acute and active stage, it is imperative to immobilize the affected joint and restrict weight-bearing to arrest the progression of joint deformity. The non-weight-bearing status of the knee NOA can be augmented via a brace, plaster, or total contact cast (TCC). Assistive devices such as crutches or wheelchair mobilization should be encouraged to aid the non-weight-bearing status. A non-weight-bearing period of 3 months has been recommended [28]. Adjunctive pharmacological therapy and low-intensity ultrasound may be useful.

The primary goal of treatment of foot NOA is to improve the quality of life, maintain a stable plantigrade foot that is suitable for ambulation, minimize permanent foot deformity, and prevent ulceration and infection. The affected foot should be immobilized in an irremovable total TCC, and/or a controlled ankle motion (CAM) walker, which helps to redistribute and reduce pressures on the plantar foot while allowing ambulation.

Duration and intensity of offloading (non-weight-bearing versus weight-bearing, nonremovable versus removable devices) are guided by clinical markers of healing such as edema, hyperemia, and temperature [30] and imaging assessments (conventional radiographs or MRI). Following this acute stage, various specialized devices are prescribed such as prescriptive shoes, boots, or other weight-bearing braces to prevent recurrence or ulceration on subsequent deformities.

7.7.3 Pharmacological Therapy

The treatment guidelines are largely guided by professional opinion rather than the highest level of clinical evidence-based recommendations. Since NOA is a rare disease, only a few randomized trials with smaller sample sizes are available.

The main principles of medical treatment of NOA are (1) antiresorptive therapy, (2) anabolic therapy, and (3) bone growth stimulation.

7.7.3.1 Antiresorptive Therapy

Excessive bone turnover has been observed in patients with active NOA. Therefore, antiresorptive therapies such as oral and intravenous bisphosphonates, intranasal calcitonin, and denosumab have been used as therapeutic strategies for a long time. Bisphosphonates may help the acute phase of NOA as they inhibit osteoclastic reabsorption. Jude et al. [29] reported that a single dose of pamidronate leads to a reduction in bone turnover, symptoms, and disease activity in diabetic patients with active NOA. Patients intolerant to oral bisphosphonates such as pamidronate and alendronate may benefit from intravenous zoledronic acid therapy. Intranasal calcitonin is another antiresorptive agent that has been studied in NOA and has a safer profile in renal failure. There is little or no conclusive evidence to recommend the use of bisphosphonates in NOA.

7.7.3.2 Anabolic Therapy

Teriparatide (recombinant human parathyroid hormone 1–34) is often recommended for the treatment of severe osteoporosis because it stimulates bone formation and may potentially enhance fracture healing. Rastogi et al. [30] demonstrated the favorable role of Teriparatide in increasing foot bone modeling in chronic NOA in diabetes. In a double-blind placebo-controlled trial, intervention with Teriparatide did not reduce time to resolution or enhance fracture healing of NOA. There was no additional favorable effect of the below-knee casting in achieving earlier resolution of active NOA in diabetes patients [31]. Larger randomized and appropriately blinded trials are therefore needed to investigate the role of Teriparatide in NOA.

7.7.4 Bone Growth Stimulation

Ultrasonic bone stimulation and direct current electrical bone growth stimulators have shown a promising effect, especially in patients undergoing arthrodesis. It helps in the healing of fresh fractures and acts as an adjunct therapy in patients with acute NOA [32]. There is however limited evidence and no good quality follow-up studies have validated these methods as an adjunct therapy.

7.7.5 Surgical Management

Neuropathic joints may need multiple staged reconstructive surgeries over time. The decision to perform surgical intervention remains controversial, during acute as well as chronic phases of NOA. This is because of several factors such as patient comorbidities, poor bone quality, compliance with non-weight-bearing, presence of skin ulceration, perceived risk of infection, and extent of the deformity and disability. Surgery is indicated for resection of infected bone (osteomyelitis), removal of bony prominences (exostectomy) to relieve bony pressures and for correcting deformities. This is combined with accommodative bracing [33].

Surgical interventions of shoulder NOA including arthroplasty or arthrodesis may have a limited role with poorer outcomes and a high risk of recurrence [34]. Joint debridement is rarely performed as a palliative measure. There is an increased risk of infection following shoulder arthrodesis [35].

In knee NOA, surgical treatment is considered in patients with severe instability, soft tissue laxity, and bony destruction. The surgical treatment of choice has classically been arthrodesis, which is commonly achieved using an intramedullary nail [36]. The patella, along with the entire synovium is usually excised.

In foot NOA, surgical intervention is generally avoided during the active inflammatory phase because of the higher risk of wound infection or failure of fixation [37]. Simon SR et al. [38] reported that early correction of deformity combined with arthrodesis and extended period of non-weight-bearing results in an improved quality of life. Achilles tendon lengthening procedure is meant to reduce forefoot pressure and restore the alignment of the ankle/hindfoot to midfoot and forefoot, combined with arthrodesis to improve pain and instability [39]. The presence of ulceration is a sign of poor prognosis and is associated with a higher risk of bone infection and amputation in the future [40, 41].

7.7.6   Novel/Experimental Therapies for Neuropathic Osteoarthropathy

Current research is exploring the inflammatory pathways involved in osteoclast activation including various inflammatory cytokines such as TNF-α, IL-1, IL-6, and the Osteoprotegerin-RANKL-RANK axis responsible for the osteoclast maturation. These could be the potential targets for future immunomodulatory therapy.

Petrova NL et al. [42] have demonstrated TNF-α modulated RANKL-mediated osteoclastic resorption in vitro in acute NOA and suggested that the addition of an anti-TNF agent may have a beneficial role in the treatment of NOA in the future. Denosumab, a fully human monoclonal antibody to the receptor activator of nuclear factor-κB ligand (RANKL), has shown promising results in the management of osteoporosis and bone metastatic disease. The preliminary results of a small open-label, pilot study of a single dose of Denosumab showed favorable results in active NOA [43]. Busch-Westbroek et al. also reported that a single dose of Denosumab resulted in a significant reduction of the total average time for treatment by contact plastering and the resolution time of fractures on imaging in acute NOA of the foot [44].

A combination of platelet-rich concentrate and a small amount of autologous bone marrow aspirate administered while performing arthrodesis was found to be effective in high-risk diabetic patients with NOA [45, 46].

7.8   Conclusion

Despite advancements in medical research, neuropathic osteoarthropathy remains a poorly understood disease. Educating patients and healthcare personnel, early recognition, prompt offloading and immobilization of the affected limb in acute NOA, maintaining a stable plantigrade foot free of infection and ulcerations in chronic NOA, and optimum control of comorbid conditions are the mainstay of therapy. Judicious use of laboratory and radiological investigations is recommended to exclude NOA mimics. High-quality research is warranted to develop convenient and highly predictive biochemical, genetic markers, and newer radiological modalities to identify patients who are at a higher risk of developing NOA.

References

1. Schoots IG, Slim FJ, Busch-Westbroek TE, Maas M. Neuro- osteoarthropathy of the foot-radiologist: friend or foe? Semin Musculoskelet Radiol. 2010;14:365–76.
2. Ergen FB, Sanverdi SE, Oznur A. Charcot foot in diabetes and an update on imaging. Diabet Foot Ankle. 2013;4:21884.

3. McEwen LN, Ylitalo KR, Herman WH, Wrobel JS. Prevalence and risk factors for diabetes-related foot complications in translating research into action for diabetes (TRIAD). J Diabetes Complicat. 2013;27(6):588–92.
4. Eichenholtz SN. Charcot joints. Springfield: Charles C. Thomas; 1966.
5. Kiss J, Martin JR, McConnell F. Angiographic and lymphangiographic examination of neuropathic knee joints. J Can Assoc Radiol. 1968;19:19–24.
6. Jeffcoate WJ, Game F, Cavanagh PR. The role of proinflammatory cytokines in the cause of neuropathic osteoarthropathy (acute Charcot foot) in diabetes. Lancet (London, England). 2005;366:2058–61. https://doi.org/10.1016/S0140-6736(05)67029-8.
7. Baumhauer JF, O'Keefe RJ, Schon LC, Pinzur MS. Cytokine-induced osteoclastic bone resorption in charcot arthropathy: an immunohistochemical study. Foot Ankle Int. 2006;27:797.
8. Zhao H-M, Diao J-Y, Liang X-J, Zhang F, Hao D-J. Pathogenesis and potential relative risk factors of diabetic neuropathic osteoarthropathy. J Orthop Surg Res. 2017;12:142. https://doi.org/10.1186/s13018-017-0634-8.
9. Witzke KA, Vinik AI, Grant LM, et al. Loss of RAGE defense: a cause of Charcot neuroarthropathy? Diabetes Care. 2011;34(7):1617–21. https://doi.org/10.2337/dc10-2315.
10. Pitocco D, Zelano G, Gioffre G, Di Stasio E, Zaccardi F, Martini F, et al. Association between osteoprotegerin G1181C and T245G polymorphisms and diabetic charcot neuroarthropathy: a case-control study. Diabetes Care. 2009;32:1694–7. https://doi.org/10.2337/dc09-0243.
11. Bruhn-Olszewska B, Korzon-Burakowska A, Wegrzyn G, Jakobkiewicz-Banecka J. Prevalence of polymorphisms in OPG, RANKL and RANK as potential markers for Charcot arthropathy development. Sci Rep. 2017;7:501. https://doi.org/10.1038/s41598-017-00563-4.
12. Pasquier J, Thomas B, Hoarau-Vechot J, Odeh T, Robay A, Chidiac O, et al. Circulating microparticles in acute diabetic Charcot foot exhibit a high content of inflammatory cytokines, and support monocyte-to-osteoclast cell induction. Sci Rep. 2017;7:16450. https://doi.org/10.1038/s41598-017-16365-7.
13. Jones EA, Manaster BJ, May DA, Disler DG. Neuropathic osteoarthropathy: diagnostic dilemmas and differential diagnosis. Radiographics. 2000;20 Spec No(Suppl_1):S279–93.
14. Chan RLS, Chan CH, Chan HF, Pan NY. The many facets of neuropathic arthropathy. BJR Open. 2019;1:20180039.
15. Standaert C, Cardenas DD, Anderson P. Charcot spine as a late complication of traumatic spinal cord injury. Arch Phys Med Rehabil. 1997;78:221–5.
16. Kapila A, Lines M. Neuropathic spinal arthropathy: CT and MR findings. J Comput Assist Tomogr. 1987;11:736–9.
17. Brant-Zawadzki M, Burke VD, Jeffrey RB. CT in the evaluation of spine infection. Spine. 1983;8:358–64.
18. Rosenberg ZS, Shankman S, Steiner GC, Kastenbaum DK, Norman A, Lazansky MG. Rapidly destructive osteoarthritis: clinical, radiographic and pathologic features. Radiology. 1992;182:213–6.
19. Johnson JT. Neuropathic injuries of the hip. Clin Orthop Relat Res. 1993;90:29–32.
20. Tully JG Jr, Latteri A. Paraplegia, syringomyelia tarda and neuropathic arthrosis of the shoulder: a triad. Clin Orthop. 1978;134:244–8.
21. Santiesteban L, Zuckerman JD. Neuropathic arthropathy of the glenohumeral joint: a review of the literature. Bull NYU Hosp Jt Dis. 2018;6:88–99.
22. Stewart N, Karpik K. Syringomyelic neuropathic arthropathy of the elbow. N Z Med J. 2016;129:87.
23. Ergen FB, Sanverdi SE, Ozmur A. Charcot foot in diabetes and an update on imaging. Diabet Foot Ankle. 2013;21:884.
24. Sella EJ, Barrette C. Staging of Charcot, neuroarthropathy along the medial column of the foot is the diabetic patient. J Foot Ankle Surg. 1999;38:34–40.
25. Osterhoff G, Boni T, Berli M. Recurrence of acute Charcot neuropathic osteoarthropathy after conservative treatment. Foot Ankle Int. 2013;34:359–64.
26. Frykberg RG, Zgonis T, Armstrong DG, et al. Diabetic foot disorders. A clinical practice guideline (2006 revision). J Foot Ankle Surg. 2006;45:61–6.

27. Rosskopf AB, Berli M. The role of radiological imaging for treatment of Charcot foot. Sprunggelenk. 2018;16:99–108.
28. Lee L, Blume PA, Sumpio B. Charcot joint disease in diabetes mellitus. Ann Vasc Surg. 2003;17:571–80.
29. Jude EB, Selby PL, Burgess J, et al. Bisphosphonates in the treatment of Charcot neuroarthropathy: a double-blind randomised controlled trial. Diabetologia. 2001;44:2032–7.
30. Rastogi A, Hajela A, Prakash M, Khandelwal N, Kumar R, Bhattacharya A, Mittal BR, Bhansali A, Armstrong DG. Teriparatide (recombinant human parathyroid hormone [1-34]) increases foot bone remodeling in diabetic chronic Charcot neuroarthropathy: a randomized double-blind placebo-controlled study. J Diabetes. 2019;11(9):703–10. https://doi.org/10.1111/1753-0407.12902. Epub 2019 Feb 13. PMID: 30632290.
31. Petrova NL, Donaldson NK, Bates M, et al. Effect of recombinant human parathyroid hormone (1-84) on resolution of active Charcot neuro-osteoarthropathy in diabetes: a randomized, double-blind, placebo-controlled study [published correction appears in Diabetes Care. 2021 Nov;44(11):2642]. Diabetes Care. 2021;44(7):1613–21. https://doi.org/10.2337/dc21-0008.
32. Kane WJ. Direct current electrical bone growth stimulation for spinal fusion. Spine (Phila Pa 1976). 1988;13(3):363–5.
33. Catanzariti AR, Mendicino R, Haverstock B. Ostectomy for diabetic neuroarthropathy involving the midfoot. J Foot Ankle Surg. 2000;39:291–300.
34. Atalar AA, Sungur M, Demirhan M, Özger H. Neuropathic arthropathy of the shoulder associated with syringomyelia: a report of six cases. Acta Orthop Traumatol Ture. 2010;44:328–36.
35. Clare DJ, Wirth MA, Groh GL, Rockwood CA Jr. Shoulder arthrodesis. J Bone Joint Surg Am. 2001;83-A:593–600.
36. Vince KG, Cameron HU, Hungerford DS, et al. What would you do? Case challenges in knee surgery. J Arthroplasty. 2005;20:44–50.
37. Wukich DK, Sung W. Charcot arthropathy of the foot and ankle: modern concepts and management review. J Diabetes Complicat. 2009;23:409–26.
38. Simon SR, Tejwani SG, Wilson DL, Santner TJ, Denniston NL. Arthrodesis as an early alternative to nonoperative management of Charcot arthropathy of the diabetic foot. J Bone Joint Surg Am. 2000;82-A:939–50.
39. Hastings MK, Mueller MJ, Sinacore DR, Salsich GB, Engsberg JR, Johnson JE. Effects of a tendo-Achilles lengthening procedure on muscle function and gait characteristics in a patient with diabetes mellitus. J Orthop Sports Phys Ther. 2000;30:85–90.
40. Ahmadi ME, Morrison WB, Carrino JA, Schweitzer ME, Raikin SM, Ledermann HP. Foot with and without superimposed osteomyelitis: MR imaging characteristics. Radiology. 2006;238:622–31.
41. Marmolejo VS, Arnold JF, Ponticello M, Anderson CA. Charcot foot: clinical clues, diagnostic strategies, and treatment principles. Am Fam Physician. 2018;97(9):594–9.
42. Petrova NL, Petrov PK, Edmonds ME, Shanahan CM. Inhibition of TNF-α reverses the pathological resorption pit profile of osteoclasts from patients with acute Charcot osteoarthropathy. J Diabetes Res. 2015;2015:917945. https://doi.org/10.1155/2015/917945.
43. Shofler D, Hamedani E, Seun J, Sathananthan A, Katsaros E, Liggan L, Kang S, Pham C. Investigating the use of Denosumab in the treatment of acute Charcot neuroarthropathy. J Foot Ankle Surg. 2021;60(2):354–7. https://doi.org/10.1053/j.jfas.2020.09.018. Epub 2020 Dec 2. PMID: 33472754.
44. Busch-Westbroek TE, Delpeut K, Balm R, Bus SA, Schepers T, Peters EJ, Smithuis FF, Maas M, Nieuwdorp M. Effect of single dose of RANKL antibody treatment on acute Charcot neuro-osteoarthropathy of the foot. Diabetes Care. 2018;41(3):e21–2. https://doi.org/10.2337/dc17-1517. Epub 2017 Dec 22. PMID: 29273577.
45. Brodsky JW. The diabetic foot. In: Coughlin MJ, Mann RA, Saltzmann CL, editors. Surgery of the foot and ankle. St. Louis: Mosby; 2006. p. 1281–368.
46. Pinzur MS. Use of platelet-rich concentrate and bone marrow aspirate in high-risk patients with Charcot arthropathy of the foot. Foot Ankle Int. 2009;30(2):124–7. https://doi.org/10.3113/FAI-2009-0124. PMID: 19254506.

Cheiroarthropathy and Other Musculoskeletal Manifestations of Diabetes

8

Koshy Nithin Thomas and Durga Prasanna Misra ⓘ

8.1 Introduction

Diabetes mellitus is one of the commonest metabolic diseases worldwide. It is particularly widely prevalent in Asia. It is well recognized that long-standing diabetes mellitus can affect numerous organ systems including the musculoskeletal system. These features are protean and include arthropathy, tenosynovitis, capsulitis, spinal ligament ossification, and entrapment neuropathies. Though at first glance, the primary pathology might appear less sinister than inflammatory musculoskeletal disorders, such as rheumatoid arthritis or spondyloarthritis, it is no less debilitating and considerably impacts the quality of life. As the prevalence of diabetes worldwide is on the rise, it shall inevitably increase the burden of these disorders presenting to healthcare. For clinicians, knowledge of these manifestations is necessary to enable early identification of these disorders and the prompt institution of appropriate treatment. In this chapter, we have discussed the various rheumatological manifestations of diabetes, with a focus on diabetic cheiroarthropathy (Table 8.1).

K. N. Thomas · D. P. Misra (✉)
Department of Clinical Immunology and Rheumatology, Sanjay Gandhi Postgraduate Institute of Medical Sciences (SGPGIMS), Lucknow, India
e-mail: dpmisra@sgpgi.ac.in

Table 8.1 Prevalence of musculoskeletal manifestations of diabetes mellitus

Musculoskeletal features of diabetes mellitus	Prevalence [reference number]
Adhesive capsulitis	11–30% [4]
Diabetic cheiroarthropathy	8–76% [8, 23]
Dupuytren's syndrome	20–63% [16]
Carpel tunnel syndrome	11–30% [14]
Flexor tenosynovitis	5–20% [14]
Diffuse idiopathic skeletal hyperostosis	13–40% [14, 23]
Neuropathic arthropathy	2.9% [23]

8.2 Diabetic Cheiroarthropathy

Derived from the Latin word "chiro" which means hands, diabetic cheiroarthropathy is a syndrome of limited mobility of the joints of the hands. Other synonymous terminologies are "syndrome of limited joint mobility" or "stiff hand" syndrome. An early description of this syndrome by Lundbeck in 1957 reported palmar fascial contractures in patients with diabetes who presented with a stiffness of their hands [1]. Subsequently, Jung et al. described a series of patients with concurrent flexor contractures of the fingers associated with carpal tunnel syndrome [2]. Presently, diabetic cheiroarthropathy is defined as contractures of the fingers without demonstrable involvement of the palmar fascia [3].

Cohort studies have demonstrated that diabetic cheiroarthropathy can precede overt microvascular complications of diabetes. In a cohort of 309 children with type 1 diabetes followed up over 16 years, a higher proportion of individuals with cheiroarthropathy eventually developed microvascular complications when compared with those without cheiroarthropathy (83% vs 25%, respectively) [4]. In another cohort, the adjusted odds ratio (for confounding factors of age, gender, disease duration, and diabetes control) of cheiroarthropathy was 1.60 (95% confidence interval 1.14–2.24) in the presence of neuropathy and 1.45 (95% confidence interval 0.99–2.11) in the presence of retinopathy [5]. However, this study used the term diabetic cheiroarthropathy for the classical description as well as for Dupuytren's contracture, adhesive capsulitis, and other involvement of the upper limb associated with diabetes [5]. Microvascular pathology has been observed in other musculoskeletal manifestations associated with diabetes such as Dupuytren's contracture [6].

Cohort studies have demonstrated a prevalence of diabetic cheiroarthropathy in up to 55% of patients with type 1 DM and 76% of patients with type 2 DM [7]. More recent literature has reported the prevalence of prayer sign in 22% of patients with diabetes [5]. While this might be due to an improvement in overall glycaemic control with time, it could also be due to the differences in techniques used for case identification in different studies. The latter study reported an association of cheiroarthropathy with a longer duration of diabetes, worse diabetes control (based on HbA1c), the presence of microvascular complications such as retinopathy and neuropathy, and the deposition of glycated end products detected by skin intrinsic fluorescence [5]. There was no significant difference in the proportion of patients with diabetic cheiroarthropathy when treated with intensive or conventional insulin therapy. However, other musculoskeletal manifestations of diabetes such as adhesive capsulitis, Dupuytren's contracture, and flexor tenosynovitis were considerably reduced in the group receiving intensive insulin therapy (as opposed to conventional insulin therapy) [5]. Somewhat contrary to these observations, another recent study reported that cheiroarthropathy was commoner in prediabetes (47%) when compared with type 1 (28%) or type 2 (27%) diabetes. In this cross-sectional study, the presence of prediabetes, associated neuropathy, and higher fasting blood glucose were associated with greater odds of cheiroarthropathy [8].

Diabetes mellitus leads to the deposition of advanced glycation end products (AGE) in various tissues of the body. Collagen fibers contain an abundance of the amino acids lysine and hydroxylysine which undergo nonenzymatic glycation in the presence of a hyperglycemic milieu. Following this, there occurs an increased cross-linking of collagen. Such cross-linked collagen is less amenable to natural degradation processes by collagenases. Also, altered metabolism via the aldose reductase and sorbitol dehydrogenase pathways in collagen results in physical alterations of collagen structure [3]. Deposition of AGE is hypothesized to be the central mechanism driving the pathogenesis of diabetic cheiroarthropathy. AGEs are present in greater quantities in established diabetes mellitus, although they have also been observed in those with prediabetes [9]. A dysregulation of matrix metalloproteinases has also been observed in type 1 diabetes [10], which further results in an imbalance in the turnover of connective tissue. Such an imbalance clinically manifests as stiff joints and thickened skin which results in the phenotype of diabetic cheiroarthropathy.

Patients with diabetic cheiroarthropathy often complain of hand stiffness or a weak grip. While the condition is generally painless, associated peripheral distal sensory neuropathy due to diabetes mellitus might result in pain. Contractures are asymptomatic, to begin with, usually starting in the proximal interphalangeal (PIP) joints with a greater affection of lateral fingers initially but eventually progressing to affect all digits of the hand. While the metacarpophalangeal and the PIP joints are the most severely affected, the distal interphalangeal joints might also be involved. Resulting contractures limit flexion as well as extension. The classical picture of the *prayer sign* is a consequence of the fact that the palms and fingers cannot be approximated when the two palms are opposed together with the wrists fully extended (Fig. 8.1). Another related clinical sign is the *tabletop sign*, which denotes the inability to lay fingers and palms flat on a table. At a later stage of the disease, proximal joints such as the wrists, elbow, and other large joints might also be involved [3]. Ultrasonographic imaging of the hands reveals a characteristic finding of flexor tendon sheath thickening. Enhancement of the affected tendon sheaths might also be visualized on magnetic resonance imaging.

The skin of the fingers might also be affected by a thickened waxy texture. Such a finding has been eponymously described as *diabetic sclerodactyly*. This can mimic the skin thickening associated with systemic sclerosis however the absence of Raynaud's phenomenon or nail fold capillaroscopy changes of systemic sclerosis as well as a positive history of diabetes mellitus are distinguishing features. When the syndrome of limited hand joint mobility is associated with adhesive capsulitis or

Fig. 8.1 Prayer sign in diabetic cheiroarthropathy— Limited hand joint mobility with an inability to oppose the palmar surfaces of both hands (image provided courtesy of Professor Vikas Agarwal, SGPGIMS, Lucknow, India)

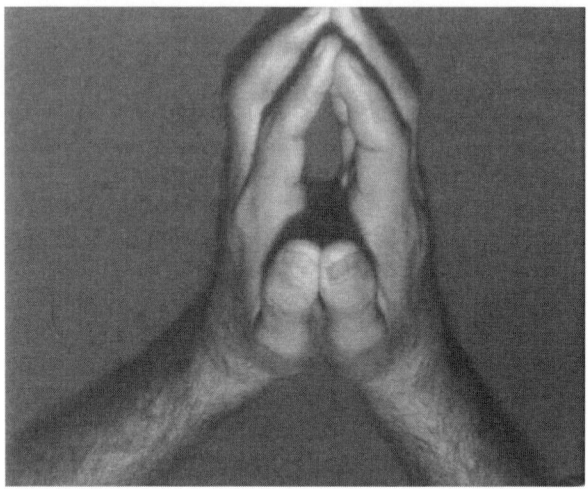

frozen shoulder on the same side, it has been described as shoulder hand syndrome. This might be confused with complex regional pain syndrome or reflex sympathetic dystrophy, another musculoskeletal syndrome found to be associated with diabetes mellitus [11].

Diabetic cheiroarthropathy is associated with considerable disability. Those with diabetic cheiroarthropathy have considerably worse disability scores in the upper limbs when compared with those without [6, 9].

8.3 Adhesive Capsulitis

Colloquially referred to as *frozen shoulder*, adhesive capsulitis is associated with considerable disability and functional limitation in patients with diabetes. While commonly associated with diabetes, other etiologies include shoulder injuries, stroke involving the upper limb of the same side, or ischemic heart disease. Diabetes mellitus increases the risk of developing adhesive capsulitis. This entity has been reported in 11–30% of individuals with diabetes mellitus as opposed to only 2–10% of those without diabetes [4]. The anatomical pathology in adhesive capsulitis involves a thickening of the capsule of the shoulder joint resulting in a reduction in the glenohumeral joint space and diminished shoulder mobility [4].

Individuals with adhesive capsulitis generally have shoulder pain lasting more than a month. They are unable to exert pressure or lie on the affected shoulder. Clinical examination reveals diminished mobility in at least three planes for the affected shoulder [12]. A greater degree of limitation has been observed for external rotation and abduction of the shoulder [13]. An affliction of both shoulders has been observed in 10–30% of individuals with adhesive capsulitis and diabetes mellitus. Such individuals also develop adhesive capsulitis at a younger age. Once established, adhesive capsulitis in diabetic individuals lasts longer than in those without diabetes [14]. While older age and a longer duration of diabetes mellitus are associated with a greater risk of adhesive capsulitis, an association has not been observed with diabetes control reflected by HbA1c (even though studies have shown that intensive insulin therapy leads to an improvement in musculoskeletal manifestations of diabetes). A cohort of more than 400 patients with diabetes mellitus reported a greater prevalence of adhesive capsulitis in type 2 diabetes (22%) as opposed to type I diabetes (10%) [4].

Classically, three phases of adhesive capsulitis have been described in the literature. Initial symptoms of shoulder pain and stiffness (the so-called *freezing* phase) are followed by predominant restriction of shoulder joint mobility (the so-called *frozen* phase) and a gradual improvement in mobility and pain over the longer term (the so-called *thawing* phase) [13]. While adhesive capsulitis has been traditionally considered to be self-limiting, less than one-half of patients recover normal shoulder joint function when followed up over 4 years [15].

8.4 Dupuytren's Contracture

Dupuytren's contracture classically presents with limited hand mobility resulting from thickening and tethering of the affected palmar fascia, more often involving the ulnar (medial) two fingers. The prevalence of Dupuytren's contracture in those with diabetes ranges from 20 to 63%. Conversely, 13–39% of individuals with Dupuytren's contracture have concomitant diabetes mellitus. Clinical examination reveals palpable nodules on the palmar surface which later coalesce to form thickened cord-like fascia. Contracture results in flexion at predominantly the metacarpophalangeal joint but also the proximal interphalangeal joint. Dupuytren's contracture can coexist with diabetic cheiroarthropathy. For reasons that are not yet clear, Dupuytren's contracture associated with diabetes mellitus is less severe than in those without diabetes (such as that associated with smoking, alcohol abuse, chronic intake of antiepileptic drugs, or human immunodeficiency virus infection) [16].

8.5 Flexor Tenosynovitis

Patients with diabetes mellitus have a greater prevalence of flexor tenosynovitis (5–20%) than those without (1–2%). A proliferation of fibrous tissue in tendon sheaths of individuals with diabetes mellitus results in decreased space for the movement of the tendon within these sheaths [16]. This results in a stenosing tenosynovitis which clinically manifests as *trigger finger*, i.e., locking of the finger in a flexed position due to the limited space for movement of the tendon within the tendon sheath [16]. The pathology involves degeneration and disorganization of collagen fibers in the flexor tendon sheath. This tendinopathy in diabetes is thought to be related to decreased new vessel formation partly contributed by a reduction in the expression of vascular endothelial growth factor [17]. Females have a greater risk of developing this complication. There is a greater propensity to involve multiple fingers and affect both hands. Flexor tenosynovitis is often coexistent with diabetic cheiroarthropathy or carpal tunnel syndrome [16]. A recent systematic review reported increased odds of associated tendinopathy in those with diabetes mellitus (odds ratio 3.67, 95% confidence interval 2.71–4.97) as well as greater odds of diabetes mellitus in those with tendinopathy (odds ratio 1.28, 95% confidence interval 1.10–1.49) [18].

8.6   Carpel Tunnel Syndrome

Compressive or entrapment neuropathy of the median nerve in the carpal tunnel in patients with diabetes can result from a proliferation of the tendon sheath or the flexor retinaculum. While 11–16% of patients with diabetes mellitus have carpal tunnel syndrome, 5–8% of those with carpal tunnel syndrome have associated diabetes mellitus. In such patients, a differential diagnosis for carpal tunnel syndrome is primary axonal neuropathy of the median nerve as a sequela of diabetes. Patients with carpal tunnel syndrome present with nocturnal pain and paraesthesias in the median nerve distribution. Over time, thenar muscle atrophy and weakness of hand-grip might ensue. Clinical signs suggestive of carpal tunnel syndrome include the Tinel's sign (Fig. 8.2) and Phalen's sign (Fig. 8.3). Demonstration of axonopathy of the median nerve on a nerve conduction study as well as an anatomical depiction of

Fig. 8.2 Tinel's sign: paraesthesias develop in the median nerve distribution of the hand on tapping the flexor aspect of the wrist

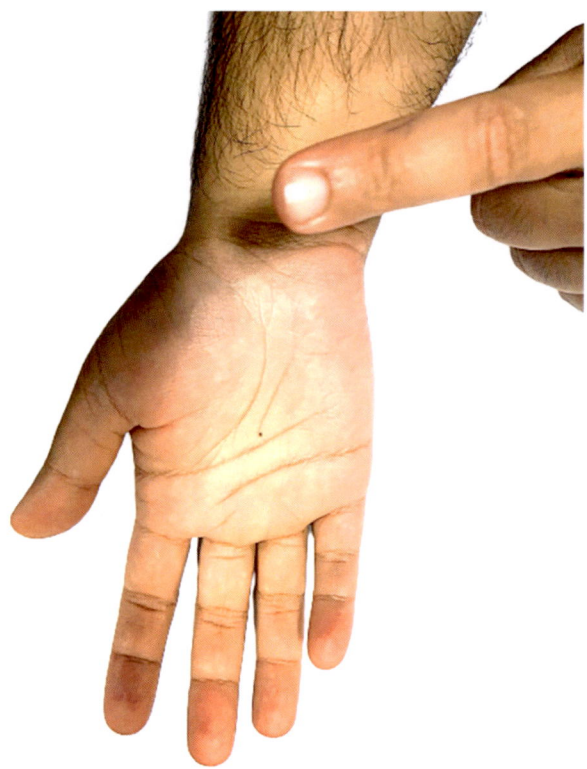

Fig. 8.3 Phalen's sign: occurrence of paraesthesias in the median nerve distribution of the hand following hyperflexion of the wrist for a minute

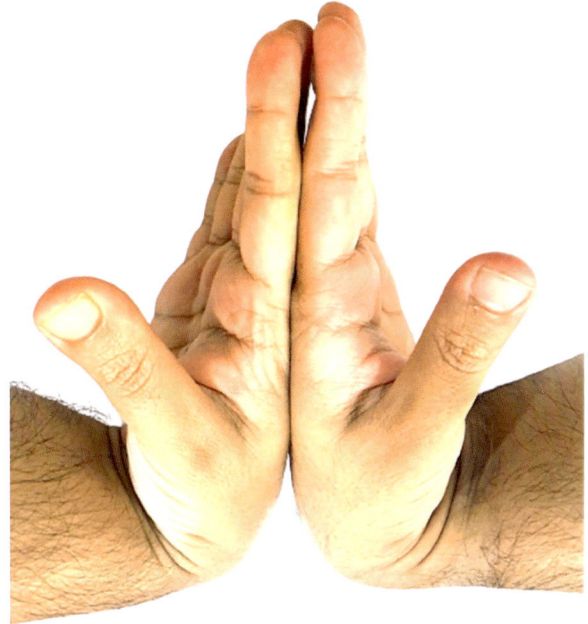

median nerve compression in the carpal tunnel using ultrasound or less commonly magnetic resonance imaging enables the diagnosis of this condition. Such imaging modalities have a sensitivity ranging from 64 to 96% for the diagnosis of carpal tunnel syndrome [14].

8.7   Reflex Sympathetic Dystrophy

Reflex sympathetic dystrophy or complex regional pain syndrome refers to paraesthesias, hyperalgesia, swelling, subcutaneous edema, and atrophy in long-standing cases limited to the upper or lower limb. Diabetes mellitus is a commonly associated etiology, although trauma to the site where reflex sympathetic dystrophy occurs is another important etiology [19].

8.8   Hand Osteoarthritis

A cross-sectional epidemiological study from the Netherlands evaluated 3585 individuals aged at least 55 years for the relationship between body weight, diabetes mellitus, and hypertension with osteoarthritis of the hand. This study reported a greater odds of hand osteoarthritis in patients with diabetes aged between 55 and 62 years (odds ratio 1.9, 95% confidence interval 1.0–3.8), but not in other age groups. The concomitant presence of diabetes, hypertension, and overweight status was associated with greater odds of hand osteoarthritis when compared with those without this combination of disease phenotypes (odds ratio 2.3, 95% confidence interval 1.3–3.9). Body mass index is associated with a greater risk of hand osteoarthritis involving the proximal interphalangeal joint, metacarpophalangeal joint, and distal interphalangeal joint but not for the thumb base [20].

8.9   Diffuse Idiopathic Skeletal Hyperostosis

Abnormal calcification of the interspinous ligaments (Fig. 8.4) often associated with overgrowth of bones at the edges of joints without an underlying disorder of bone mineralization results in a phenotype of diffuse idiopathic skeletal

Fig. 8.4 Flowing syndesmophytes in the dorsolumbar spine in an individual with diffuse idiopathic skeletal hyperostosis associated with diabetes mellitus

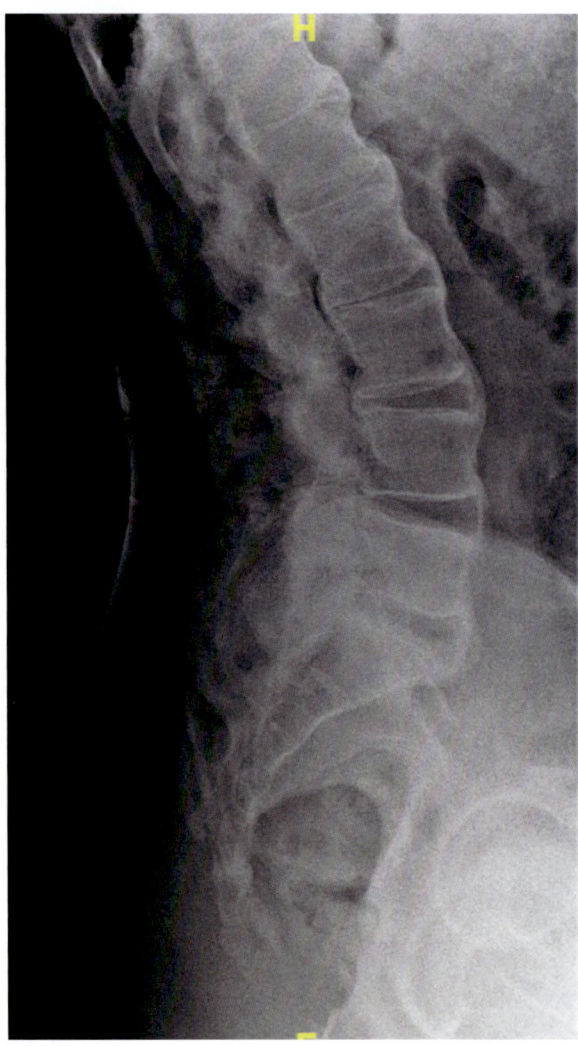

hyperostosis. This results in restricted spinal mobility without painful spinal movements per se, which is an important clue to differentiate this entity from spondyloarthropathy. This syndrome is more common in individuals with type 2 diabetes mellitus (13–40%) when compared to the general population (2.2–3.5%) [14, 21].

8.10 Diabetic Myonecrosis

Localized muscle infarction consequent to microvascular disease in a long-standing poorly controlled diabetes mellitus is termed diabetic myonecrosis. It can present with severe, usually localized, muscular pain. Common sites afflicted are the quadriceps muscle and calf muscles. A differential diagnosis of pyomyositis should be excluded (pyomyositis would have a collection of pus in the muscle which is demonstrable on imaging and grows microorganisms on cultures). Clinicians should be aware that idiopathic inflammatory myopathy involves proximal muscles and is usually not painful. Painful femoral neuropathy due to diabetes (diabetic amyotrophy) should be excluded; this condition can be associated with Charcot's arthropathy in the lower limb joints. Magnetic resonance imaging demonstrates iso or hypointensity on T1 weighted images along with hyperintensity on T2 weighted short tau inversion recovery images, without a demonstrable pus collection in the muscle [22].

8.11 Neuropathic Arthropathy

Neuropathy is a common accompaniment of long-term diabetes mellitus. Neuropathic arthropathy or Charcot's arthropathy results from a loss of proprioception resulting in joint damage due to excessive loading of the joint. Neuropathic arthropathy in the context of diabetes often affects the ankle and foot. It can present with destructive painless arthropathy [14].

8.12 Treatment

Since musculoskeletal pathologies associated with diabetes mellitus are mostly a consequence of the deposition of advanced glycation end products in soft tissue, control of hyperglycemia remains crucial to treat as well as prevent these complications. This principle is epitomized by a case series in the 1980s of four patients with type 1 diabetes mellitus, which reported improvement in skin thickness following the use of an insulin pump to enhance glycemic control [24]. Beyond this, there exist few specific treatments. Management of these conditions relies on a multidisciplinary approach including physical therapies, intralesional injections of corticosteroids, and surgical release in extreme situations.

8.12.1 Diabetic Cheiroarthropathy

Physical therapies to actively and passively stretch involved hands, coupled with the use of orthotic devices to improve or preserve hand function remain the mainstay of the treatment of diabetic cheiroarthropathy. Symptomatic analgesia using non-steroidal anti-inflammatory drugs where the pain is a predominant complaint, for a short duration keeping in mind the absence of any concomitant renal failure before using such medications, remains the predominant form of pharmacotherapy for this situation [14]. Specific therapies for diabetic cheiroarthropathy are lacking [14].

8.12.2 Adhesive Capsulitis

Non-steroidal anti-inflammatory drugs provide short-term analgesia, although their use is not backed by randomized controlled trials [15, 25].

A systematic review of 18 randomized clinical trials evaluated the evidence base for the use of various therapies in adhesive capsulitis. Intra-articular glucocorticoid injections in the standard doses had strong evidence for their effectiveness in the short-term (up to 3 months) and moderate evidence for their intermediate-term effectiveness (4–6 months). Laser therapy was also an effective short-term treatment. Gradual shoulder joint mobilization was effective both in the short and long term, with or without concomitant physical therapy. Suprascapular nerve block was associated with potential benefits when compared to no therapy, glucocorticoid injections, or acupuncture. Oral glucocorticoids used in varying doses from 10 to 40 mg daily prednisolone equivalent doses for 3–4 weeks had a short-term benefit when compared to no treatment [25]. Another recent systematic review reported short-term (but not long-term) pain relief with intra-articular glucocorticoids. However, this therapy effectively improved the passive range of shoulder movements in both the short as well as long-term (up to 24 weeks) [15].

8.12.3 Trigger Finger

General measures include hand mobilization exercises and physiotherapy [14].

Intralesional glucocorticoid therapy (in the standard doses for hand joint injections) is commonly used however has limited success rates in individuals with diabetes mellitus when compared with those without diabetes (49% and 76%, respectively) [26]. Another concern with intralesional glucocorticoids for trigger fingers is the high recurrence rate (48–78%). Furthermore, a randomized controlled trial failed to provide evidence for the amelioration of the requirement for surgical release with glucocorticoid injection [27]. Limited literature suggests that up-front surgical release might be more cost-effective than intralesional glucocorticoids preceding such surgical release for trigger fingers [28].

8.12.4 Dupuytren's Contracture

Physical therapies including hand exercises have limited benefits for this condition [14].

Surgical release remains the treatment of choice, more so when associated with flexion of more than 30° at the metacarpophalangeal joint. Fasciotomies (via needle, percutaneous, or open route) or open fasciectomy are the various options. However, these procedures are prone to recurrence and there remain chances of injury to tendons or accompanying nerves or blood vessels in a large proportion of cases [29]. Emerging therapeutic options include the intralesional injection of collagenase clostridium histolyticum. In a recent randomized controlled trial, this treatment with three injections administered monthly was associated with improvement in 64% vs 6.8% in those receiving placebo [30].

8.12.5 Carpal Tunnel Syndrome

General measures include analgesia with short courses of non-steroidal anti-inflammatory drugs or pregabalin/gabapentin [14].

Injections of glucocorticoid around the compressed median nerve (in the standard doses for wrist joint injections), now enhanced by ultrasonographic guidance, provide short-term relief in a majority of individuals. The use of a wrist splint during times of acute worsening is useful. In refractory cases, surgical release of the entrapped median nerve is helpful [14].

8.12.6 Other Conditions

Diabetic myonecrosis generally improves with rest and anti-inflammatory agents. Reflex sympathetic dystrophy is managed with analgesics along with pregabalin, short courses (up to 4 weeks) of oral corticosteroids or intravenous bisphosphonate injections for 3–6 months. Hand osteoarthritis is managed with exercises and rehabilitation to retain hand function for daily activities. DISH requires spinal extension exercises to maintain spinal mobility Management of the neuropathic joint is difficult and includes off-loading of the joint, symptomatic analgesia, and bisphosphonates. Surgical intervention to fuse the affected joint might be required, although results are not always encouraging when the neuropathy is advanced [14, 22].

8.13   Conclusion

Musculoskeletal syndromes associated with diabetes mellitus result in considerable disability. Most of these conditions have no definitive therapy. Attaining optimal glycemic control is imperative to prevent as well as treat any established musculoskeletal features of diabetes mellitus. Judicious use of physical therapies and intralesional corticosteroid administration are important therapeutic adjuncts.

References

1. Lundbaek K. Stiff hands in long-term diabetes. Acta Med Scand. 1957;158(6):447–51. https://doi.org/10.1111/j.0954-6820.1957.tb15511.x.
2. Jung Y, Hohmann TC, Gerneth JA, Novak J, Wasserman RC, D'Andrea BJ, et al. Diabetic hand syndrome. Metabolism. 1971;20(11):1008–15.
3. Kapoor A, Sibbitt WL. Contractures in diabetes mellitus: the syndrome of limited joint mobility. Semin Arthritis Rheum. 1989;18(3):168–80.
4. Rosenbloom AL, Silverstein JH, Lezotte DC, Richardson K, McCallum M. Limited joint mobility in childhood diabetes mellitus indicates increased risk for microvascular disease. N Engl J Med. 1981;305(4):191–4.
5. Larkin ME, Barnie A, Braffett BH, Cleary PA, Diminick L, Harth J, et al. Musculoskeletal complications in type 1 diabetes. Diabetes Care. 2014;37(7):1863–9.
6. Kischer CW, Speer DP. Microvascular changes in Dupuytren's contracture. J Hand Surg. 1984;9(1):58–62.
7. Starkman HS, Gleason RE, Rand LI, Miller DE, Soeldner JS. Limited joint mobility (LJM) of the hand in patients with diabetes mellitus: relation to chronic complications. Ann Rheum Dis. 1986;45(2):130–5.
8. Gokcen N, Cetinkaya Altuntas S, Coskun Benlidayi I, Sert M, Nazlican E, Sarpel T. An overlooked rheumatologic manifestation of diabetes: diabetic cheiroarthropathy. Clin Rheumatol. 2019;38(3):927–32.
9. Jiménez IU, Díaz-Díaz E, Castro JS, Ramos JP, León MC, Alvarado Ríos JA, et al. Circulating concentrations of advanced glycation end products, its association with the development of diabetes mellitus. Arch Med Res. 2017;48(4):360–9.
10. Thrailkill KM, Bunn RC, Moreau CS, Cockrell GE, Simpson PM, Coleman HN, et al. Matrix metalloproteinase-2 dysregulation in type 1 diabetes. Diabetes Care. 2007;30(9):2321–6.
11. Arkkila PE, Kantola IM, Viikari JS, Ronnemaa T. Shoulder capsulitis in type I and II diabetic patients: association with diabetic complications and related diseases. Ann Rheum Dis. 1996;55(12):907–14.
12. Pal B, Anderson J, Dick WC, Griffiths ID. Limitation of joint mobility and shoulder capsulitis in insulin- and non-insulin-dependent diabetes mellitus. Rheumatology. 1986;25(2):147–51.
13. Reeves B. The natural history of the frozen shoulder syndrome. Scand J Rheumatol. 1975;4(4):193–6.
14. Al-Homood IA. Rheumatic conditions in patients with diabetes mellitus. Clin Rheumatol. 2013;32(5):527–33.
15. Wang W, Shi M, Zhou C, Shi Z, Cai X, Lin T, et al. Effectiveness of corticosteroid injections in adhesive capsulitis of shoulder: a meta-analysis. Medicine (Baltimore). 2017;96(28):e7529.
16. Smith LL, Burnet SP, McNeil JD. Musculoskeletal manifestations of diabetes mellitus. Br J Sports Med. 2003;37(1):30–5. https://doi.org/10.1136/bjsm.37.1.30.
17. Abate M, Schiavone C, Salini S. Neoangiogenesis is reduced in chronic tendinopathies of type 2 diabetic patients. Int J Immunopathol Pharmacol. 2012;25(3):757–61. https://doi.org/10.1177/039463201202500322.
18. Ranger TA, Wong AMY, Cook JL, Gaida JE. Is there an association between tendinopathy and diabetes mellitus? A systematic review with meta-analysis. Br J Sports Med. 2016;50(16):982–9.
19. Marshall AT. Reflex sympathetic dystrophy. Rheumatology. 2000;39(7):692–5.

20. Dahaghin S, Bierma-Zeinstra SMA, Koes BW, Hazes JMW, Pols HAP. Do metabolic factors add to the effect of overweight on hand osteoarthritis? The Rotterdam Study. Ann Rheum Dis. 2007;66(7):916–20.
21. Misra DP, Chengappa KG, Jain VK, Negi VS. Talonavicular and Naviculocuneiform joint involvement in diffuse idiopathic skeletal hyperostosis. J Clin Rheumatol. 2017;23(2):119. https://doi.org/10.1097/RHU.0000000000000507.
22. Gupta R, Mohindra N, Agarwal V. A rare cause of focal myopathy in diabetes. Indian J Rheumatol. 2013;8:190–1.
23. Agrawal RP, Gothwal S, Tantia P, Agrawal R, Rijhwani P, Sirohi P, et al. Prevalence of rheumatological manifestations in diabetic population from North-West India. J Assoc Physicians India. 2014;62(9):788–92.
24. Lieberman LS, Rosenbloom AL, Riley WJ, Silverstein JH. Reduced skin thickness with pump administration of insulin. N Engl J Med. 1980;303(16):940–1.
25. Favejee MM, Huisstede BMA, Koes BW. Frozen shoulder: the effectiveness of conservative and surgical interventions—systematic review. Br J Sports Med. 2011;45(1):49–56.
26. Stahl S, Kanter Y, Karnielli E. Outcome of trigger finger treatment in diabetes. J Diabetes Complicat. 1997;11(5):287–90.
27. Baumgarten KM, Gerlach D, Boyer MI. Corticosteroid injection in diabetic patients with trigger finger: a prospective, randomized, controlled double-blinded study. J Bone Joint Surg Am. 2007;89(12):2604–11.
28. Luther GA, Murthy P, Blazar PE. Cost of immediate surgery versus non-operative treatment for trigger finger in diabetic patients. J Hand Surg. 2016;41(11):1056–63.
29. Abate M, Schiavone C, Salini V, Andia I. Management of limited joint mobility in diabetic patients. Diabetes Metab Syndr Obes. 2013;6:197–207. https://doi.org/10.2147/DMSO.S33943.
30. Hurst LC, Hotchkiss RN, Smith TM. Injectable collagenase Clostridium histolyticum for Dupuytren's contracture. N Engl J Med. 2009;361(10):968–79.

Hemochromatosis Arthropathy

Patrick D. W. Kiely

9.1 Introduction

Genetic hemochromatosis (GH) is an autosomal recessive disorder in which dysfunctional iron homeostasis leads to excess tissue iron deposition and organ dysfunction [1, 2]. In Northern European populations mutations of the *HFE* gene on chromosome 6 are responsible for the majority of cases of GH, with substitution of tyrosine (Y) for cysteine (C) at position 282 (C282Y) or aspartic acid (D) for histidine (H) at position 63 (H63D) of the HFE protein being the most frequent abnormalities. The gene frequencies are common, with approximately 10% of the UK population of northern European ancestry carrying one mutation of the *HFE* gene, and 0.5% carrying two mutations. Collectively, mutations of the *HFE* gene are classified as causing Type 1 Hemochromatosis (Table 9.1). Penetrance to the clinical phenotype of iron overload is low, almost exclusively restricted to the C282Y homozygous mutation, and only occurring in approximately 10–30% with this genotype. Iron loading is more common in men, for example, reported in 28.4% of men compared to 1.2% of women over the age of 40 years [4], and in 11% of postmenopausal women [5]. A recent analysis of morbidity in 2890 people of European descent aged 40–70 years with the C282Y homozygous genotype, from the UK Biobank cohort, found GH to be diagnosed in 21.7% of men and 9.8% of women [6].

P. D. W. Kiely (✉)
Department of Rheumatology, St. George's University Hospitals NHS Foundation Trust, London, UK

Institute of Medical and Biomedical Education, St. George's University of London, London, UK
e-mail: patrick.kiely@nhs.net

Table 9.1 Type 1 Hemochromatosis *HFE* gene mutations and prevalence in people of North European ancestry. (Reprinted with permission from [3])

Genotype	Prevalence
H63D/WT	1 in 8
C282Y/WT	1 in 12–15
C282Y/H63D	1 in 40
H63D/H63D	1 in 42
C282Y/C282Y	1 in 250–300

WT wild type

9.2 Pathophysiology

The mechanism of iron loading is a consequence of a reduction in the hormone hepcidin, which degrades ferroportin, and is the sole inhibitor of iron release from iron-exporting cells, such as the duodenal enterocyte, hepatocyte, and macrophage [2, 7, 8]. Hepcidin deficiency therefore leads to unchecked iron absorption from the gut and release from internal recycling. Hepcidin deficiency can also occur as a consequence of mutations in non-*HFE* genes such as hemojuvelin (*HJV*), hepcidin (*HAMP*), and transferrin receptor-2 (*TfR2*) genes. These are much rarer than the *HFE* mutations and are classified as Type 2A, 2B, and 3 Hemochromatosis, respectively [7, 8].

Plasma iron excess saturates transferrin, leading to the accumulation of non-transferrin bound iron (NTBI). This is taken up by parenchymal cells, especially the liver, heart, and pancreas. NTBI is toxic, through the generation of reactive oxygen species, causing organ dysfunction and damage [7, 8]. The triad of hepatic fibrosis, diabetes, and skin pigmentation leading to the term "bronze diabetes" has been well described in advanced cases. Other features include cardiomyopathy, hypopituitarism, hypogonadism, osteoporosis, and hepatocellular carcinoma, with dysfunction being a direct consequence of the amount of iron deposition [7]. Male participants with the C282Y homozygous genotype from the UK Biobank cohort were found to have a significantly higher odds ratio of liver disease (O.R. 4.3, 2.99–6.18), osteoporosis (O.R. 2.3, 1.49–3.57), rheumatoid arthritis (O.R. 2.23, 1.51–3.30), osteoarthritis (O.R. 2.01, 1.71–2.36), and diabetes (O.R. 1.52, 1.18–1.98) versus participants with no C282Y mutations [6]. Similarly in a large Swedish cohort the hazard ratio of any non-septic arthritis, including OA, was significantly raised amongst GH patients compared to matched population controls (H.R. 2.38, 2.14–2.64) and specifically for osteoarthritis (H.R. 2.43, 2.15–2.74), crystal arthritides (H.R. 3.08, 2.19–4.32), and rheumatoid arthritis (H.R. 1.58, 1.16–2.17) [9].

9.3 Diagnostic Delay in Genetic Hemochromatosis

Frustratingly for patients, there is often a long delay between onset of symptoms and diagnosis, leading to several years of unnecessary reversible features, and potentially irreversible consequences of sustained iron overload. Early recognition and diagnosis are therefore important, as a normal life expectancy is preserved if treatment is started before hepatic cirrhosis becomes established, ideally before ferritin rises to over 1000 µg/L [4, 8, 10]. The commonest symptoms reported at diagnosis are fatigue, and joint pain [10–13], often first occurring around the end of the fourth decade and widely reported from large surveys to predate the diagnosis of GH by many years. These symptoms are insufficiently characteristic to raise early suspicion, and hence a delay invariably occurs before the diagnosis is considered and investigations initiated. In an American postal questionnaire survey, with 2851 GH respondents, the mean age of symptom onset was 41 years, occurring for an average of 10 years before the diagnosis was made [13]. In a UK patient survey of 470 GH respondents, attributable symptoms were reported to have been present for a mean 8.1 years before diagnosis [10]. A study of 199 patients with GH and iron overload found joint pain in 53% at diagnosis, preceding the diagnosis by a mean 9.0 ± 10 years [14], and a separate cohort of 306 patients reported joint pain in 51.5% at diagnosis with a mean interval of 8.6 years between the onset of pain and diagnosis of GH [10].

Where there is a family history of the condition, detection of elevated transferrin saturation (>45%) and ferritin (>300 µg/L in men, >200 µg/L in pre-menopausal women) will reveal iron overload and lead to an early diagnosis. For other patients, detection of iron overload may be serendipitous, for example as a consequence of random testing or part of a non-specific well-person health screen. However, for over 50% of patients, recognition of symptoms and signs is required to initiate measurement of iron indices and then gene analysis [11, 12]. Without easily identifiable symptoms it is estimated that for every patient diagnosed with GH, there are 8–10 undiagnosed and unaware of their risk [12]. Although the frequencies of *HFE* gene mutations are relatively high in north European populations, especially Celtic, the low penetrance to iron overload means that widespread population screening is not undertaken, although this stance is contested [6].

9.4   Clinical Features of Hemochromatosis Arthropathy

From an early stage, the majority of GH patients report joint symptoms [2, 10, 11, 14–16], ranging from 51.5 to 77% of patients at diagnosis in 5 EU cohorts totaling 1247 patients, for example in 77% of a group of 62 GH patients attending a specialist hemochromatosis arthropathy clinic, in 76% of 470 GH respondents to a questionnaire [11], and 53% of 199 patients assessed in 7 EU centers [14]. In a large UK survey, 87% of 1998 respondents said they had ever experienced arthritis or joint pain [12].

Richette compared symptoms in GH patients to controls and found significantly increased frequency of pain in multiple joints including hand (O.R. 17.2, 10.3–28.9), wrist (O.R. 12.2, 6.4–22.4), ankle (O.R. 11.3, 6.3–20.0), hip (O.R. 9.3, 5.3–16.2) and knee (O.R. 6.3, 4.3–9.2) [10]. Arthropathy has been reported to be significantly associated with high ferritin at presentation with a threshold of peak ferritin >1000 µg/L conferring increased risk [4, 10, 15, 17, 18]. The prevalence of joint pain rises after diagnosis, irrespective of de-ironing treatment, for example from 53 to 72% of a cohort of 199 northern European patients within 10 years of diagnosis [14], and from 51.5 to 86.9% of a cohort of 306 French patients [10].

Whilst there are no classification criteria for the arthropathy of hemochromatosis, the features are well described. Superficially patients have the clinical characteristics of osteoarthritis (OA) [11, 14, 15, 19, 20], with bony swelling, tenderness and painful loss of range of movement of affected joints, whereas synovial swelling is less frequently seen [14, 21]. The characteristics that distinguish hemochromatosis arthropathy (HA) from primary generalized OA are summarized in Table 9.2. GH patients have a phenotype of "accelerated OA" with onset at a younger than expected age in the absence of trauma or biomechanical deformity and a high rate of joint replacement surgery [9, 21]. The characteristic age of onset of joint symptoms is in the fourth and fifth decades, and it is not uncommon for a patient to be diagnosed with GH after arthroplasty for rapidly progressive arthropathy, especially of the hip.

Affected joints include those typically affected by OA, such as hip, knee, proximal and distal interphalangeal, and first carpometacarpal. Characteristically, two joint regions not usually involved in OA are over-represented in HA, providing important phenotypic features from a diagnostic perspective, these being the second and third metacarpophalangeal (MCP) and ankle joints [11, 14, 21–26]. In one series the first joints reported to be affected were the MCP and the ankles followed by the knee and hip [11]. The distribution of affected joints in established HA in four series is shown in Table 9.3, with the MCP, PIP, DIP, wrist, hip, knee, and ankle joints all frequently affected. Of note, although second and third MCP disease is characteristically reported, the arthropathy of hemochromatosis can affect all MCP joints and all other joint regions within the hand [11].

The term "iron fist" has been coined to describe the appearance of the clenched fingers in patients with second and third MCP joint involvement. The inability to fully flex the second and third MCP joints result in the flexed proximal interphalangeal (PIP) joints of the same fingers being raised above the level of the PIP joints of

Table 9.2 Characteristics that distinguish hemochromatosis arthropathy from primary generalized osteoarthritis. (Reprinted with permission from [3])

Disease characteristics	Hemochromatosis arthropathy	Primary generalized osteoarthritis
Gender prevalence	Male > Female	Female > Male (knee, hand)
Age of onset	Fourth and fifth decades	Sixth decade and older
Trauma, biomechanical deformity	Unusual	Common (hip, knee, ankle)
Frequently affected joints	MCP, PIP, hip, knee, ankle	Hip, knee, first CMC, PIP, DIP
Osteophytes	Exuberant	Present
Subchondral cysts	Large and numerous	Present
Progression to arthroplasty	Higher likelihood can be rapid	Usually slow

MCP metacarpophalangeal, *PIP* proximal interphalangeal, *DIP* distal interphalangeal, *CMC* carpometacarpal

Table 9.3 Distribution of affected joints in Hemochromatosis arthropathy, % of affected patients

Joint region	Richardson et al- 1 ($n = 62$)	Richardson et al- 2 ($n = 470$)	Sahinbegovic et al. ($n = 199$)	Hemochromatosis UK ($n = 1481$)
PIP	64.5	47	51.7[a]	69.3[b]
Knee	64	42	59.4	32.6
Ankle	61	35	32.9	28.6
MCP	60	46	51.7[a]	69.3[b]
Hip	48	26	26.6	56.8
DIP	43.5	42		
Wrist	34	52	11.9	46.9[c]
MTP	30.5	25		43.7[d]
Shoulder	27.5	20	14.7	
1st CMC	22.5	59		
Elbow	19	11		
Midfoot	10	13		

Richardson et al-1, $n = 62$, Haemochromatosis arthropathy cases, symptoms or signs, physician observed [11]

Richardson et al-2, $n = 470$, Genetic haemochromatosis, UK national patient survey, self-reported joint involvement [11]

Sahinbegovic et al., $n = 199$, Genetic haemochromatosis cases, symptoms or signs, physician observed [14]

Haemochromatosis UK, $n = 1481$, Genetic haemochromatosis UK national patient survey, self-reported joint involvement [12]

[a] Recorded as "fingers"

[b] Recorded as knuckles

[c] Recorded as hand or wrist

[d] Recorded as feet

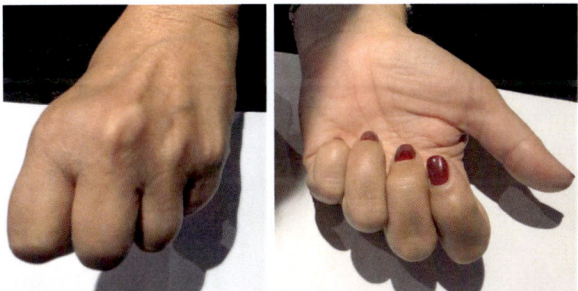

Fig. 9.1 Photograph of a patient with C282Y homozygous hemochromatosis arthropathy involving the second and third MCP joints. This demonstrates the "iron fist" sign, in which the inability to fully flex the second and third MCP joints results in the flexed proximal interphalangeal (PIP) joints of the same fingers to be raised above the level of the PIP joints of the fourth and fifth fingers, and the fingertips are not able to touch the palm

the fourth and fifth fingers, and the fingertips may not touch the palm (Fig. 9.1). Focussing on the ankle, recognition of OA is important, as this entity is rare in the absence of trauma [27, 28], and when encountered should raise the suspicion of GH [11].

Whilst most cases of HA are described in patients with iron overload and the C282Y homozygous *HFE* mutation, arthropathy is also described in patients with the lesser *HFE* mutations and not necessarily in patients with significant or any iron overload [29]. A report from the Melbourne Collaborative Cohort of persons of north European descent aged 40–69 found MCP arthropathy in 20% of 144 patients with the compound heterozygous *HFE* mutation (C282Y/H63D) and 15.7% of 108 people with the H63D homozygous or heterozygous *HFE* mutations [4].

Histological studies of hemochromatotic joints are restricted to small series or isolated cases [30, 31]. In 15 patients with GH, synovial histological features from knee, hip, ankle, wrist, and phalangeal samples were very similar to a control group with OA, except for more synovial hemosiderin deposition associated with infiltrating neutrophils and increased sublining layer CD68-positive macrophages [32].

9.5   Imaging Features of Hemochromatosis Arthropathy

Plain radiographs show features of OA, with subcortical cysts, joint space narrowing, and osteophytes [21]. Chondrocalcinosis is reported in up to 50% of cases [15], most frequently seen in the wrist and knee [10, 21]. Calcification can be seen in both hyaline and fibrocartilage and can be widespread, including the acetabular labrum, symphysis pubis and intervertebral discs [21]. The concept of accelerated OA is supported by characteristic exuberant osteophytes giving the term "hooks" in association with the MCP joints and elsewhere. A comparison with hand OA has shown more severe radiographic changes in GH patients at the MCP and wrist joints but less so in first carpometacarpal, PIP, and DIP joints [33]. The combination of prominent subcortical cysts and large osteophytes should raise suspicion of GH, especially at the second and third MCP joints and ankles.

Ultrasound of the MCP joints in two patients with early and late GH has been reported to show a grade 2 power Doppler signal in the synovium, consistent with synovial inflammation [34, 35]. A comparison of US features between HA and OA patients found similar greyscale and power Doppler signal scores on an overall assessment of multiple joints, and significantly more prevalent cartilage abnormalities and calcium pyrophosphate dehydrate deposition in the HA patients [26].

MRI features of the ankle in GH patients confirm the concept of accelerated OA with significantly larger and more extensive cysts/bone marrow lesions, osteophytes, and full-thickness cartilage loss compared to primary OA controls [36].

Illustrative examples of plain radiographic, CT, and MRI appearances of these features, and a 3D-reconstructed CT of the hand of a patient with the C282Y homozygous genotype are shown in Figs. 9.2, 9.3, 9.4, 9.5, 9.6, and 9.7.

Fig. 9.2 X-ray of the hands and wrists of a patient with C282Y hemochromatosis arthropathy demonstrating the involvement of the first carpometacarpal, metacarpophalangeal and proximal interphalangeal joints, with multiple subchondral cysts, joint space narrowing and hook osteophytes at the third metacarpophalangeal joints

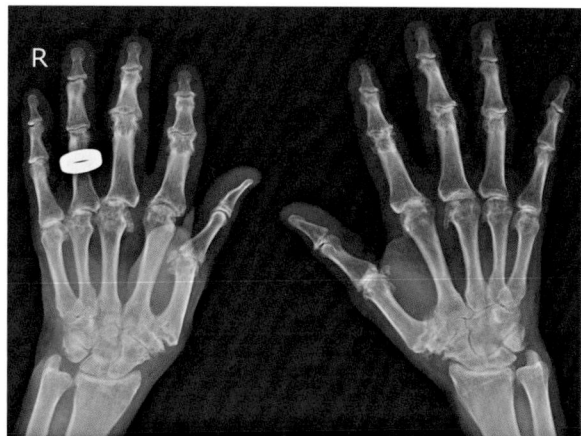

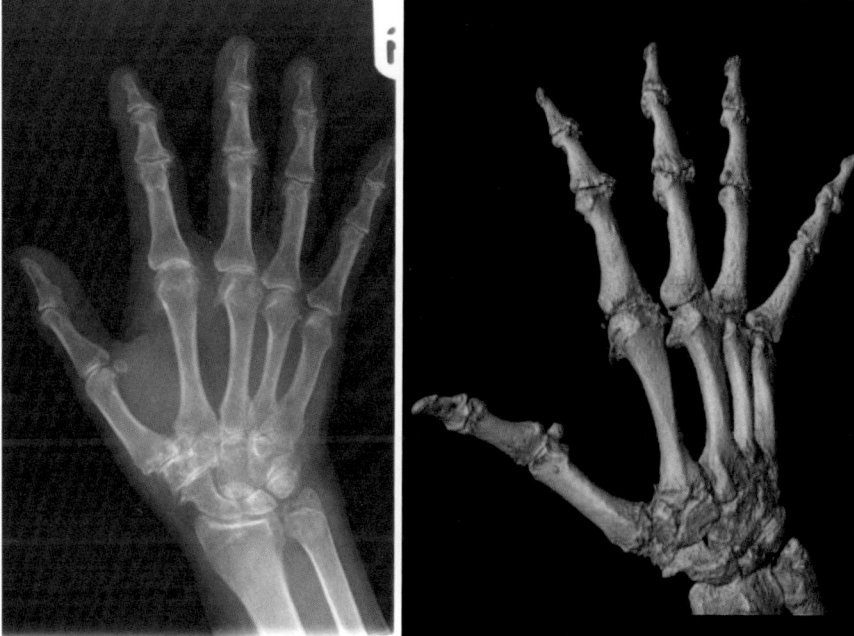

Fig. 9.3 X-ray and 3D-reconstructed CT scan of the right hand of a patient with C282Y homozygous hemochromatosis arthropathy, showing widespread features including hook osteophytes at the second and third metacarpophalangeal joints, and also joint space narrowing, subchondral cysts and osteophytes at the scapho-trapezium, first carpometacarpal, proximal and distal interphalangeal joints. (Reprinted with permission from [3])

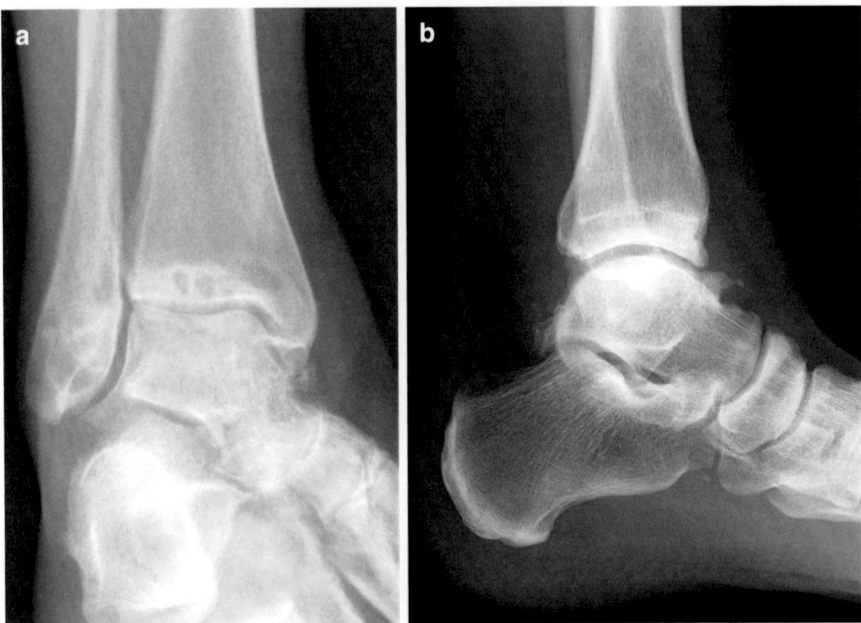

Fig. 9.4 X-rays of the ankle of two patients with C282Y homozygous hemochromatosis arthropathy showing (**a**) prominent large distal tibia subchondral cysts, and (**b**) large hook-like anterior and posterior talus osteophytes

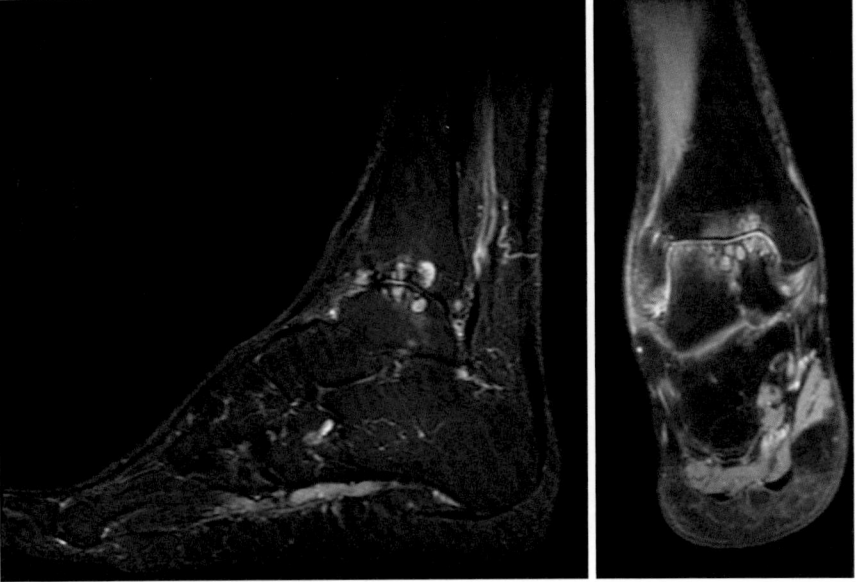

Fig. 9.5 Sagittal and coronal short-tau inversion recovery MR images showing tibial plafond and talar dome subchondral bone marrow lesions consisting mainly of cysts with surrounding ill-defined edema, in a patient with C282Y homozygous hemochromatosis arthropathy. (Reprinted with permission from [3])

Fig. 9.6 Sagittal CT scan showing talar dome subchondral cysts in a patient with C282Y heterozygous hemochromatosis arthropathy

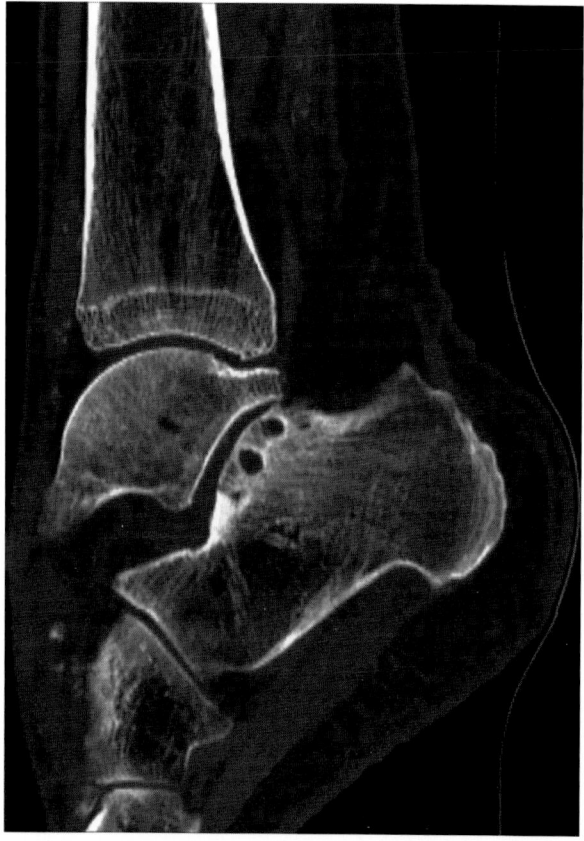

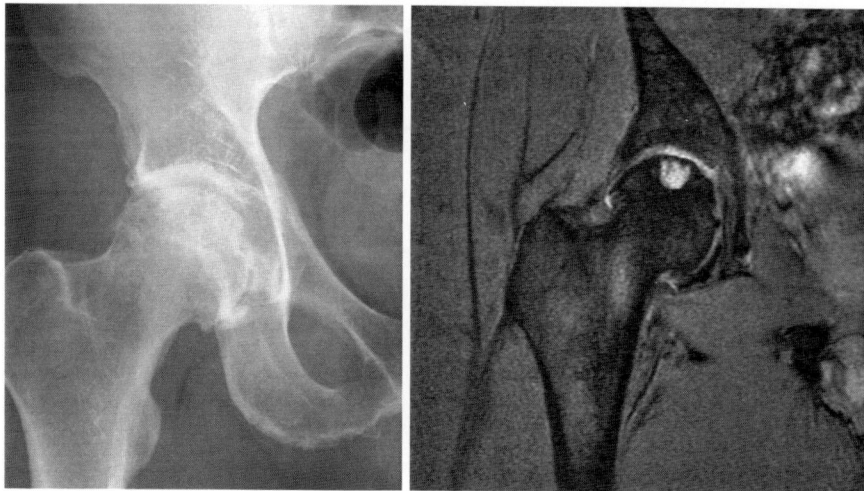

Fig. 9.7 X-ray and MR image showing a large femoral head subchondral cyst in a patient with C282Y homozygous hemochromatosis arthropathy

9.6   Management

Management of GH is centered on iron depletion by venesection, termed "de-ironing." If commenced early this is effective at avoiding or preventing the progression of many organ-based manifestations, such as hepatic and cardiac disease, and reversing others, such as hepatic fibrosis [7, 37, 38]. General health also improves, including fatigue for many patients [8]. Pre-venesection serum ferritin <1000 µg/L is taken to be a marker of good prognosis [4, 15], and ideally all cases should be detected and commenced on a venesection program before this threshold is exceeded.

In contrast, the response of joint symptoms to de-ironing is poor. In the UK Hemochromatosis survey of 1998 respondents with GH, 48.7% reported persistent pain following de-ironing. A beneficial effect on joint symptoms has been reported in a minority of cases, 12–20% in three series [10, 11, 14]. Furthermore, patients may develop joint symptoms in previously unaffected joints after entering maintenance therapy despite low total body iron levels [10, 11, 14, 21].

Management of arthropathy focuses on strategies to protect joints from biomechanical strain and physical damage, and symptom control. Attention to gait and the provision of neutralizing orthotics is particularly useful. Hindfoot pronation is very common and if uncorrected may lead to aggravated disease in the ankle and subtalar joints, and also abnormal load-bearing throughout the legs with back, hip, and knee pain as a consequence.

There are no randomized trials of pharmaceutical agents in HA, and so therapeutic decisions are pragmatic and based on approaches for osteoarthritis. Pain relief may be provided by simple opioid, non-steroidal anti-inflammatory, and neuropathic analgesics, individually or in combinations. Typically paracetamol or a codeine-based compound preparation may be started on an as-required basis escalating to regular use and stronger preparations such as transdermal buprenorphine if necessary. Cox-2 selective anti-inflammatory agents, such as etoricoxib, can be very effective, taken at night if there is predominant morning stiffness. As chronic pain often results in a state of pain sensitization, with reduced pain thresholds [39], neuropathic agents such as low dose pregabalin and amitriptyline can also be effective. Individual joint injections with corticosteroids are also very effective, repeated up to four times per year as necessary. Given the association with chondrocalcinosis, colchicine may be given for acute crystal flares and potentially for chronic pain [35], though as with all analgesics, this lacks evidence from formal trials.

Without disease-modifying therapies, inevitably "joint failure" from advanced cartilage loss, bone damage, and intractable pain occurs. This may be alleviated by surgical intervention, either joint fusion or arthroplasty. Richette reported an increased risk of arthroplasty of the knee (O.R. 5.3, 1.1–25.6) and hip (O.R. 5.2, 2.2–11.9) compared to matched controls [10], and similarly Elmberg reported increased hazard ratios of hip (2.88, 2.39–3.47), knee (2.14, 1.58–2.88) and ankle (10.54, 5.69–19.52) replacement amongst GH patients in a Swedish population survey [9]. Predictors of arthroplasty were found to be a higher radiographic score in 2nd/3rd MCP joints, female sex, and chondrocalcinosis [10]. No trials have compared surgical outcomes in GH patients with OA controls, but anecdotally outcomes are good.

9.7 Unmet Needs

Our understanding of HA is in its infancy compared to many other rheumatic diseases. The pathogenic processes that stem from *HFE* mutations to arthropathy are incompletely understood, and whilst excess iron is toxic to parenchymal tissues, whether it is this which leads to HA is in question [3, 29]. Uncertainty arises from the observation of the progression of arthropathy to new joints after de-ironing, and the finding of phenotypically classical HA in patients without a history of iron overload (or other manifestations of GH), in cases with the C282Y homozygous and lesser *HFE* mutations [23, 24, 29, 40]. Furthermore, the finding of an increased risk of rheumatoid arthritis, a completely unrelated arthropathy from a pathogenic perspective, in population studies with GH [9], the C282Y [6] or H63D [41] mutation is unexpected if an iron centric view of the effects of the *HFE* mutation on joints is taken. Instead, it adds to the circumstantial evidence that there may be a separate, iron-independent, influence of *HFE* mutations on cartilage or bone homeostasis.

Current management strategies are purely supportive, protecting joints and ameliorating symptoms. Given the inability of de-ironing to improve the symptoms or progression of HA in the majority of cases, there is a need for the development of disease-modifying therapies. This will require evidence of efficacy from clinical trials, which at present would be undermined by a lack of classification criteria for HA, to standardize enrolment.

9.8 Conclusion

In summary, HA is a very prevalent feature of GH, often predating diagnosis and progressing despite de-ironing therapy. It is recognizable as an OA-like phenotype, with accelerated features including early age of onset, rapidly progressive course, and florid OA features on X-ray and MRI, especially subcortical cysts and large osteophytes. Involvement of the second and third MCP and ankle joints is a distinctive feature and should prompt measurement of transferrin saturation and ferritin in undiagnosed cases, though phenotypic HA can occur without iron overload.

Acknowledgments Tables 9.1 and 9.2 and Figs. 9.3 and 9.5 were fully or partially published in Kiely PDW. Haemochromatosis arthropathy—a conundrum of the Celtic curse. J R Coll Physicians Edinb 2018; 48: 233-8.

References

1. Janssen MC, Swinkels DW. Hereditary haemochromatosis. Best Pract Res Clin Gastroenterol. 2009;23:171–88.
2. Pietrangelo A. Genetics, genetic testing, and management of haemochromatosis: 15 years since hepcidin. Gastroenterology. 2015;149:1240–51.
3. Kiely PDW. Haemochromatosis arthropathy—a conundrum of the celtic curse. J R Coll Physicians Edinb. 2018;48:233–8.

4. Allen KJA, Gurrin LC, Constantine CC, Osborne NJ, Delatycki MB, Nicoll AJ, et al. Iron-overload-related disease in HFE hereditary hemochromatosis. N Engl J Med. 2008;358:221–30.
5. Rossi E, Jeffrey GP. Clinical penetrance of C282Y homozygous HFE haemochromatosis. Clin Biochem Rev. 2004;3:183–90.
6. Pilling LC, Tamosauskaite J, Jones G, Wood AR, Jones L, Kuo C-L, et al. Common conditions associated with hereditary haemochromatosis genetic variants: cohort study in UK biobank. BMJ. 2019;364:k5222.
7. Brissot P, Pietrangelo A, Adams PC, de Graaff B, McLaren CE, Loreal O. Haemochromatosis. Nat Rev Dis Primers. 2018;4:18016.
8. Powell LW, Seckington RC, Deugnier Y. Haemochromatosis. Lancet. 2016;388:706–16.
9. Elmberg M, Hultcrantz R, Simard JF, Carlsson A, Askling J. Increased risk of arthropathies and joint replacement surgery in patients with genetic hemochromatosis: a study of 3,531 patients and their 11,794 first degree relatives. Arthritis Care Res. 2013;65:678–85.
10. Richette P, Ottaviani S, Vicaut E, Bardin T. Musculoskeletal complications of hereditary hemochromatosis: a case control study. J Rheumatol. 2010;37:2145–50.
11. Richardson A, Prideaux A, Kiely P. Haemochromatosis: unexplained metacarpophalangal or ankle arthropathy should prompt diagnostic tests: findings from two UK observational cohort studies. Scand J Rheumatol. 2016;46:69–74.
12. Living with the impact of iron overload. https://www.haemochromatosis.org.uk/Handlers/Download.ashx?IDMF=c519f05d-d656-4ec3-8edf-7cbf39bb57d4.
13. McDonnell SM, Preston BL, Jewell SA, Barton JC, Edwards CQ, Adams PC. A survey of 2851 patients with hemochromatosis. Symptoms and response to treatment. Am J Med. 1999;106:619–24.
14. Sahinbegovic E, Dallos T, Aigner E, Axmann R, Manger B, Englbrecht M, et al. Musculoskeletal disease burden of hereditary hemochromatosis. Arthritis Rheum. 2010;62:3792–8.
15. Carroll GJ, Breidahl WH, Bulsara MK, Olynyk JK. Hereditary haemochromatosis is characterised by a clinically definable arthropathy that correlates with iron load. Arthritis Rheum. 2011;63:286–94.
16. Brissot P, Ball S, Rofail D, Cannon H, Jin JW. Hereditary haemochromatosis: patient experiences of the disease and phlebotomy treatment. Transfusion. 2011;51:1331–8.
17. Valenti L, Fracanzani AL, Rossi V, et al. The hand arthropathy of hereditary haemochromatosis is strongly associated with iron overload. J Rheumatol. 2008;35:153–8.
18. Harty LC, Lai D, Connor S, et al. Prevalence and progress of joint symptoms in hereditary hemochromatosis and symptomatic response to venesection. J Clin Rheumatol. 2011;17:220–2.
19. Husar-Memmar E, Stadlmayr A, Datz C, Zwerina J. HFE-related haemochromatosis: an update for the rheumatologist. Curr Rheumatol Rep. 2014;16:393–9.
20. Guggenbuhl P, Brissot P, Loreal O. Haemochromatosis: the bone and the joint. Best Pract Res Clin Rheumatol. 2011;25:649–64.
21. Dymock IW, Hamilton EBD, Laws JW, Williams R. Arthropathy of haemochromatosis. Ann Rheum Dis. 1970;29:469–76.
22. Schmid H, Struppler C, Braun GS, et al. Ankle and hindfoot arthropathy in hereditary hemochromatosis. J Rheumatol. 2003;30:196–9.
23. Carroll GJ. Primary osteoarthritis in the ankle joint is associated with finger metacarpophalangeal osteoarthritis and the H63D mutation in the HFE gene: evidence for a haemochromatosis-like polyarticular osteoarthritis phenotype. J Clin Rheumatol. 2006;12:109–13.
24. Becerra-Fernandez E, Panopalis P, Menard HA. Idiopathic hindfoot problems as an early rheumatologic manifestation of hereditary haemochromatosis type I. Arthritis Rheum. 2011;63(Suppl):S762.
25. Davies MB, Saxby T. Ankle arthropathy of hemochromatosis: a case series and review of the literature. Foot Ankle Int. 2006;27:902–6.
26. Dejaco C, Stadlmayr A, Duftner C, Trimmel V, Husic R, Krones E, et al. Ultrasound verified inflammation and structural damage in patients with hereditary haemochromatosis-related arthropathy. Arthritis Res Ther. 2017;19:243–52.

27. Saltzman CL, Salamon ML, Blanchard GM, et al. Epidemiology of ankle arthritis. Report of a consecutive series of 639 patients from a tertiary orthopaedic center. Iowa Orthop J. 2005;25:44–6.

28. Valderrabano V, Horisberger M, Russell I, Dougall H, Hintermann B. Etiology of ankle osteo-arthritis. Clin Orthop Relat Res. 2009;467:1800–6.

29. Alizadeh BZ, Njajou OT, Hazes JMW, Hofman A, Slagboom PE, Pols HAP, et al. The H63D variant in the HFE gene predisposes to arthralgia, chondrocalcinosis and osteoarthritis. Ann Rheum Dis. 2007;66:1436–42.

30. Van Vulpen LFD, Roosendaal G, van Asbeck BS, et al. The detrimental effects of iron on the joint: a comparison between haemochromatosis and haemophilia. J Clin Pathol. 2015;68:592–600.

31. Papakonstantinou O, Mohana-Borges AVR, Campell L, et al. Hip arthropathy in a patient with primary hemochromatosis: MR imaging findings with pathologic correlation. Skeletal Radiol. 2005;34:180–4.

32. Heiland GR, Aigner E, Dallos T, et al. Synovial immunopathology in haemochromatosis arthropathy. Ann Rheum Dis. 2010;69:1214–9.

33. Dallos T, Sahinbegovic E, Stamm T, Aigner E, Axmann R, Stadlmayr A, et al. Idiopathic hand osteoarthritis vs. haemochromatosis arthropathy—a clinical, functional and radiographic study. Rheumatology. 2013;52:910–5.

34. Oke AR, Wong E, McCrae F, Young-Min S. Hereditary hemochromatosis arthropathy and Doppler ultrasound findings of synovitis. Rheumatology. 2017;56:1240–1.

35. Hum R, Ho P. Hereditary haemochromatosis presented as a case of rheumatoid arthritis. Rheumatology Advances in Practice. 2017; https://doi.org/10.1093/rap/rkx010.004.

36. Elstob A, Ejindu V, Heron C, et al. Haemochromatosis arthropathy: MRI hindfoot characteristics; a case-control study. Clin Radiol. 2018;73:323.e1–8.

37. Niederau C, Fischer R, Purschel A, et al. Long-term survival in patients with hereditary haemochromatosis. Gastroenterology. 1996;110:1107–19.

38. Falize L, Guillygomarc'h A, Perrin M, et al. Reversibility of hepatic fibrosis in treated genetic hemochromatosis: a study of 36 cases. Hepatology. 2006;44:472–7.

39. Sofat N, Ejindu V, Kiely PDW. What makes osteoarthritis painful? The evidence for local and pain processing. Rheumatology. 2011;50(12):2157–65. https://doi.org/10.1093/rheumatology/ker283.

40. Ross JM, Kowalchuk RM, Shaulinsky J, et al. Association of heterozygous hemochromatosis C2828Y gene mutation with hand osteoarthritis. J Rheumatol. 2003;30:121–5.

41. Li J, Zhu Y, Singal DP. HFE gene mutations in patients with rheumatoid arthritis. J Rheumatol. 2000;27:2074–7.

Skeletal Fluorosis

10

Subramanian Shankar and Vivek Vasdev

10.1 Introduction

The first documentation of the effect of fluoride on human health can be traced back to the late nineteenth century when it was detected in different concentrations in teeth, bones, and other tissues in humans [1]. Fluorine came to be regarded as an essential microelement when the presence of fluorides in teeth was found to be protective against microbial attack and decay, especially in childhood. However, excessive intake was seen to be associated with detrimental effects on skeletal tissue and other organ systems. Chronic endemic fluorosis is now recognized as a major health issue that is prevalent in India and 50 other Asian and African countries [2].

Skeletal fluorosis is a result of excess fluoride intake over a long period through consumption of drinking water, food products, and industrial pollutants. The clinical manifestations often mimic arthritis and skeletal fluorosis can easily be mistaken for rheumatoid arthritis, osteoarthritis, or seronegative spondyloarthropathy in the initial phases [3, 4].

The minimum requirement of fluoride in diet is not well established but at a daily intake in excess of 6 mg, adverse effects on the bones have been observed [5–7]. The absorption of fluoride from drinking water has been shown through many epidemiological studies as the major cause of fluorosis. According to the World Health Organization (WHO), a concentration above 1.5 mg/L in drinking water leads to adverse effects of fluoride (Fig. 10.1) [8]. In India alone, as many as 62 million people (including six million children) are estimated to have serious health issues due to consumption of water contaminated with fluoride [9].

S. Shankar (✉)
O/o DGAFMS, New Delhi, India

V. Vasdev
Armed Forces Medical College, Pune, India

© The Author(s), under exclusive license to Springer Nature
Switzerland AG 2022
V. Ravindran et al. (eds.), *Rarer Arthropathies*, Rare Diseases of the Immune
System, https://doi.org/10.1007/978-3-031-05002-2_10

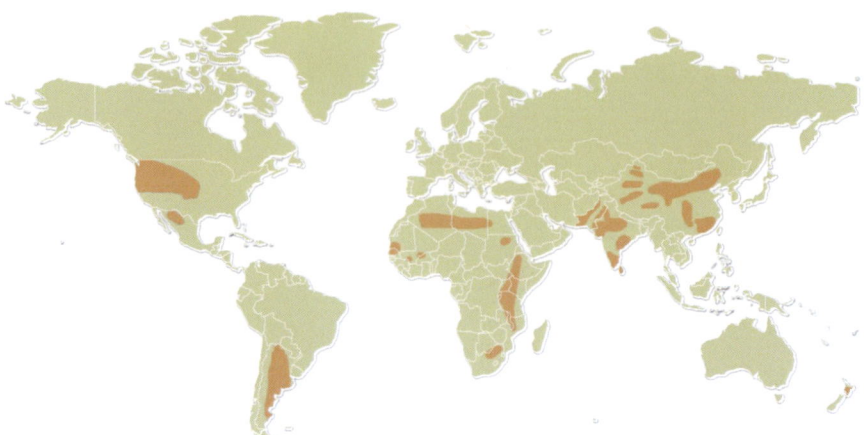

Fig. 10.1 Fluoride in groundwater (>1.5 mg/L), a worldwide distribution. (Adapted from WHO data)

10.2   Fluorine in Nature

Fluorine, a highly reactive gas at room temperature, is found in nature either as fluoride or as a complex with other elements [10]. The accumulation of fluoride in the environment occurs gradually from various sources like volcanic discharges, industrial by-products, and dissolution of minerals. These complexes settle into the soil of neighboring areas and eventually reach groundwater. Fluorine is found in about 300 different kinds of minerals, prominent among them being fluorspar (CaF_2), fluorapatite ($Ca_5(PO_4)_3F$), topaz ($Al_2(SiO_4)(F,OH)_2$), and cryolite (Na_3AlF_6). The volcanic regions that have a high content of fluoride include Iceland, Sicily, the East African Rift, China, South India, and New Zealand [11]. Fluoride is also produced by industries during processes such as aluminum smelting, ceramic and glass production, fertilizer production, and coal burning. These are released into groundwater or as fumes in the environment. Fluoride released in the air travels some distance before settling back into the soil or water. Fluoride-rich industrial emissions therefore can thus cause higher fluoride exposure even in areas that are located at a fair distance from the site of origin [12, 13].

The fluoride–metal compounds also get distributed into the soil and are subsequently absorbed by the microbes and plants. Some of the highest fluoride-accumulating plants are spinach, grapes, tomato, tea, and elderberry [14]. Some plants such as tea accumulate fluorides as they age and in some populations, heavy tea consumption is therefore considered to be the primary mechanism of fluoride toxicity among adults [15]. In many developed countries, the source of fluoride exposure is government-instituted fluoridated water, toothpaste, dental gel, and varnish [16]. At times fluorosis can be iatrogenic. Drugs such as NSAIDs, Voriconazole, etc., contain fluoride and their overuse can lead to chronic fluorosis [17]. In children, calcium deficiency has been linked to juvenile fluorosis [18].

10.3 Pathogenesis

Fluoride affects a wide variety of cells and tissues apart from the skeletal system including renal, endothelial, gonadal, red blood cells, and neurological cells. However, the most severe form of toxicity due to chronic fluoride intake is skeletal fluorosis. It is estimated that an average person needs to ingest 6–10 mg of fluorides daily for a minimum of 10 years to develop skeletal fluorosis [19]. The rate of fluoride accumulation is higher in children and adults with chronic kidney disease [2].

10.3.1 Effects of Fluoride on Bone Minerals

Fluoride forms fluorapatite by substituting for the hydroxyl group in hydroxyapatite, which then gets incorporated into the bone during the process of bone formation and mineralization (Fig. 10.2) [20]. It has been observed that fluoride increases the compactness and stability of the crystal lattice. The mixture of hydroxyapatite and fluorapatite has been found to have more stability and resistance to resorption compared to either of the two, individually [21].

The commencement of mineralization however is late. This results in the increased formation of osteoid. The mineralization profile of bone tilts towards more dense and mature fractions where the concentration of fluoride appears to be high.

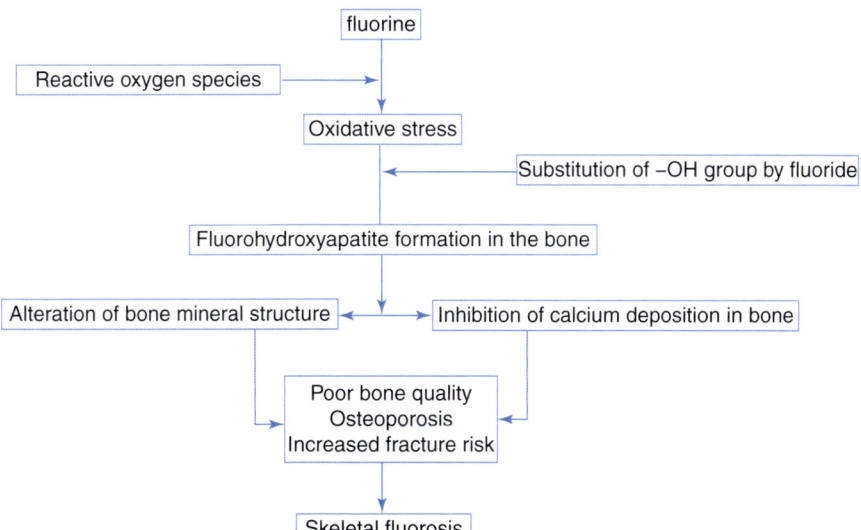

Fig. 10.2 Pathogenesis of fluorosis

10.3.2 Effects of Fluoride on Bone Cells

Fluoride appears to have an effect on bone cells at serum levels much higher than what would be achieved through the consumption of fluoridated water only [22]. In fluorotic individuals and those exposed to fluoride therapy, there is an increase in bone mass. Fluoride appears to have a mitogenic effect on osteoblasts. However, these osteoblasts appear flattened and show moderate activity instead of being cuboidal, plump, and extremely secretory. Therefore, it appears that, while fluoride has mitogenic properties and promotes the differentiation of precursors of osteoblast, it is, to an extent, noxious to individual osteoblast at those concentrations.

The overall effect of fluoride, nevertheless, is an increase in the bone formation. Some evidence from in vitro studies suggests that on exposure to sodium fluoride, resorption lacunae decrease in number and there is also a reduction in the quantity of resorbed bone per osteoclast. Eventually, there is an increase in bone mass, which explains the interest in the therapeutic use of fluoride for osteoporosis [23].

10.3.3 Effects of Fluoride on Bone Architecture

In patients with osteoporosis, therapeutic administration of moderate doses of fluoride produces a marked rise in bone mass. The parameters of bone formation which include osteoid volume, surface, and width are elevated implying an increase in the volume of trabecular bone. Studies assessing the effect on the mechanical properties of bone by moderate to high doses of fluoride have revealed a decline in mechanical strength despite an unchanged or increased amount of bone [24].

10.3.4 Effects of Fluoride on Collagen-Mineral Interface

The collagen and fluorapatite interface appears to be weaker compared to the native hydroxyapatite. This has also been shown to have a deleterious effect on the mechanical properties of the bone [25]. It appears that the physicochemical and biological effects of fluoride on the collagen-mineral interface act to negatively affect the physical properties of bone.

Overall, it appears that fluoride has a complex effect on the bone which is dose-dependent and leads to alterations in the amount and structure of bone along with the mineral-collagen interface. The result is a change in the mechanical properties of bone, and by extension, to the fracture risk. Clinical techniques, such as dual-energy X-ray absorptiometry or histomorphometry only show increased bone density and mass and fail to accurately assess the risk of fracture in such cases [24].

Overall effect of fluoride on mechanical properties based on animal studies suggests a dose-dependent effect. There is an improvement with increasing fluoride content to a certain point, followed by severe compromise of mechanical properties as the concentrations of fluoride rise [20, 24].

10.3.5 Skeletal Fluorosis

The term skeletal fluorosis encompasses a spectrum of deleterious effects due to chronic exposure to high levels of fluoride on the skeleton. These include changes in architecture, mineralization, remodeling, and mechanical qualities of bone. There is an increase in the volume of cancellous bone which is radiologically observed as osteosclerosis along with an increase in cortical bone width and porosity. Remodeling in fluorotic bone is skewed in favor of formation which is characterized by increased newly formed bone (osteoid) parameters that include width, perimeter, and volume. The increase in osteoid is due to decreased mineral apposition rate and increased mineralization lag time [26, 27].

There seems to be a strong genetic influence on the development of skeletal fluorosis. In one study, despite high concentrations of fluoride in the drinking water (1.2–8.9 ppm), the occurrence of skeletal fluorosis was around 40%, which varied with not just the concentration of fluorides but also the population [26].

The association between genetic polymorphism and the pattern of skeletal fluorosis has been confirmed by several genetic epidemiological studies among individuals residing in the same community and sharing the same environmental conditions. These studies have underlined that genetic variants in candidate genes (such as glutathione S-transferase P1, matrix metallopeptidase 2, vitamin D receptor, prolactin, and myeloperoxidase) may amplify the risk of endemic fluorosis among exposed individuals [28].

Increased fluoride concentration in bone is associated with an increase in mineralization in fluoride-treated humans, animal models, and fluorotic bone [29]. However, this increased mineralization is linked with certain characteristic defects which include enlarged lacunae and "mottled osteons" (circum-lacunar mineralization defects) and linear formation defects seen in cancellous bone [30].

Consequently, despite increased mineralization, there is decreased mechanical integrity due to excessive fluoride exposure [24]. A similar decline has been seen in the mechanical properties of bone in patients treated with fluoride as a therapy for osteoporosis [31].

10.3.6 Histopathology

A significant surge in parameters of osteoid formation and trabecular bone volume is appreciated in skeletal fluorosis on histomorphometric study after double labeling with tetracycline. Another histomorphometric analysis of under-calcified transiliac biopsy sections taken from patients suffering from skeletal fluorosis revealed thickening of cortex with marrow cavity narrowing, reduced resorption of bone, and virtually absent osteoclasts. An obvious increase in bone surfaces lined by osteoids and in some studies, evidence of resorption has also been described [32].

Other histological findings reported include osteocondensation along with an increase in osteoid width, formation defects in bone, and an extended osteoblast perimeter. These changes may give a pseudo-osteomalacia appearance. Other qualitative abnormalities suggestive of skeletal fluorosis include a hypo-mineralized halo, surrounding defects of apposition, and periosteocytic deficiencies of mottled appearance [32].

10.4 Clinical Features

Excessive fluoride intake affects the body in many ways. In children, fluoride toxicity mainly manifests in the form of dental fluorosis. However, cases of skeletal fluorosis in the pediatric age group are also seen. Skeletal fluorosis is mainly seen in adults possibly because the metabolic activity of the bone for remodeling is relatively high in children which prevents the retention of fluorides in the bone [33]. Skeletal fluorosis is frequently asymptomatic initially. Patients complain of vague pains in small joints of the hand or feet and lower back. Stiffness of joints with a declined range of motion, weakness of muscle, and chronic fatigue may also occur [9, 33]. The United States Public Health Service has divided skeletal fluorosis based on symptoms and radiology (Table 10.1) [4, 34].

The presence of dental fluorosis helps in making the diagnosis of skeletal fluorosis. Dental fluorosis results from exposure to high fluoride intake in childhood (<12 years age), which corresponds to a period of permanent teeth mineralization [4, 35]. As the disease progresses, bones and joints become increasingly weaker, making movements hard and painful. The fusion of vertebrae also takes place in many areas of the vertebral column leading to kyphosis and restriction of spinal movements. The symptoms of reduced spinal mobility first appear in the cervical spine. The neck movements are restricted along all axes and eventually the head and neck become fixed. The thoracic spine is next to get affected and leads to kyphotic

Table 10.1 Phases of skeletal fluorosis

Phases	Symptomatology	Radiological findings
Preclinical phase	Asymptomatic	Slightly increased bone density
Phase 1	Sporadic pain, stiffness of joints	Osteosclerosis of pelvis and vertebral column
Phase 2	Chronic joint pain, arthritic symptoms	Slight calcification of ligaments, increased osteosclerosis/cancellous bones; with/without osteoporosis of long bones
Phase 3	Limitation of joint movement	Calcification of ligaments/neck, vertebral column; crippling deformities/spine and major joints; muscle wasting; neurological defects/compression of spinal cord

posture apart from the pain and stiffness. Ultimately the entire vertebral column gets fused and becomes fixed with complete loss of rotatory and other spinal movements.

Peripheral joints also get affected. In the upper extremities, elbows and shoulders are commonly affected with pain and decreased mobility. The patient is unable to carry out overhead movements and cannot rotate the shoulders. Small joints of hands, although become painful, retain mobility and do not develop deformities. In lower limbs, the hip and knee are affected commonly. Scissors gait due to bilateral hip involvement forces the patient to use crutches or sticks for support while ambulating. In the knees, progressive loss of mobility is seen with complete loss of movements seen in the late stages. Varus deformities are commonly seen, but valgus deformities have also been reported [33]. The flexion contracture of lower limbs and limitation of expansion of the chest wall may also occur. Ultimately, the patient becomes crippled, with a significantly amplified risk of fracture.

Certain clinical tests of spinal mobility, e.g., coin test, chin test, and stretch test, are commonly used in making a diagnosis of skeletal fluorosis. These tests however are nonspecific and have to be interpreted with an appropriate background while making the diagnosis of skeletal fluorosis (Table 10.2) [9].

Approximately 10% of patients suffering from skeletal fluorosis have neurological complications [36]. It occurs due to mechanical compression of the spinal cord and exiting nerve roots subsequent to osteophytosis, reduced anteroposterior diameter of the spinal canal and intervertebral foramina, sclerosis of vertebral column, and ossification of spinal ligaments. Ossification of the ligamentum flavum and posterior longitudinal ligament causing myelopathy has also been described in cases of skeletal fluorosis and are mostly located in the lower thoracic part of the spinal cord [37]. The radiculomyelopathy seen in fluorosis is progressive and characterized by muscle wasting and spastic paraparesis or quadriparesis [38]. Signs of involvement of long tracts, urinary bladder incontinence, and flexor spasms have also been described. Cranial nerve palsies have also been reported in skeletal fluorosis. Usually, the compression of the eighth nerve within the sclerosed auditory canal causes progressive high-frequency perceptive deafness.

Fluorosis has been linked to anemia, premature births, stillbirths, and abortions. It has also been linked to thyroid hormone abnormalities in children, hypertension, renal failure, and iodine deficiency disorders [39].

Table 10.2 Clinical tests for skeletal fluorosis

Test	Description
Coin test	Inability to lift a coin from the floor without flexing a large joint of lower limb
Chin test	Inability to touch chest with chin
Stretch test	Inability to abduct shoulders, flex elbows, and touch the back of the head

10.5   Diagnosis

There are no diagnostic criteria for skeletal fluorosis. The diagnosis is made based on the history of residence in an area endemic to fluorosis, consumption of fluorine-rich substances for a long duration, clinical features, skeletal imaging, and certain biochemical chemical tests showing high serum or urine.

10.5.1 Laboratory Investigations

10.5.1.1   Fluoride or Fluorine Levels
The diagnosis of skeletal fluorosis can be established by the detection of increased fluorine in the blood, urine, or bone tissue. Normally, blood fluorine values are less than 0.05 mg/L and those above 0.2 mg/L are associated with an increased risk of bone fluorosis [2].

The best indicators of fluoride intake are urinary fluoride levels which are best assessed in a 24-h sample as the fluoride concentration is not constant throughout the day. Normal urinary fluoride concentration varies from 0.1 to 2.0 ppm and levels above it indicate high fluoride intake [40]. The gold standard is a quantitative analysis of fluoride in bone ash [2].

10.5.1.2   Sialic Acid/Glycosaminoglycan (SA/GAG) Ratio
SA and GAG are bone matrix molecules whose levels are deranged in skeletal fluorosis. The SA:GAG ratio is decreased by approximately 30% in skeletal fluorosis whereas the values are higher in conditions like osteoarthritis, spondyloarthritides, and osteoporosis [41].

10.5.2 Imaging

10.5.2.1   Radiographs
Imaging features along with the epidemiological data usually suffices to diagnose skeletal fluorosis (Fig. 10.3). A radiological classification for skeletal fluorosis has been postulated by Roholm which categorizes the radiological changes into three stages characterized by thick trabeculations (stage 1), loss of trabeculations and regular contour of bone with discrete calcification of soft tissue insertions (stage 2), and finally densification of the skeleton with irregular cortical thickening and reduction in the medullary cavity (stage 3) [2].

10.5.2.2   Radionuclide Scan
It shows a high turnover state in the axial and appendicular skeleton. Increased tracer uptake may be seen between forearm bones and along with the attachments of ligaments. This modality is seldom used and carries the risk of high radiation exposure and nonspecificity. Moreover, it is not readily available [42].

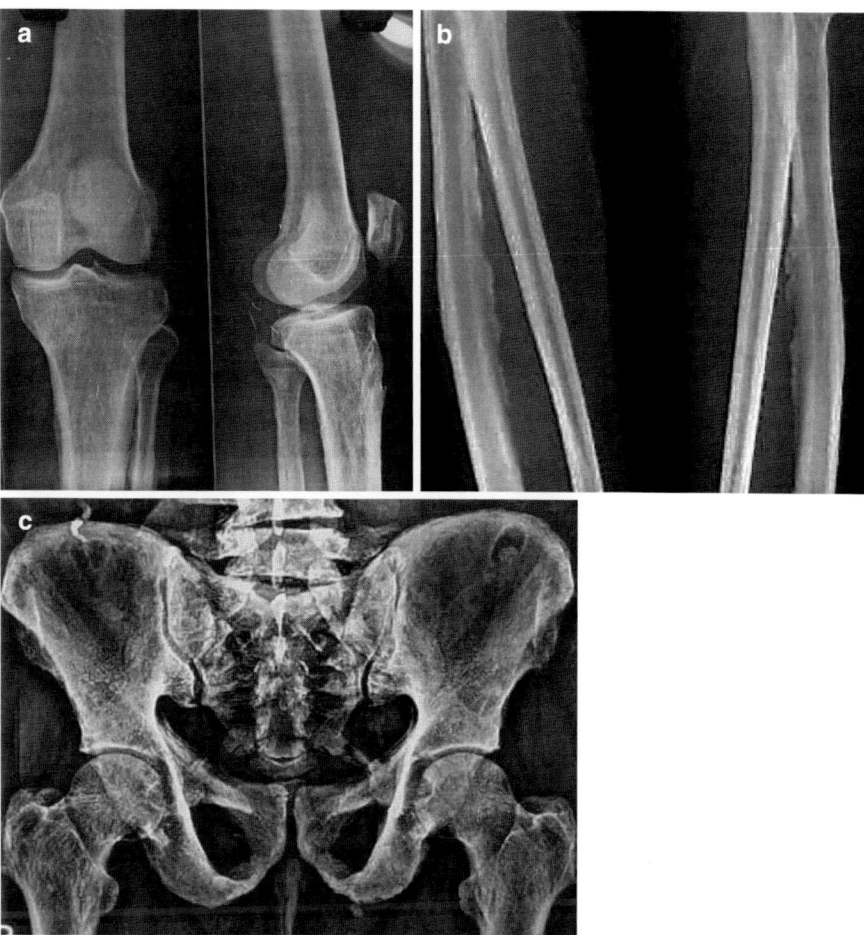

Fig. 10.3 (a) X ray knee of the patient and (b) X ray forearm of the patient depicting ossification of the interosseous membrane. Osteosclerosis of forearm bones can also be appreciated. (c) X ray pelvis depicting sacrospinous ligament ossification and trabecular thickening of bones. (Image courtesy Dr. Sandeep Supehia)

10.6   Differential Diagnosis

Skeletal fluorosis is characterized by the triad of osteocondensation, osteophytosis, and ligamentous calcification. These are most obvious on radiographs of the pelvis and spine. However, these findings are not specific and can be seen in multiple other conditions. These features should be interpreted in the background of epidemiology and endemicity of fluorosis in a given geographical area. Multiple other conditions that may mimic skeletal fluorosis need consideration and are mentioned in Table 10.3.

Table 10.3 Differential diagnosis of skeletal fluorosis

Osteocondensation	Osteophytosis	Ligamentous calcification
Skeletal metastasis, myelofibrosis, mastocytosis, sickle cell disease, renal osteodystrophy, Paget's disease, hypoparathyroidism	Spondyloarthropathy, diffuse idiopathic skeletal hyperostosis (DISH), acromegaly, and neuropathic osteoarthropathy	Idiopathic Paget's disease DISH

10.7 Treatment

The treatment is mainly symptomatic as there is no specific treatment. In the case of children between 6 and 12 years of age, the combination of calcium, vitamin C, and vitamin D3 appears to cause regression of signs of skeletal fluorosis. Some radiological studies have revealed the possible reversibility of skeletal fluorosis lesions many years after the end of fluoride exposure [43].

As there are no pharmacological agents approved to treat skeletal fluorosis, restriction of the consumption of high fluoride intake is an important aspect of the management of skeletal fluorosis. Surgical procedures such as decompressive laminectomy may be needed in selected cases of myelopathy due to ossification of the ligamentum flavum and/or posterior longitudinal ligament. The risks and benefits of such intervention must be deliberated upon, considering the quality of the remodeled bone and the risk of hemorrhage. The long-term outcome of surgical procedures is poor in such cases [38].

10.8 Prevention

Preventive actions are of great significance which includes water defluoridation and nutritional intervention [44]. Studies have shown that apart from exposure to excess fluorides, the health and nutritional status, content of calcium and magnesium, and antioxidants in the food also play a role in the development of skeletal fluorosis. Calcium and magnesium content reduces the bioavailability and toxicity of fluorides [36]. Since the main source of fluoride intake is the consumption of fluoride-rich groundwater, various defluoridation techniques have been developed and effectively used [45].

10.8.1 Defluoridation

As the major mode of fluoride entry into the body is through consumption of water, defluoridation of drinking water is an important step to prevent the development and progression of skeletal fluorosis. There are multiple modalities available to carry out the defluoridation of water. These modalities have their advantages and disadvantages. A summary has been provided in Table 10.4.

Table 10.4 Defluoridation techniques

Properties and methods	Chemicals required	Cost	Removal efficiency	Principle of working
Coagulation-precipitation	Lime and alum	Low	Medium	Charge neutralization of colloids is done by adding chemicals followed by the formation of flocs precipitate
Ion exchange	Synthetic chemicals like cation and anion exchange resins	High	High	Synthetic chemicals, namely, anion and cation exchange resins have been used for fluoride removal
Membrane	No chemical	High	High	Through a layer which acts as a barrier controlling transport of selective particles from other sides
Adsorption	No chemicals	Medium	High	Transport of fluoride ions to the adsorbent surface or adsorption of fluoride ions on to the active adsorbent surface
Electro-coagulation	No chemical addition externally	High	Very high	Electrolytic process which generates coagulant by oxidizing anodic plate

10.9   Conclusion

Fluorosis is a major public health issue in many nations due to excessive fluoride ingestion. Predominantly affecting the skeletal system, it presents a diagnostic dilemma as it mimics multiple other conditions. In an endemic area, the diagnosis is predominantly clinical. There is no specific treatment and prevention remains the best option to tackle this condition.

References

1. Kanduti D, Sterbenk P, Artnik and. Fluoride: a review of use and effects on health. Mater Sociomed. 2016;28:133. https://doi.org/10.5455/MSM.2016.28.133-137.
2. Sellami M, Riahi H, Maatallah K, Ferjani H, Bouaziz MC, Ladeb MF. Skeletal fluorosis: don't miss the diagnosis! Skeletal Radiol. 2020;49:345–57. https://doi.org/10.1007/S00256-019-03302-0.
3. Kumar S, Kakar A, Gogia A, Byotra SP. Skeletal fluorosis mimicking seronegative spondyloarthropathy: a deceptive presentation. Trop Doct. 2011;41:247–8. https://doi.org/10.1258/TD.2011.110117.
4. Shukla A. Skeletal fluorosis mimicking seronegative arthritis. Indian J Rheumatol. 2016;11:171. https://doi.org/10.4103/0973-3698.187413.
5. Karimzade S, Aghaei M, Mahvi AH. Investigation of intelligence quotient in 9-12-year-old children exposed to high- and low-drinking water fluoride in West Azerbaijan Province, Iran. Fluoride. 2014;47:9–14.

6. Aghaei M, Karimzade S, Yaseri M, Khorsandi H, Zolfi E, Mahvi AH. Hypertension and fluoride in drinking water: case study from West Azerbaijan, Iran. Fluoride. 2015;48:252–8.

7. Aghaei M, Derakhshani R, Raoof M, Dehghani M, Mahvi AH. Effect of fluoride in drinking water on birth height and weight: an ecological study in Kerman Province, Zarand county, Iran. Fluoride. 2015;48:160–8. https://doi.org/10.13140/RG.2.1.2919.0484.

8. Shanthi M, Thimma Reddy BV, Shivani K. Health impact to different concentrations of fluoride in drinking water of South India. Int J Sci Stud. 2014;2:2–5.

9. Arlappa N, Aatif Qureshi ISR. Fluorosis in India: an overview. Int J Res Dev Health. 2013;1:97–102.

10. Johnston NR, Strobel SA. Principles of fluoride toxicity and the cellular response: a review. Arch Toxicol. 2020;94:1051–69. https://doi.org/10.1007/S00204-020-02687-5.

11. D'Alessandro W. Human fluorosis related to volcanic activity: a review. WIT Trans Biomed Health. 2006;10:21–30. https://doi.org/10.2495/ETOX060031.

12. Monfort E, García-Ten J, Celades I, Gazulla MF, Gomar S. Evolution of fluorine emissions during the fast firing of ceramic tile. Appl Clay Sci. 2008;38:250–8. https://doi.org/10.1016/J.CLAY.2007.03.001.

13. Walna B, Kurzyca I, Bednorz E, Kolendowicz L. Fluoride pollution of atmospheric precipitation and its relationship with air circulation and weather patterns (Wielkopolski National Park, Poland). Environ Monit Assess. 2013;185:5497. https://doi.org/10.1007/S10661-012-2962-9.

14. Jacobson JS, Weinstein LH, Mccune DC, Hitchcock AE. The accumulation of fluorine by plants. J Air Pollut Control Assoc. 1966;16:412–7. https://doi.org/10.1080/00022470.1966.10468494.

15. Cao J, Zhao Y, Liu J, Xirao R, Danzeng S, Daji D, et al. Brick tea fluoride as a main source of adult fluorosis. Food Chem Toxicol. 2003;41:535–42. https://doi.org/10.1016/S0278-6915(02)00285-5.

16. Pretty IA. High fluoride concentration toothpastes for children and adolescents. Caries Res. 2016;50(Suppl 1):9–14. https://doi.org/10.1159/000442797.

17. Thekkudan SF, Kumar P, Nityanand S. Voriconazole-induced skeletal fluorosis in an allogenic hematopoietic stem cell transplant recipient. Ann Hematol. 2016;95:669–70. https://doi.org/10.1007/S00277-016-2603-4.

18. Kurdi MS. Chronic fluorosis: the disease and its anaesthetic implications. Indian J Anaesth. 2016;60:157–62. https://doi.org/10.4103/0019-5049.177867.

19. Whitford GM. The metabolism and toxicity of fluoride. Monogr Oral Sci. 1996;16 Rev 2:1–153. https://doi.org/10.1016/0300-5712(92)90111-o.

20. Chachra D, Vieira APGF, Grynpas MD. Fluoride and mineralized tissues. Crit Rev Biomed Eng. 2008;36:183–223. https://doi.org/10.1615/CRITREVBIOMEDENG.V36.I2-3.40.

21. Grynpas MD. Fluoride effects on bone crystals. J Bone Miner Res. 1990;5(Suppl 1):S169–75. https://doi.org/10.1002/JBMR.5650051362.

22. Turner CH, Boivin G, Meunier PJ. A mathematical model for fluoride uptake by the skeleton. Calcif Tissue Int. 1993;52:130–8. https://doi.org/10.1007/BF00308322.

23. Okuda A, Kanehisa J, Heersche JNM. The effects of sodium fluoride on the resorptive activity of isolated osteoclasts. J Bone Miner Res. 1990;5(Suppl 1):S115–20. https://doi.org/10.1002/JBMR.5650051381.

24. Turner CH, Garetto LP, Dunipace AJ, Zhang W, Wilson ME, Grynpas MD, et al. Fluoride treatment increased serum IGF-1, bone turnover, and bone mass, but not bone strength, in rabbits. Calcif Tissue Int. 1997;61:77–83. https://doi.org/10.1007/S002239900299.

25. Thurner PJ, Erickson B, Turner P, Jungmann R, Lelujian J, Proctor A, et al. The effect of NaF in vitro on the mechanical and material properties of trabecular and cortical bone. Adv Mater. 2009;21:451–7. https://doi.org/10.1002/ADMA.200801204.

26. Choubisa SL, Choubisa L, Choubisa DK. Endemic fluorosis in Rajasthan. Indian J Environ Health. 2001;43:177–89.

27. Chachra D, Turner CH, Dunipace AJ, Grynpas MD. The effect of fluoride treatment on bone mineral in rabbits. Calcif Tissue Int. 1999;64:345–51. https://doi.org/10.1007/S002239900630.

28. Liu Q, Liu H, Yu X, Wang Y, Yang C, Xu H. Analysis of the role of insulin signaling in bone turnover induced by fluoride. Biol Trace Elem Res. 2016;171:380–90. https://doi.org/10.1007/S12011-015-0555-5.

29. Boivin G, Chavassieux P, Chapuy MC, Baud CA, Meunier PJ. Skeletal fluorosis: histomorphometric analysis of bone changes and bone fluoride content in 29 patients. Bone. 1989;10:89–99. https://doi.org/10.1016/8756-3282(89)90004-5.

30. Boivin G, Duriez J, Chapuy MC, Flautre B, Hardouin P, Meunier PJ. Relationship between bone fluoride content and histological evidence of calcification defects in osteoporotic women treated long term with sodium fluoride. Osteoporos Int. 1993;3:204–8. https://doi.org/10.1007/BF01623677.

31. Søgaard CH, Mosekilde L, Richards A, Mosekilde L. Marked decrease in trabecular bone quality after five years of sodium fluoride therapy—assessed by biomechanical testing of iliac crest bone biopsies in osteoporotic patients. Bone. 1994;15:393–9. https://doi.org/10.1016/8756-3282(94)90815-X.

32. Tamer MN, Kale Köroğlu B, Arslan Ç, Akdoğan M, Köroğlu M, Çam H, et al. Osteosclerosis due to endemic fluorosis. Sci Total Environ. 2007;373:43–8. https://doi.org/10.1016/J.SCITOTENV.2006.10.051.

33. Ramkumar G, Shanmugasundaram P. A study on crippling in skeletal fluorosis. Int J Cur Res Rev. 2014;6:26–30.

34. Pramanik S, Saha D. The genetic influence in fluorosis. Environ Toxicol Pharmacol. 2017;56:157–62. https://doi.org/10.1016/J.ETAP.2017.09.008.

35. Teotia SP, Teotia M, Singh KP. Highlights of forty years of research on endemic skeletal fluorosis in India. In: 4th international workshop on fluorosis prevention and defluoridation of water; 2004 Mar 2, pp. 107–125.

36. Patil MM, Lakhkar BB, Patil SS. Curse of fluorosis. Indian J Pediatr. 2018;85:375–83. https://doi.org/10.1007/S12098-017-2574-Z.

37. Meena C, Dwivedi S, Rathore S, Gonmei Z, Toteja GS, Bala K, et al. Assessment of skeletal fluorosis among children in two blocks of rural area, Jaipur District, Rajasthan, India. Asian J Pharm Clin Res. 2017;10:322–5. https://doi.org/10.22159/AJPCR.2017.V10I9.19993.

38. Kumar H, Boban M, Tiwari M. Skeletal fluorosis causing high cervical myelopathy. J Clin Neurosci. 2009;16:828–30. https://doi.org/10.1016/J.JOCN.2008.08.028.

39. Susheela AK, Toteja GS. Prevention & control of fluorosis & linked disorders: developments in the 21st century—reaching out to patients in the community & hospital settings for recovery. Indian J Med Res. 2018;148:539–47. https://doi.org/10.4103/IJMR.IJMR_1775_18.

40. Gupta N, Gupta N, Chhabra P. Image diagnosis: dental and skeletal fluorosis. Perm J. 2016;20:e105–6. https://doi.org/10.7812/TPP/15-048.

41. Jha M, Susheela AK, Krishna N, Rajyalakshmi K, Venkiah K. Excessive ingestion of fluoride and the significance of sialic acid: glycosaminoglycans in the serum of rabbit and human subjects. J Toxicol Clin Toxicol. 1982;19:1023–30. https://doi.org/10.3109/15563658208992537.

42. Chaoke L, Rongdi J, Shouren C. Epidemiological analysis of endemic fluorosis in China. J Environ Sci Health Part C. 1997;15:123–38. https://doi.org/10.1080/10590509709373493.

43. Wang W, Kong L, Zhao H, Dong R, Li J, Jia Z, et al. Thoracic ossification of ligamentum flavum caused by skeletal fluorosis. Eur Spine J. 2007;16:1119–28. https://doi.org/10.1007/S00586-006-0242-0.

44. Khairnar MR, Dodamani AS, Jadhav HC, Naik RG, Deshmukh MA. Mitigation of fluorosis—a review. J Clin Diagn Res. 2015;9:ZE05–9. https://doi.org/10.7860/JCDR/2015/13261.6085.

45. Ingle N, Dubey H, Kaur N, Sharma I. Defluoridation techniques: which one to choose. J Health Res Rev. 2014;1:1. https://doi.org/10.4103/2394-2010.143315.

Ochronosis

11

Darpan Thakare and Vikas Agarwal

11.1 Introduction

Alkaptonuria is a rare, autosomal recessive disorder of tyrosine metabolism with a worldwide prevalence of one case per 250,000–1,000,000 births [1]. It is reported to be more prevalent in Slovakia, the Dominican Republic, and Jordan with the highest prevalence in Slovakia (1 in 19,000) [2]. The earliest description of ochronosis comes from an Egyptian mummy dating back to 1500 B.C. The radiological examination of this mummy was suggestive of ochronosis, and a spectroscopic examination of the pigment obtained from a punch biopsy confirmed the presence of a homogentisic acid-derived polymer. The term alkaptonuria was first used in 1859 by Boedeker to describe the discoloration of urine due to a reducing compound. Virchow named the condition Ochronosis (meaning "yellow disease" in Greek) because the connective tissues appeared ochre (yellow) on the microscopic examination due to the accumulation of this pigment. It was one of the first disorders in humans found to conform with the principles of Mendelian recessive inheritance [3].

11.2 Pathogenesis

Alkaptonuria results from the deficiency of homogentisate 1,2-dioxygenase (HGD) enzyme (Fig. 11.1), predominantly produced by hepatocytes in the liver and in the kidneys, it is responsible for the breakdown of homogentisic acid; an intermediate in the tyrosine degradation pathway. Inability to convert homogentisic acid to maleylacetoacetic acid (MAA) results in the accumulation of homogentisic acid in collagenous tissues and the product of its oxidation, benzoquinone, causes tissue injury.

D. Thakare · V. Agarwal (✉)
Department of Clinical Immunology and Rheumatology, Sanjay Gandhi Postgraduate
Institute of Medical Sciences, Lucknow, Uttar Pradesh, India

© The Author(s), under exclusive license to Springer Nature
Switzerland AG 2022
V. Ravindran et al. (eds.), *Rarer Arthropathies*, Rare Diseases of the Immune
System, https://doi.org/10.1007/978-3-031-05002-2_11

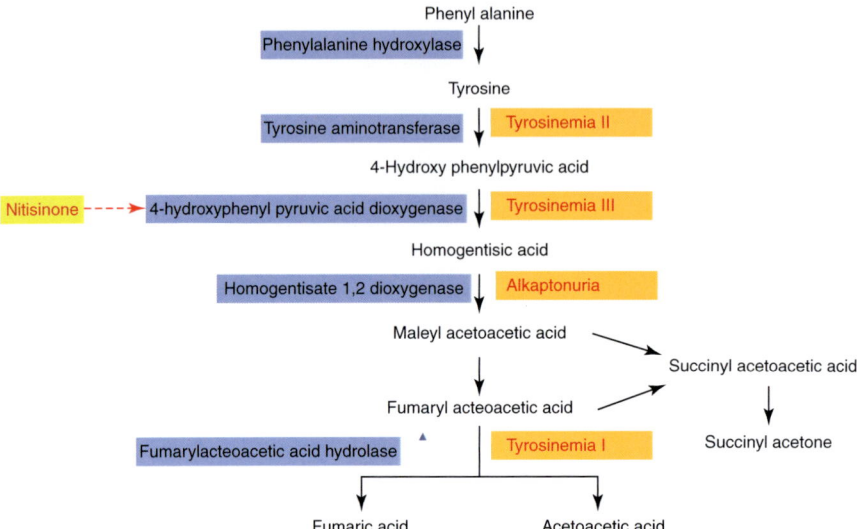

Fig. 11.1 Defects in metabolism of phenylalanine leading to various tyrosine metabolism disorders

Although homogentisic acid is rapidly cleared from the body by the kidneys, it also slowly accumulates within the various tissues of the body.

As a result of the deposition of oxidized homogentisic acid in deeper layers of articular cartilage, the cartilage loses its elasticity and becomes brittle, eventually leading to fragmentation and the formation of loose bodies. Small cartilage fragments may adhere atop the synovial membrane leading to thickening, fibrosis, and chondromatosis [4]. Large segments of cartilage may disappear leading to bony ankylosis, osteophytes, and subchondral cysts formation.

11.3   Clinical Features

Alkaptonuria presents with a classic clinical triad of homogentisic aciduria, ochronosis, and ochronotic arthropathy, with each feature presenting at various stages in life. The initial symptom that occurs in infancy is homogentisic aciduria, a characteristic black discoloration of urine due to homogentisic acid oxidation that occurs after urine has been standing or can be induced by alkalization, leading to 21% of the patients being diagnosed before the age of 1 year [5].

Ochronosis develops due to the accumulation of benzoquinone, both intra- and extra-cellularly in the connective tissues. This manifestation is usually observed from the third to fifth decades of life. Ochronosis is typically seen in ear cartilage (Fig. 11.2) and eyes (Fig. 11.3). Cutaneous pigmentation can also be seen on ala of nose, face, palms (Fig. 11.4) and soles, cheeks, buccal mucosa, axilla, and inguinal

Fig. 11.2 Greyish-black
discoloration of the ear
pinna in a middle-aged
patient

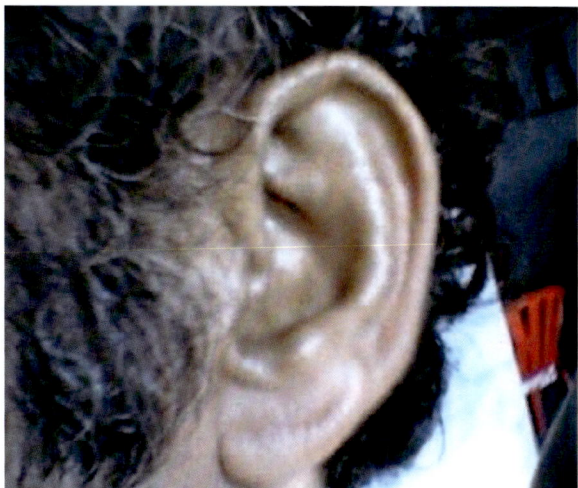

Fig. 11.3 Greyish black
discoloration of the sclera
in a middle-aged patient

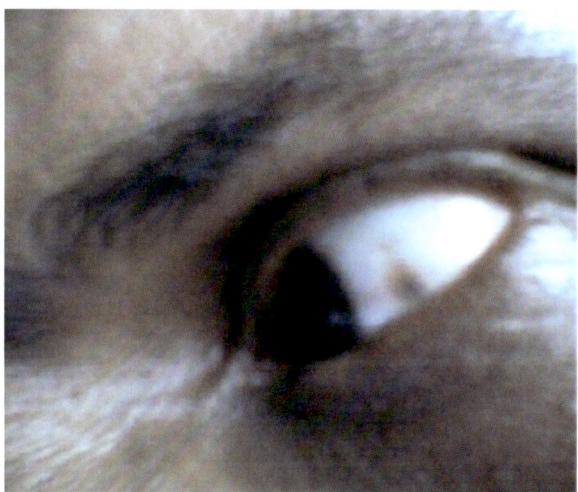

areas. Less common manifestations include cardiovascular involvement with aortic valve stenosis, often requiring surgical replacement [6], asymptomatic nephrolithiasis, and prostatic calculi.

Ochronotic arthropathy usually starts between the ages of 40 and 50 years. There is a gender predilection towards men with a ratio of 2:1 [7]. Lumbar pain is usually the initial musculoskeletal manifestation, with the patient complaining of stiffness, usually not severe and can be misdiagnosed as an early form of ankylosing spondylitis. There is gradual loss of lumbar and cervical lordosis, progressive kyphoscoliosis, disc prolapse that may result in spinal stenosis, and myelopathy. In advanced stages, the contours of the spine deform with irregular spinous processes and

Fig. 11.4 Greyish-black
discoloration of the palms
in a middle-aged patient

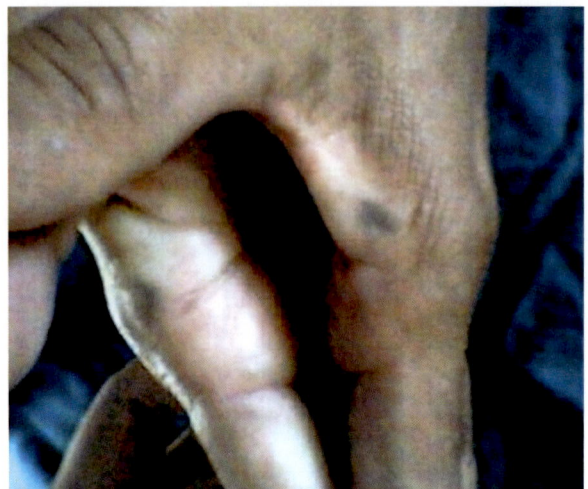

Fig. 11.5 Forward flexion
deformity of neck in a
middle- aged patient with
Ochronosis

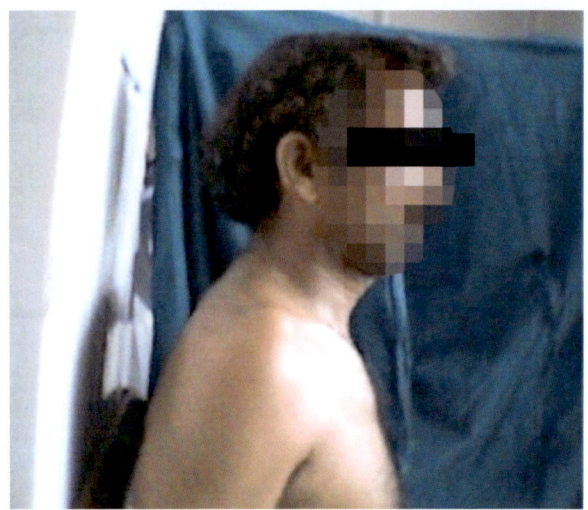

complete ankylosis of the whole lumbar and thoracic spine. As a result of degenerative changes at the vertebral endplates and narrowing of intervertebral space, body height decreases by up to 8 cm over 20 years. Although there may be forward protrusion of the head as a result of neck deformity (Fig. 11.5), the cervical spine maintains its mobility for a relatively long time despite significant changes.

Peripheral joint involvement occurs about 10 years after spinal changes. It predominantly affects large joints in the order of knees (64%) (Fig. 11.6), shoulders (42%), hips (35%), while the small joints are generally spared [8]. The

Fig. 11.6 Bilateral swollen knees in a middle aged patient with Ochronosis

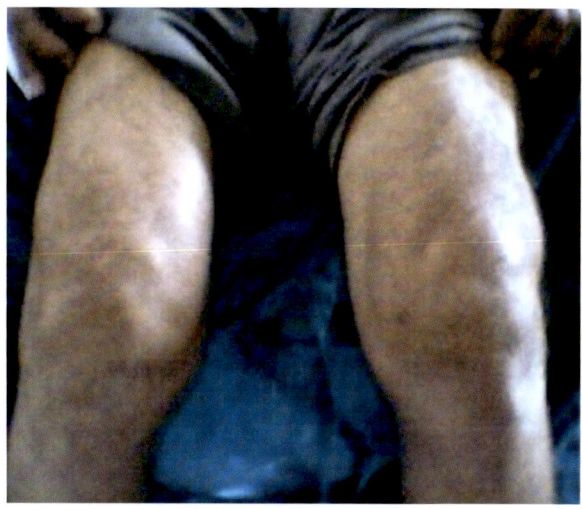

arthropathy closely resembles osteoarthritis, clinically presents with a mechanical type of pain and swelling, and there is a minor inflammatory component. One-third of the patients have an effusion, which is yellowish and remains unchanged even after prolonged standing in the air, suggesting a small concentration of homogentisic acid. The production of multiple, loose osteochondral bodies is characteristic of ochronotic arthropathy and is a sign of ochronotic chondromatosis [9]. Additionally, osteophytes and subchondral cysts are also formed. The joints gradually become stiff and deformed, needing surgical management [10].

Tendons are also affected in ochronosis because of their high collagen content. The patellar and Achilles tendon are the most affected. Several cases of spontaneous tendon and ligament rupture have been reported [11]. Osteoporosis, long bone fractures [6], and osteonecrosis of long bones are also reported in ochronosis.

11.4 Investigations

Elevated levels of homogentisic acid in the urine, blood, and other tissues can be determined by specific enzymatic and colorimetric tests, direct spectrophotometric methods, high-performance liquid chromatographic testing, and molecular techniques. Other simple urinary studies include darkening of urine with the addition of sodium hydroxide, black reaction with ferric chloride, and blackening of emulsion paper with the addition of alkali to the urine.

11.5   Imaging

Radiographic findings in Ochronotic arthropathy are summarized in Box 11.1.

Box 11.1 Radiographic Findings of Ochronotic Arthropathy

Axial involvement

   Vertebral-body osteoporosis

   Intervertebral disc calcification

   Intervertebral disc space narrowing with vacuum phenomenon

   Small or absent osteophytosis

   Loss of lumbar lordosis

Peripheral joint and involvement

   Joint-space narrowing

   Bony eburnation

   Collapse and fragmentation (osteochondral loose bodies)

   Small osteophytes

   Tendon involvement with ruptures or calcifications

11.5.1 Spinal Disease

The disease often affects the lumbar spine initially. Calcification of multiple intervertebral discs is the hallmark finding in ochronosis (Fig. 11.7). The earliest feature seen is the vacuum disc phenomenon with narrowing of the intervertebral disc space. Advanced changes include ossification of the disc, osteophytosis, loss of disc height with eventual collapse, and fusion of adjacent vertebrae. Calcification of the intervertebral disc can help differentiate this from other causes of back pain.

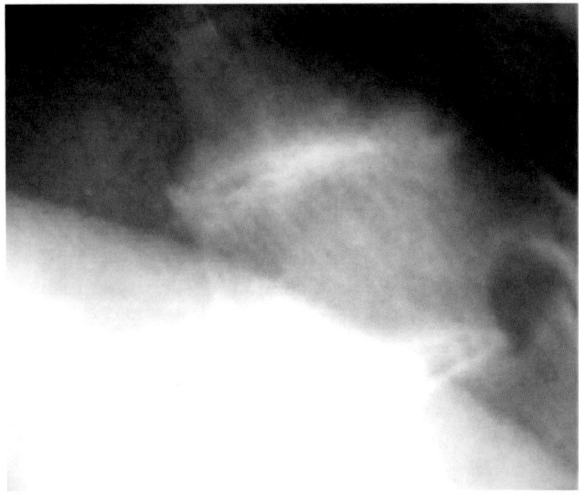

Fig. 11.7 Intervertebral disc calcification with narrowing of the disc space in the lumbar vertebra

Fig. 11.8 Asymmetrically reduced joint space in knee joint in a patient with Ochronosis

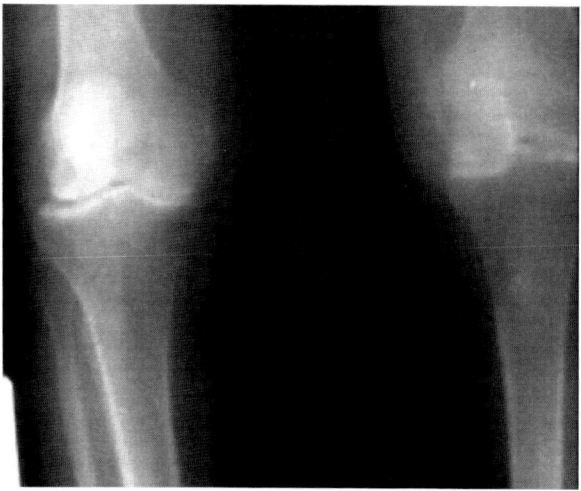

Changes seen in ankylosing spondylitis such as calcification of the intervertebral ligaments, syndesmophytes, erosions, and sacroiliitis are rare. Magnetic resonance imaging (MRI) findings include uniform loss of intervertebral disc height with central intradiscal low T1 and T2 signals, corresponding to intradiscal calcification and multilevel disc prolapse which mirrors the characteristic radiographic changes of ochronosis.

11.5.2 Peripheral Joint Disease

Ochronosis involves the large weight-bearing joints, often sparing small joints. Radiographic findings include joint space narrowing and subchondral sclerosis (Fig. 11.8), which often resembles osteoarthritis. However, osteophytes are less commonly seen and this helps distinguish ochronotic arthropathy from osteoarthritis. Full-thickness erosions of articular cartilage up to the subchondral bone and subchondral cysts can occur in advanced cases. Involvement of the shoulders and hips are more severe, with osteochondral bodies. Tendinous calcification and ossification may occur.

11.6 Differential Diagnosis

The diagnosis of ochronosis may be difficult because it resembles ankylosing spondylitis and osteoarthritis. The differences between ochronotic arthropathy, ankylosing spondylitis, osteoarthritis are summarized in Tables 11.1 and 11.2. It can resemble rheumatoid arthritis during acute presentations although small joints are often not affected.

Table 11.1 Differences between ochronotic arthropathy and ankylosing spondylitis

	Ochronotic arthropathy	Ankylosing spondylitis
Axial involvement		
Calcification of intervertebral discs	Dense	Mild
Multiple vacuum discs	Common	Rare
Syndesmophytes	Minimal, Broad	Significant, Thin and vertical
Apophyseal joint disease	Mild	Severe
Ossification of ligaments	Minimal	Significant
Erosion and fusion of sacroiliac joints	Absent	Present
Peripheral joint involvement		
Joint-space loss	Symmetrical or asymmetrical	Symmetrical
Osteophytes	Scanty	None
Intra-articular osseous bodies, fragmentation	Prominent	None

Table 11.2 Differences between ochronotic arthropathy and osteoarthritis

	Ochronotic arthropathy	Osteoarthritis
Peripheral joint involvement		
Joints involved	Knees, shoulders, hips, elbows, and ankles	Hips, knees, hands
Narrowing of joint space	Symmetrical or asymmetrical	Asymmetrical space narrowing
Osteophytes	Scanty	Prominent
Intra-articular osseous bodies, fragmentation	Prominent	Sparse
Axial involvement		
Osteophytes	Sparse	Prominent
Discal calcification	Dense	Mild
Multiple vacuum discs	Common	Rare
Syndesmophytes	Minimal, Broad	None
Apophyseal joint disease	Mild	Mild to severe

Disc calcifications must be distinguished from diffuse idiopathic skeletal hyperostosis (DISH), juvenile idiopathic arthritis, calcium pyrophosphate dihydrate crystal deposition disease (CPPD), Klippel-Feil syndrome, and congenital and acquired fusions of the spine.

11.7 Management

Several therapies have been tried with little success. There is no approved treatment for alkaptonuria. The management remains palliative and involves physiotherapy, joint replacement surgery, and pain control using paracetamol, anti-inflammatory drugs, opioids, anticonvulsants, local anesthetics, gabapentin, acupuncture, and nerve block [12]. Ascorbic acid is believed to reduce the conversion of homogentisic acid to benzoquinone via oxidation. However, its efficacy has not been demonstrated and it was found to increase homogentisic acid production, contributing to the formation of renal oxalate stones [13]. Similarly, low-protein diet, dietary restriction of tyrosine and phenylalanine have also not proven effective [13].

One promising therapy includes Nitisinone which inhibits the 4-hydroxyphenylpyruvate dioxygenase enzyme (Fig. 11.1), an enzyme involved in the conversion of hydroxyphenylpyruvate to HGA. Reduction in HGA levels may decrease the disease severity of Alkaptonuria. Nitisinone has been shown to decrease urinary and blood levels of HGA by over 99.7%. Nitisinone decreased the All Alkaptonuria Severity Score Index (AKUSSI) from baseline and led to slower disease progression [14]. In another study, a 2 mg dose of Nitisinone was reported not only to slow down the clinical progression of alkaptonuria but also to arrest the progression of eye and ear Ochronosis [15]. It is unknown whether early treatment before the development of musculoskeletal symptoms would be beneficial [16].

Since Alkaptonuria is caused by a deficiency of an enzyme, it is natural that enzyme replacement would be an ideal therapy for ochronosis. However, increased tyrosine levels following Nitisinone therapy may lead to keratopathy and eye symptoms, alterations in cognitive functions, and a rise in transaminases [17].

11.8 Conclusion

Ochronosis is a rare, hereditary, metabolic disorder with a rapidly progressive, disabling, degenerative joint disease. In childhood, investigation of simple observation that the color of urine turns dark brown or black on exposure to air or discoloration of the skin overlying cartilages external ear or sclera, either by the patient or the parents, may lead to early diagnosis. In adulthood, degenerative joint diseases of large joints and the spine may clinch the diagnosis with typical intervertebral disc calcifications. Clinicians need to be aware of the clinical phenotype of this rare genetic disease. Nitisinone currently holds promise to treat patients with Alkaptonuria.

References

1. Phornphutkul C, Introne WJ, Perry MB, Bernardini I, Murphey MD, Fitzpatrick DL, et al. Natural history of alkaptonuria. N Engl J Med. 2002;347(26):2111–21.
2. Ranganath L, Taylor AM, Shenkin A, Fraser WD, Jarvis J, Gallagher JA, et al. Identification of alkaptonuria in the general population: a United Kingdom experience describing the challenges, possible solutions and persistent barriers. J Inherit Metab Dis. 2011;34(3):723–30.
3. Scriver CR. Garrod's Croonian lectures (1908) and the charter 'inborn errors of metabolism': albinism, alkaptonuria, cystinuria, and pentosuria at age 100 in 2008. J Inherit Metab Dis. 2008;31(5):580–98.
4. Borman P, Bodur H, Cılız D. Ochronotic arthropathy. Rheumatol Int. 2002;21(5):205–9.

5. Peker E, Yonden Z, Sogut S. From darkening urine to early diagnosis of alkaptonuria. Indian J Dermatol Venereol Leprol. 2008;74(6):700.
6. Fisher AA, Davis MW. Alkaptonuric ochronosis with aortic valve and joint replacements and femoral fracture: a case report and literature review. Clin Med Res. 2004;2(4):209–15.
7. Rovenský J, Urbánek T, Stančikova M. The clinical picture of alkaptonuria and ochronosis. Reumatologia. 2012;50(4):324–35.
8. Ventura-Ríos L, Hernandez Díaz C, Gutiérrez-Pérez L, Bernal-González A, Pichardo-Bahena R, Cedeño-Garcidueñas A, et al. Ochronotic arthropathy as a paradigm of metabolically induced degenerative joint disease. A case-based review. Clin Rheumatol. 2016;35:1389–95.
9. Radiologic features of lumbar spine in ochronosis in late stages|SpringerLink [Internet]. [cited 2021 Oct 23]. https://link.springer.com/article/10.1007/s10067-005-0033-0.
10. Meschini C, Cauteruccio M, Oliva MS, Sircana G, Vitiello R, Rovere G, et al. Hip and knee replacement in patients with ochronosis: clinical experience and literature review. Orthop Rev. 2020;12(Suppl 1):8687.
11. Alkaptonuria, ochronosis, and ochronotic arthropathy. [Internet]. [cited 2021 Oct 23]. https://reference.medscape.com/medline/abstract/14978662.
12. Ranganath LR, Jarvis JC, Gallagher JA. Recent advances in management of alkaptonuria (invited review; best practice article). J Clin Pathol. 2013;66(5):367–73.
13. Wolff JA, Barshop B, Nyhan WL, Leslie J, Seegmiller JE, Gruber H, et al. Effects of ascorbic acid in alkaptonuria: alterations in benzoquinone acetic acid and an ontogenic effect in infancy. Pediatr Res. 1989;26(2):140–4.
14. Ranganath LR, Psarelli EE, Arnoux JB, et al. Efficacy and safety of once-daily nitisinone for patients with alkaptonuria (SONIA 2): an international, multicentre, open-label, randomised controlled trial. Lancet Diabetes Endocrinol. 2020;8(9):762–72.
15. Ranganath LR, Khedr M, Milan AM, et al. Nitisinone arrests ochronosis and decreases rate of progression of alkaptonuria: evaluation of the effect of nitisinone in the United Kingdom National Alkaptonuria Centre. Mol Genet Metab. 2018;125(1–2):127–34.
16. Ranganath LR, Timmis OG, Gallagher JA. Progress in alkaptonuria—are we near to an effective therapy? J Inherit Metab Dis. 2015;38(5):787–9.
17. Wolffenbuttel BHR, Heiner-Fokkema MR, van Spronsen FJ. Preventive use of nitisinone in alkaptonuria. Orphanet J Rare Dis. 2021;16(1):343.

Arthritis in Tuberculosis

12

Ashok Kumar and Kushagra Gupta

12.1 Introduction

Tuberculosis (TB) is the most common infectious cause of death around the world, only being surpassed by Covid-19 in 2020 [1]. It is one of the oldest diseases known to infect humans, with evidence of skeletal involvement found in some of the earliest human settlements and mummies dating back 9000 years [2]. Diagnosing mycobacterial infections of the musculoskeletal system is often a challenging task due to the rarity of the disease, lack of specific signs and symptoms, and difficulty in obtaining a microbiological or tissue diagnosis. Musculoskeletal (MSK) manifestations of TB can have a significant impact on the quality of life of the patient. The use of anti- tumor necrosis factor (TNF) therapy in the recent era has led to an increase in the incidence of TB in rheumatology practice. A high index of suspicion is the key to making a diagnosis in the appropriate clinical setting.

12.2 Epidemiology

The estimated global incidence of TB in 2019 was ten million. In the same year, TB caused 1.4 million deaths, making it the most common infectious cause of death [1]. Musculoskeletal TB accounts for 1–3% of the overall TB burden [3]. About one-third of the world's population is infected with TB, creating a large global reservoir [4]. The demography of TB varies among different regions depending on socioeconomic factors. In developed countries where TB is non-endemic, infection mainly affects the elderly with compromised immune systems like those living in old age homes, homeless people, prisoners, alcoholics, and immigrants from endemic regions. There is a latency between the primary infection and onset of skeletal

A. Kumar (✉) · K. Gupta
Department of Rheumatology, Fortis Flt. Lt. Rajan Dhall Hospital, New Delhi, India

© The Author(s), under exclusive license to Springer Nature Switzerland AG 2022
V. Ravindran et al. (eds.), *Rarer Arthropathies*, Rare Diseases of the Immune System, https://doi.org/10.1007/978-3-031-05002-2_12

infection which may last up to several years suggesting reactivation of latent infection. In developing countries where TB is endemic, children and young to middle-aged adults are more commonly affected and the disease usually occurs within a year of onset of primary infection.

12.3   Pathogenesis

Mycobacterium tuberculosis (M. tuberculosis) is the most common organism causing mycobacterial infections. More than 50 other different species have been discovered, which form part of the M. tuberculosis complex, which includes M. Tuberculosis, M. bovis, M. africanum, M. microti, and many others. Nontuberculous mycobacteria (NTM) also referred to as atypical mycobacteria are mycobacteria other than M. tuberculosis and M. leprae. In tuberculosis, primary infection occurs via inhalation of aerosolized bacilli. Lungs are the site of primary infection. After acquiring the bacilli, the development of the disease depends on the host immune factors. In the lungs, TB bacilli are phagocytosed by macrophages however some of the mycobacteria survive and grow intracellularly. These mycobacteria rupture the macrophages and spread in the body via the hematogenous route and get seeded in various tissues such as synovium and bone. Initially, the adaptive immune system may limit the spread of the infection through the formation of granulomas. CD4 and CD8 cells play an important role in this step by recruiting macrophages via the release of interferon-ɣ. At this stage, the host starts to show a positive reaction to tuberculin in vivo and the evidence of sensitized T cell mediated release of interferon-gamma in vitro. Mycobacteria may remain dormant for life in this stage or there may be reactivation of "latent infection" whenever immunity is compromised by causes such as advancing age, malnutrition, HIV infection, and chronic kidney disease.

Occasionally, TB may occur by the contiguous spread. Examples include the extension of pulmonary parenchymal infection in the upper lobes to the atlantoaxial joint and TB osteomyelitis spilling into the neighboring diarthrodial joints like the knee.

Once the TB bacillus is reactivated, the nature of the disease depends on the host-parasite interaction. This can be of two types; caseous exudative type and granular type. The exudative type is characterized by abscess formation, sinus discharge, and bone destruction and is usually associated with constitutional symptoms. It is more commonly seen in the younger age group. On the other hand, the granulomatous type is indolent and less destructive and more commonly seen in adults. The clinical picture encountered often lies somewhere on the spectrum between the two types. The course of tuberculous infection is insidious and progression is slow as compared to bacterial infection. This may be due to the inability of mycobacteria to produce collagenase enzyme [5].

12.4   Risk Factors

Various factors may predispose an individual to osteoarticular TB (Table 12.1). Studies have shown ethnic differences in the host immunity to TB [6]. Environmental factors like poverty, education, and unemployment are major determinants in the

Table 12.1   Risk factors for Osteoarticular tuberculosis

Environmental factors
• Poor socioeconomic status
• Crowding
• Low education
• Poor access to healthcare
• Unemployment (poor treatment compliance)
Immunocompromised state
• HIV infection
• Malnutrition
• Chronic kidney disease
• Smoking
• Diabetes mellitus
• Liver cirrhosis
• Pneumoconiosis
Local joint and tissue factors
• History of trauma
• Surgical trauma
• Rheumatoid arthritis, SLE, Sjogren syndrome
• Gout
• Sickle cell disease
• Prosthetic joints
Drugs
• Anti-tumor necrosis factor drugs
• Glucocorticoids (>10 mg/day prednisolone equivalent)

epidemiology of TB as the majority of the TB burden lies in developing countries. HIV is associated with an increased incidence of TB although the introduction of antiretroviral therapy has shown a decline in TB cases. Tuberculous infection can be the first presentation of an underlying HIV infection hence HIV should be considered in the initial workup of all patients. Various other immunocompromised states as described in Table 12.1 increase the risk for TB. The use of disease-modifying anti-rheumatic drugs (DMARDs) is also associated with an increased risk for TB. Local joint and tissue factors like underlying rheumatoid arthritis, gout, prosthetic joints, and sickle cell disease make the joint more prone to secondary infections [7]. NTM infections have been associated with previous injury, puncture wounds, and orthopedic surgery.

12.5   Clinical Manifestations

The clinical spectrum of musculoskeletal manifestations of TB can be divided into four main categories as proposed by Franco-Paredes and colleagues [8].

1. Direct involvement of the musculoskeletal system
2. Emergence of TB during treatment of rheumatic disease
3. Rheumatic disorders precipitated by treatment of TB
4. Reactive immunological phenomenon in the setting of TB

12.5.1 Direct Involvement of the Musculoskeletal System

Musculoskeletal infections caused by mycobacteria are difficult to diagnose due to the indolent course and localized nature of the disease. Diagnosis is often delayed by months as the disease initially presents with nonspecific pain which may be mistaken for soft tissue rheumatism. Constitutional symptoms may be subtle or absent and inflammatory markers may be normal. Evidence of active or past infection is found in less than 50% of patients. Correct diagnosis can be established only by demonstrating the infectious agent by pathological or microbiological techniques.

Spondylitis (Pott's disease) is the most common manifestation comprising almost half of all tuberculous musculoskeletal infections, followed by arthritis and osteomyelitis. Tuberculous infection of soft tissue, including bursitis, tenosynovitis, myositis, and fasciitis, is uncommon.

12.5.1.1 Spondylitis (Pott's Disease)

TB spondylitis most commonly affects the lower thoracic and lumbar spine (Fig. 12.1a). Involvement of the cervical and upper thoracic spine is less common. The infection usually begins with inflammation of the anterior aspect of the intervertebral joint in the cancellous part of the bone. It spreads over a couple of months

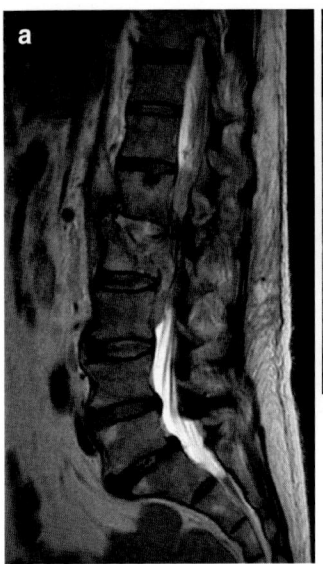
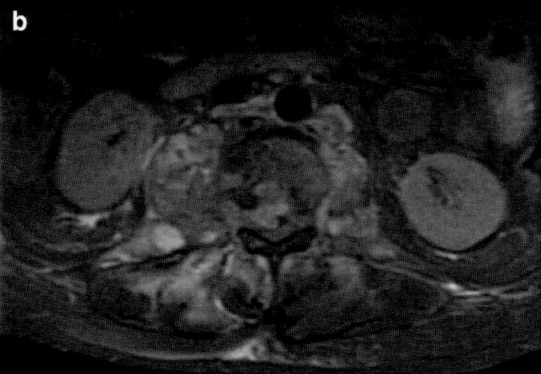

Fig. 12.1 Sagittal and axial T2 fat-suppressed images of the lumbar spine showing tuberculous spondylodiscitis at L1 L2 level. (**a**) There is an intradiscal abscess and marrow edema in both vertebrae, the superior endplate of L2 is eroded and a compression fracture of the vertebra is evident. There is also an associated anterior epidural soft tissue mass causing compression of the thecal sac. (**b**) Axial images at the same level demonstrate pedicular destruction, bilateral paravertebral abscesses (cold abscess), and an inflammatory collection in the right paraspinal muscles. (Courtesy of Dr. Shoma Mukherjee)

to involve the adjacent vertebrae. Once the adjacent vertebra is involved, the avascular disc dies and there is vertebral collapse anteriorly, leading to the formation of a gibbus deformity. This distorts the spinal canal anatomy which can cause compression of the spinal cord. The risk of spinal cord compression is maximum at the mid-thoracic level where the spinal canal is tight and can lead to paraparesis. A paravertebral abscess is a common finding which begins with an extension of infection under the anterior longitudinal ligament (Fig. 12.1b). At the cervical level, it can spread into the retropharyngeal space and affect the craniocervical junction. At the lumbar level, it can spread along the psoas muscle to present as a swelling in the inguinal or gluteal region. Occasionally, it can present as a stand-alone swelling without bony involvement.

The most common symptom is backache with localized pain and tenderness which increases on hyperextension of the spine. Pain may occur at the night and may be worse in the morning making it difficult to differentiate it from spondyloarthritis. Occasionally, pain may increase with cough or sneezing. Constitutional symptoms such as fever and weight loss may be seen in less than 40% of the patients [9]. In advanced cases, a characteristic "Alderman's gait" has been described where the patient walks with his head and chest thrown backward, protuberant abdomen, and wide-based gait to avoid jarring of the spine. Involvement of the cervical spine is rare but can present with symptoms of neck pain, dysphagia, hoarseness, torticollis and quadriparesis in advanced cases.

12.5.1.2 Arthritis

Tuberculous arthritis is the second most common presentation after Pott's spine. The classical presentation is a chronic monoarthritis affecting large weight-bearing joints, mainly hip and knee (Fig. 12.2). Other joints such as the sacroiliac joints, shoulders, elbows, wrists, ankles, and feet can also be involved (Fig. 12.3a and b). An oligoarticular or polyarticular involvement is uncommon but it is occasionally seen in the elderly, immunocompromised individuals, and children from endemic regions (where it may even be confused with juvenile idiopathic arthritis). The disease may initially start in either the synovium or the bone, but it ultimately tends to involve both parts of the joint. Patients present with pain and swelling of the joint with limitation of joint movement. The joint is usually cold to touch contrary to what is seen in bacterial septic arthritis. This is usually accompanied by a spasm of the overlying muscle to restrict joint movement to minimize the pain. Granulation tissue leads to synovial proliferation, joint effusion, and pannus formation which ultimately results in erosion of the articular cartilage leading to loss of joint space. Flexion deformities develop in long-standing disease which can be occasionally accompanied by a discharging sinus.

Hip involvement, apart from being the most common joint manifestation, is also the most difficult to diagnose and debilitating. It presents with mild to moderate pain in the groin or thigh along with difficulty bearing weight. Limping can be one of the earliest presentations, especially in children. The hip is generally held in a flexed and abducted posture at rest. Atrophy of the gluteal muscles may be seen in long-standing disease.

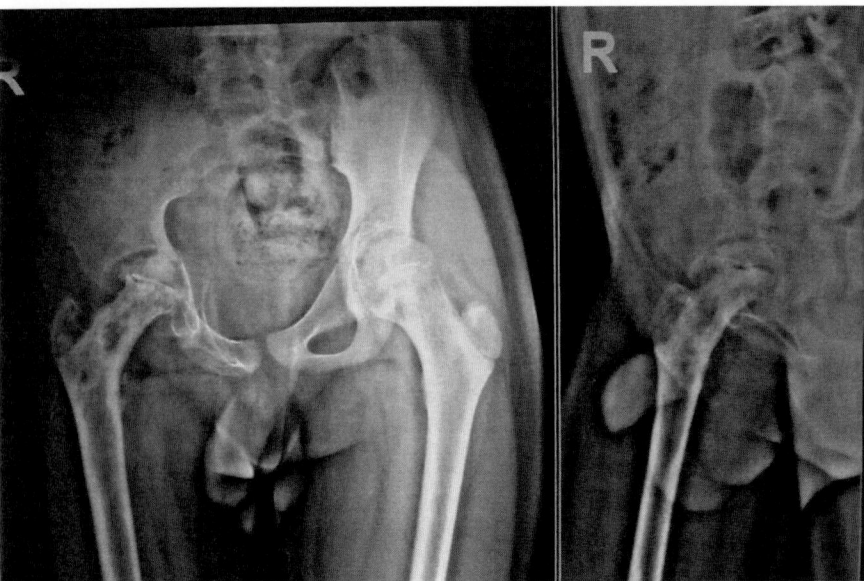

Fig. 12.2 Radiograph of the pelvis showing the destruction of the right hip following TB infection. Joint space is reduced with multiple erosions along the head of the femur. Multiple lytic lesions are also visible in the head, neck, and greater trochanter of the femur with the collapse of the head of the femur. There is also associated shortening of the affected leg. (Courtesy of Dr. Gurinder Bedi)

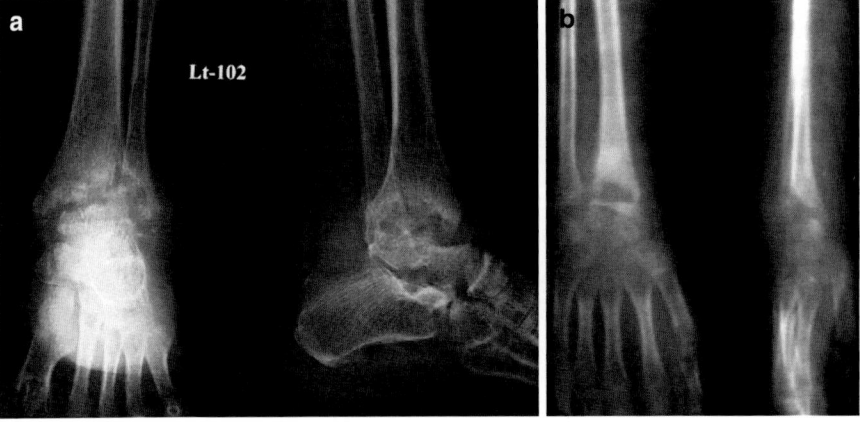

Fig. 12.3 Radiograph showing TB infection affecting ankle and wrist joints. (**a**) Reduction of joint space along with erosions and lytic lesions are seen affecting the lower end of the tibia, fibula, and talus which constitute the ankle joint. (**b**) Reduction of radiocarpal joint space and erosions are seen in the distal part of radius just proximal to the growth plate suggestive of tubercular involvement of the wrist joint. (Courtesy of Dr. Gurinder Bedi)

Sacroiliac joint involvement can be seen in up to 10% of cases involving TB of the musculoskeletal system [3]. Unilateral sacroiliitis should always raise the possibility of an infective etiology like TB or brucella, particularly where other features of spondyloarthritis are absent (Fig. 12.4). Patients usually present with unilateral buttock pain which radiates into the leg. Pain may aggravate during the night thus mimicking the pain of sacroiliitis due to spondyloarthritis. The presence of radiographic erosions, raised inflammatory markers, and a granulomatous picture on histology is often suggestive of TB.

Prosthetic joint infection is becoming more common with increased numbers of joint replacement surgeries being conducted. Usually, infection occurs due to the reactivation of latent disease in a previously destroyed joint. Removal of the prosthetic joint is often required for cure.

12.5.1.3 Osteomyelitis

Tuberculous osteomyelitis constitutes 2–3% of osteoarticular TB. Although any bone can be involved, TB commonly affects the long bones (femur and tibia) and hand bones (metacarpals, metatarsals, and phalanges) causing dactylitis (Fig. 12.5). The involvement of ribs, skull, and pelvis is also known. Seeding of bacilli occurs in the medullary cavity and the infection usually begins in the metaphysis. From there the infection can spread to the growth plate and also involve the adjacent joint. Patients usually present with pain, swelling, and discharging sinus early in the course of the disease. The involvement of growth plates in children can impair their growth, cause limb length discrepancies and deformities. The lesions are usually solitary though a multifocal presentation may be seen in children and

Fig. 12.4 STIR image of sacroiliac joint showing unilateral sacroiliitis due to TB on the right side. There is extensive involvement of both the iliac and sacral sides of the joint. Note the presence of edema in the adjoining muscles (arrows) suggesting a spread of the inflammation beyond the joint margin, highly suggestive of an infective etiology

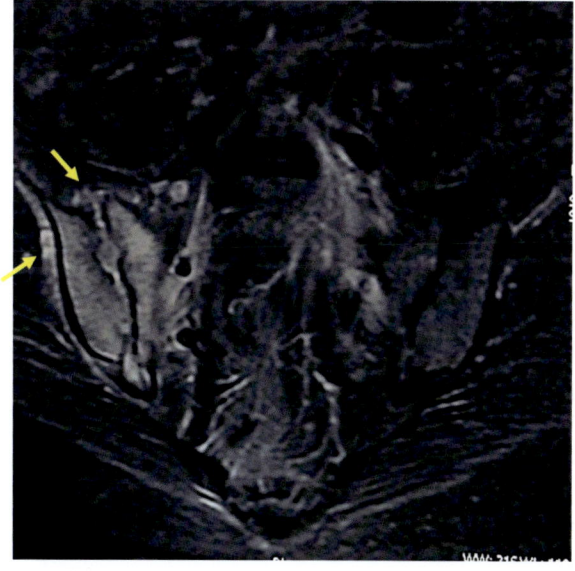

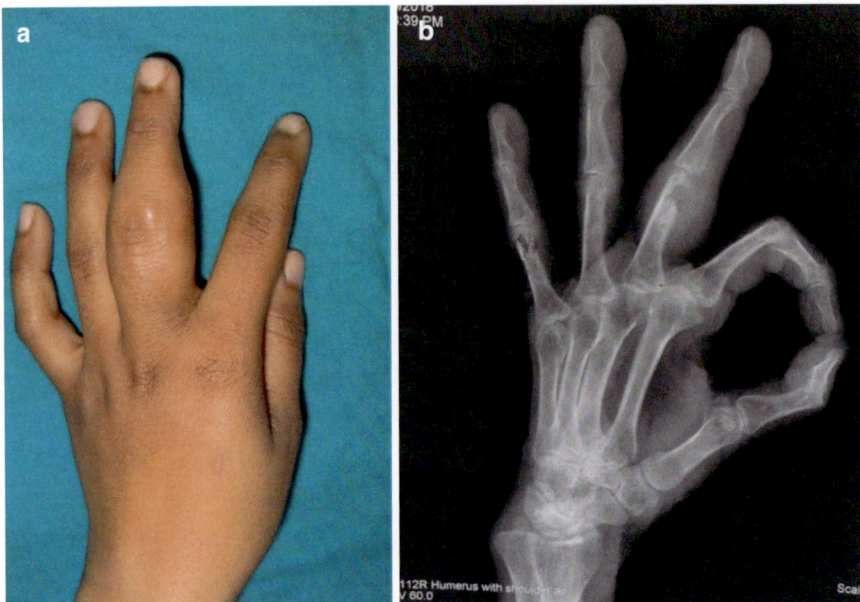

Fig. 12.5 Dactylitis affecting the left middle finger in a child due to TB. (**a**) Clinical image of left hand showing spindle sausage-like swelling involving the middle finger suggestive of dactylitis. (**b**) The corresponding radiograph shows a lytic lesion in the distal part of the proximal phalanx along with soft tissue swelling suggestive of TB (Courtesy of Dr. Gurinder Bedi)

immunocompromised individuals. Sternal osteomyelitis is known to occur after coronary bypass surgery. Lytic lesions of TB in the pubic symphysis and elbow can be mistaken for malignancy.

12.5.2 The Emergence of TB During Treatment of Rheumatic Disease

Immunosuppressive medications, required for treating systemic rheumatic diseases increase the risk of tubercular infections. TNF-alpha plays a key role in the formation and stabilization of granuloma. The use of anti-TNF drugs destabilizes the granuloma and results in the reactivation of infection. Studies have shown that TNF inhibitor use is associated with a fourfold increased risk of TB in patients with rheumatoid arthritis [10]. Among TNF inhibitors, adalimumab and infliximab are associated with a greater risk for reactivation of TB than etanercept [11, 12]. TB reactivation often occurs within a year of the onset of therapy. Screening for latent TB infection and treating it (3–6 months of isoniazid alone or isoniazid plus rifampicin) has led to a 78% reduction in TB infection [13]. For other TNF inhibitors (golimumab and certolizumab) and tocilizumab (an IL-6 receptor blocker), data regarding TB incidence has not been evaluated in randomized studies but screening for latent TB is indicated for all. Increased risk has been not been seen with the use of rituximab or abatacept [14]. Apart from biologicals, glucocorticoid use has also been shown to be a risk factor for TB reactivation. However, the risk appears to be dose-dependent and doses above 10 mg equivalent of prednisolone have been associated with an increased risk of TB [15].

12.5.3 Rheumatic Disorders Precipitated by Treatment of TB

A variety of rheumatic manifestations have been reported with anti-tuberculous therapy (ATT). Drug-induced lupus can occur with isoniazid. Presentation is mild with symptoms like fever, rash, arthralgia, and occasionally serositis. Systemic involvement is rare. ANA is positive with specificity for anti-histone antibodies. It is usually a benign self-limited condition that resolves on discontinuation of therapy. Pyrazinamide interferes with uric acid excretion and causes hyperuricemia. This hyperuricemia is mostly asymptomatic but it can occasionally precipitate gout. Fluoroquinolones are associated with tendinopathy with a higher predilection for involvement of Achilles tendon. Among patients, who develop TB on infliximab therapy, paradoxical reactions have been reported after withdrawal of infliximab [16]. They present as worsening of preexisting TB lesions or development of new lesions. The reason for this is not completely understood but it is similar to immune reconstitution inflammatory syndrome seen in patients with HIV. Escalation of therapy is generally not required though glucocorticoids may be required in severe cases.

12.5.4 Reactive Immunological Phenomenon in the Setting of TB

An immunological phenomenon associated with M. tuberculosis infection is uncommon. Poncet's disease is aseptic inflammatory arthritis primarily involving large peripheral joints such as knees, ankles, and elbows. Small joints can also be involved occasionally. It is nonerosive and can clinically present as symmetric or asymmetric, oligo or polyarticular disease. It is always associated with active pulmonary, extra-pulmonary, or miliary TB. Pathogenesis is unclear but there appears to be an immune-mediated hypersensitivity to mycobacterial antigen [17]. Tuberculin test is strongly positive and inflammatory markers may be raised. Autoantibodies are absent and there is no microbiological evidence of TB in the joints. It resolves within a few weeks of initiation of ATT. Generally, NSAIDs are sufficient for controlling the symptoms however in severe cases glucocorticoids may be required.

Rarely, reactive arthritis may occur in 0.4–0.8% of bladder cancer patients treated with intravesical BCG (Bacille Calmette-Guerin) immunotherapy [18].

Other immunological manifestations like erythema nodosum, erythema induratum, and amyloidosis have also been described in the setting of TB.

12.6 Imaging

There are no pathognomonic radiographic features that can establish a diagnosis of arthritis in TB. MRI may be useful in early disease; however, radiographic changes appear only in long-standing disease. A chest radiograph should always be obtained to rule out any evidence of coexisting pulmonary TB. Ultrasound is usually not helpful. CT scan can help establish the extent of bone destruction and aid in identifying the site for biopsy.

12.6.1 Conventional Radiography

Radiographs are normal in the early course of the disease. Spondylitis is characterized by a reduction in vertebral height with anterior wedging. There may be irregularity in the endplate and anterior vertebral margin. The classical feature of TB arthritis is the "Phemister's triad" which includes juxta-articular osteoporosis, peripheral erosions, and gradual joint space narrowing. Periarticular destruction should raise the suspicion of TB. TB osteomyelitis presents with lytic lesions in the affected bone. Periosteal reaction around lytic areas where the cortical bone is superficial like in digits, tibia, and ulna is an important feature that can help differentiate TB.

12.6.2 MRI

MRI is particularly useful to evaluate the extent of soft tissue collections and spinal cord involvement in spondylitis. Usual findings of bone marrow edema with contrast rim enhancement suggest a possibility of infection. When differentiating an infectious cause from an inflammatory cause such as in cases of unilateral sacroiliitis, a golden rule to remember is that inflammation occurring secondary to infection crosses anatomical borders. The presence of periarticular muscle edema has good accuracy for diagnosing infections (Fig. 12.4) [19].

12.7 Diagnosis

The key to making a diagnosis of TB is to have a high index of suspicion. Table 12.2 highlights the conditions in which a diagnosis of TB should be suspected [20]. Imaging and other tests may increase the suspicion of TB but histopathological and microbiological techniques are necessary for making a diagnosis. Tissue biopsy is usually required for the same.

Table 12.2 Conditions when to suspect a diagnosis of osteoarticular tuberculosis

Back pain with any of the following
• Nonmechanical pain, worse in the morning and aggravates with hyperextension of the spine
• Pain on coughing or sneezing (red flag sign)
• Presence of neurological features
• Localized tenderness with or without gibbus deformity

Monoarthritis or localized infection with any of the following
• Immigrant from an endemic region or recent visit to an endemic region
• History of TB in the past or history of contact with an active TB patient
• Presence of HIV infection or chronic renal disease
• Presence of constitutional symptoms of fever, weight loss, and night sweats
• Recent use of anti-TNF drugs or high dose GCs

Inflammatory arthritis not responding to intra-articular steroid injections

Oligo-arthritis or polyarthritis in debilitated children, elderly, or immunocompromised individuals

Dactylitis in children

GCs glucocorticoids, *HIV* human immunodeficiency virus, *TNF* tumor necrosis factor

Table 12.3 Causes of false-positive and false-negative tuberculin sensitivity test

Causes of false-positive results	Causes of false-negative results
BCG vaccination	Age > 70 years
Nontuberculous mycobacteria	Glucocorticoids (>15 mg/day prednisolone equivalent)
History of TB infection in past	HIV infection
	Hypoalbuminemia
	Azotemia
	Impaired cellular immunity
	Malnourished people
	Disseminated miliary tuberculosis
	Sarcoidosis

12.7.1 Screening Tests

Tuberculin skin test (TST) is the most widely used screening test despite having low sensitivity and specificity (~70%). A reaction of more than 10 mm is considered to be indicative of a prior exposure to mycobacterial infection. It is more helpful in the developed countries where the natural infection rate is low and routine BCG vaccination is not done as these can give rise to false-positive tests. A false-negative test may be seen in malnourished people and HIV. Table 12.3 provides a list of causes of false-positive and negative TST.

Interferon-γ release assays measure the production of IFN-γ by whole-blood mononuclear cells stimulated by specific M. tuberculosis antigens. It is more reliable than TST, especially in BCG vaccinated population and HIV infected individuals where the possibility of false-positive and negative results is high. Both these tests are useful in diagnosing latent TB infection however they cannot predict the development of disease.

12.7.2 Synovial Fluid Analysis

Synovial fluid evaluation reveals an inflammatory fluid with nonspecific features. Low glucose may favor the diagnosis [21]. The fluid may have a predominance of either polymorphs or mononuclear cells. An AFB smear is positive in only 20% of cases whereas a culture may yield results in up to 80% of cases [21]. GeneXpert MTB assay has a poor sensitivity of about 60% in synovial fluid however the specificity is high [22].

12.7.3 Biopsy and Culture

Synovial biopsy has a yield of more than 90% [21]. Bone biopsy should be obtained wherever feasible, possibly under CT guidance. In the presence of a draining sinus, culture from the discharge may be useful however growth of contaminant bacteria and fungi are common, so the results should be interpreted carefully. GeneXpert MTB assay can detect mycobacteria as well as rifampicin/isoniazid resistance. It has a high sensitivity of 82% and a specificity of almost 98% for the detection of TB in both pus and tissue [23].

12.8   Treatment

Treatment of osteoarticular TB involves a combination chemotherapy regimen to prevent the development of resistance against the drugs. First-line therapy includes four drugs, i.e., Isoniazid (H), Rifampicin (R), Pyrazinamide (Z), and Ethambutol (E) also known as HRZE therapy. They have been detailed in Table 12.4. Recommended treatment duration varies according to the TB endemicity in the region. US CDC recommends a 6–9 months course of therapy (2 months of intensive therapy with HRZE followed by 4–7 months of RH) [24]. However, in endemic regions, a minimum treatment duration of 12 months is recommended (2 months of HRZE followed by 10–16 months of HRE) for TB involving bone and joints due to increasing incidence of drug resistance and high rates of relapse [25]. Longer courses of therapy may be required in slow responders and the response is guided by improvement in clinical parameters like fever, pain, discharge, and mobility. Radiological signs of bone healing include remineralization of affected bone on X-rays. On MRI, resolution of marrow edema, fatty replacement in the marrow, and absence of contrast enhancement indicates healed lesions.

Surgical treatment is seldom indicated in the initial management of patients. Surgical debridement may be required where the response to therapy is inadequate. In the case of a prosthetic joint, removal of the prosthesis is usually necessary for the complete resolution of infection. Radiographic damage is usually irreversible. Joint replacement procedures may be required after completion of therapy where there is advanced destruction of the joint. Surgical correction may be required for kyphosis of more than 40°.

Although the incidence of initial drug resistance in osteoarticular TB is low due to the low burden of bacilli in lesions (10^5–10^6), still emergence of multidrug-resistant

Table 12.4 Drug regimens recommended for treatment of musculoskeletal tuberculosis

	Regimen of drugs	Dose	Side effects of major first-line drugs
Latent TB infection	Low endemic regions • Rifampicin alone for 4 months [4R][a] or • Isoniazid alone for 6–9 months [6H] High endemic regions • Isoniazid and rifampicin for 3 months[b] [3HR]	Rifampicin (10 mg/kg) Isoniazid (5 mg/kg)	Rifampicin—Hepatitis Isoniazid—Hepatitis, peripheral neuropathy Pyrazinamide— Hepatotoxicity, rash, arthropathy Ethambutol—Visual disturbance (optic
First-line TB therapy	Low endemic regions • 2HRZE + 4–7HR High endemic regions • 2HRZE + 10–16HRE (Substitute with FQ or AMG if there is rifampicin or isoniazid intolerance, and longer regimen is required in such a case)	Rifampicin (10 mg/kg) Isoniazid (5 mg/kg) Pyrazinamide (25 mg/kg) Ethambutol (20 mg/kg)	neuropathy, manifested as decreased visual acuity or red-green color blindness) at higher doses Streptomycin— Ototoxicity, vestibular toxicity, nephrotoxicity, electrolyte
Second-line TB therapy (organisms resistant to rifampicin and isoniazid)	Principles for second-line therapy • Intensive phase—5 drugs for 5–6 months • Continuation phase—4 drugs for 15–21 months Drug list • Levofloxacin or moxifloxacin (FQ) • Bedaquiline • Linezolid • Clofazimine • Cycloserine • Amikacin or streptomycin (AMG) (oral preferred over injectable drugs)	Use in consult with an infectious disease specialist	disturbances, local pain with IM injections Levofloxacin—GI toxicity, CNS effects, rash, dysglycemia, tendonitis, tendon rupture, QT prolongation

R Rifampicin, *H* Isoniazid, *Z* Pyrazinamide, *E* Ethambutol, *S* Streptomycin, *FQ* Fluoroquinolones, *AMG* Aminoglycosides
[a] Rifampicin based regimens are shorter and less hepatotoxic
[b] We prefer dual combination therapy in high endemic regions to prevent the drug resistance

(MDR-TB) and extremely drug-resistant (XDR-TB) variants remains a concern [26]. These variants fail to respond to first-line and second-line therapies and their incidence is evermore increasing in the population.

12.9 Conclusion

Tuberculosis is among the few rare causes of chronic arthritis, that present to a rheumatologist, which can be completely cured if treated early in the course of infection. Diagnosis of tuberculosis should be suspected in any patient presenting with chronic monoarthritis or back pain in the presence of risk factors that predispose a person to develop a tuberculous infection. Establishing the diagnosis relies on microbiological and histopathological techniques which can be challenging. Treatment lasts several months and compliance can be an issue, especially in lower socioeconomic countries. Surgery may be required for the correction of deformities in long-standing cases. There remains a large unmet need for more effective and shorter treatment regimens that can help reduce both morbidity and mortality.

References

1. Chakaya J, Khan M, Ntoumi F, et al. Global tuberculosis report 2020—reflections on the global TB burden, treatment and prevention efforts. Int J Infect Dis. 2021;113 Suppl 1(Suppl 1):S7–S12. issn:1201-9712. https://doi.org/10.1016/j.ijid.2021.02.107.
2. Hershkovitz I, Donoghue HD, Minnikin DE, et al. Detection and molecular characterization of 9,000-year-old Mycobacterium tuberculosis from a neolithic settlement in the Eastern Mediterranean. PLoS One. 2008;3(10):e3426.
3. Sharma SK, Mohan A. Extrapulmonary tuberculosis. Indian J Med Res. 2004;120(4):316–53.
4. Bloom BR. Tuberculosis—the global view. N Engl J Med. 2002;346(19):1434–5.
5. Harrington JT. Mycobacterial and fungal infections. In: Ruddy S, Harris Jr ED, Sledge CB, editors. Kelley's textbook of rheumatology. 6th ed. Philadelphia: WB Saunders; 2001. p. 1493–505.
6. Stead WW. Variation in vulnerability to tuberculosis in America today: random, or legacies of different ancestral epidemics? Int J Tuberc Lung Dis. 2001;5:807–14.
7. Hernandez-Cruz B, Sifuentes-Osornio J, Ponce-de-Leon RS, et al. Mycobacterium tuberculosis infection in patients with systemic rheumatic diseases. A case-series. Clin Exp Rheumatol. 1999;17:289–96.
8. Franco-Paredes C, Diaz-Borjon A, Senger MA, et al. The ever-expanding association between rheumatologic diseases and tuberculosis. Am J Med. 2006;119(6):470–7.
9. Fuentes Ferrer M, Gutiérrez Torres L, Ayala Ramírez O, et al. Tuberculosis of the spine. A systematic review of case series. Int Orthop. 2012;36(2):221–31.
10. Askling J, Fored CM, Brandt L, et al. Risk and case characteristics of tuberculosis in rheumatoid arthritis associated with tumor necrosis factor antagonists in Sweden. Arthritis Rheum. 2005;52(7):1986–92.
11. Tubach F, Salmon D, Ravaud P, et al.; Research Axed on Tolerance of Biotherapies Group. Risk of tuberculosis is higher with anti-tumor necrosis factor monoclonal antibody therapy than with soluble tumor necrosis factor receptor therapy: the three-year prospective French Research Axed on Tolerance of Biotherapies registry. Arthritis Rheum. 2009;60(7):1884–94.
12. Dixon WG, Hyrich KL, Watson KD, et al.; BSRBR Control Centre Consortium, Symmons DP; BSR Biologics Register. Drug-specific risk of tuberculosis in patients with rheumatoid arthritis treated with anti-TNF therapy: results from the British Society for Rheumatology Biologics Register (BSRBR). Ann Rheum Dis. 2010;69(3):522–8.
13. Carmona L, Gomez-Reino JJ, Rodriguez-Valverde V, et al. Effectiveness of recommendations to prevent reactivation of latent tuberculosis infection in patients treated with tumor necrosis factor antagonists. Arthritis Rheum. 2005;52(6):1766–72.
14. Cantini F, Niccoli L, Goletti D. Tuberculosis risk in patients treated with non-anti-tumor necrosis factor-α (TNF-α) targeted biologics and recently licensed TNF-α inhibitors: data from clinical trials and national registries. J Rheumatol Suppl. 2014;91:56–64.
15. Jick SS, Lieberman ES, Rahman MU, et al. Glucocorticoid use, other associated factors, and the risk of tuberculosis. Arthritis Rheum. 2006;55(1):19–26.
16. Garcia Vidal C, Rodriguez Fernandez S, Martinez Lacasa J, et al. Paradoxical response to anti-tuberculous therapy in infliximab-treated patients with disseminated tuberculosis. Clin Infect Dis. 2005;40(5):756–9.

17. Bhargava AD, Malaviya AN, Kumar A. Tuberculous rheumatism (Poncet's disease): a case series. Indian J Tuberculosis. 1998;45:215–9.
18. Hughes RA, Allard SA, Maini RN. Arthritis associated with adjuvant mycobacterial treatment for carcinoma of the bladder. Ann Rheum Dis. 1989;48:432–4.
19. Kang Y, Hong SH, Kim JY, et al. Unilateral sacroiliitis: differential diagnosis between infectious sacroiliitis and spondyloarthritis based on MRI findings. AJR Am J Roentgenol. 2015;205(5):1048–55.
20. Malaviya AN, Kotwal PP. Arthritis associated with tuberculosis. Best Pract Res Clin Rheumatol. 2003;17(2):319–43.
21. Mahowald ML. Chapter 128. Arthritis due to mycobacteria, fungi and parasites. In: Koopman WJ, editor. Arthritis and allied conditions. 14th ed. Philadelphia: Lippincott Williams & Wilkins; 2000.
22. Kai T, et al. Study on rapid diagnosis of knee joint tuberculosis by Xpert MTB/RIF. Chin J Antituberculosis. 2004;38(4):300–4.
23. Shen Y, Yu G, Zhong F, Kong X. Diagnostic accuracy of the Xpert MTB/RIF assay for bone and joint tuberculosis: a meta-analysis. PLoS One. 2019;14(8):e0221427.
24. American Thoracic Society, CDC, Infectious Diseases Society of America: recommendations for the treatment of tuberculosis. MMWR. 2003;52:1–77.
25. World Health Organization. Country Office for India. Index-TB guidelines: guidelines on extra-pulmonary tuberculosis in India. World Health Organization. Country Office for India; 2016. https://apps.who.int/iris/handle/10665/278953.
26. Shembekar A, Babhulkar S. Chemotherapy for osteoarticular tuberculosis. Clin Orthop. 2002;398:20–6.

Arthritis in Leprosy

13

Rasmi Ranjan Sahoo, Manesh Manoj,
and Anupam Wakhlu ⓘ

13.1 Introduction

Leprosy, also called Hansen's disease, is known since ancient times and is caused by the *Mycobacterium leprae complex* comprising *M. leprae* and *M. lepromatosis*. The bacterium multiplies extremely slowly inside the human host, which may result in disease manifestations up to 20 years after infection. The disease and its long-term complications have been associated with considerable social stigma; the disease often remains undiagnosed initially, mainly due to a lack of awareness and suspicion in an appropriate clinical context. The introduction of multidrug therapy (MDT) had led to the elimination of leprosy from several parts of the world by the year 2000. However, the disease continues to be a major public health concern in many developing countries. The relative paucity of available facilities for disease detection and eradication in the developing world has failed to control the incidence of cases and development of grade 2 disability (as defined by WHO, presence of deformities or visible damage involving hands, feet, and/or eyes) over the last decade [1]. Approximately 0.2 million cases were diagnosed across 161 countries in 2019, with major contributions from India, Brazil, Indonesia, and Bangladesh [2]. Human migration and autochthonous transmission have contributed to the emergence of the disease in other parts of the world.

Leprosy primarily affects the skin and peripheral nerves, although involvement of the upper respiratory tract and eyes are also common [3]. Skin lesions are typically hypoesthetic or anesthetic, hypopigmented or erythematous, and can present as macules, papules, plaques, or nodules. Nerve involvement is characteristic of

R. R. Sahoo · A. Wakhlu (✉)
Department of Clinical Immunology and Rheumatology, Apollomedics Super Speciality Hospitals, Lucknow, UP, India

M. Manoj
AKG Memorial Cooperative Hospital and Dr. Shenoy's Care, Kannur, Kerala, India

© The Author(s), under exclusive license to Springer Nature Switzerland AG 2022
V. Ravindran et al. (eds.), *Rarer Arthropathies*, Rare Diseases of the Immune System, https://doi.org/10.1007/978-3-031-05002-2_13

leprosy, with great auricular, ulnar, and common peroneal nerves being commonly involved. In the absence of typical skin disease, the disease poses a diagnostic dilemma to physicians. Musculoskeletal manifestations can be seen in up to three-quarters of patients and at times be the presenting manifestation [4]. Clinical manifestations indistinguishable from rheumatoid arthritis (RA), systemic lupus erythematosus (SLE), and dermatomyositis are also well-known [5, 6]. Besides, RA and leprosy can coexist.

13.2   Epidemiology

The prevalence of leprosy-related arthritis was evaluated in one large study of 1257 patients and reported a low frequency of 4.4% among the study participants [7]. A similar frequency of rheumatic manifestations was reported in an older study [8]. Acute-onset symmetric polyarthritis is the most common presentation and is often triggered by a reactional state. However, a higher frequency of joint involvement has been described in hospital-based studies and with the inclusion of patients with lepra reactions.

13.3   Pathophysiology

The pathogenic mechanisms of arthritis in leprosy include direct synovium invasion by *M. leprae, a* reactive phenomenon to mycobacterial antigens, and inflammation due to immune-complex deposition and complement breakdown, particularly in patients of erythema nodosum leprosum (ENL) [5]. Peripheral nerve involvement causing destructive arthropathy (Charcot joint) is also seen in leprosy.

13.4   Clinical Features

Joint involvement in leprosy can be broadly classified as acute oligo- and polyarthritis, chronic arthritis, and neuropathic arthropathy [4].

13.4.1 Arthritis Related to Lepra Reactions

Lepra type 1 or reversal reaction, usually occurs in borderline disease and presents either simultaneously or even after initiation of MDT [9]. Type 1 reactions may be upgrading (improvement in cellular immunity of the host, with a shift of lesions towards tuberculoid disease) or downgrading (further worsening of the immune status of the host with lack of reactivity to lepra bacilli, with a shift of lesions towards lepromatous disease) [10]. Type 2 reactional state manifests as erythema nodosum leprosum (ENL) in patients with lepromatous or borderline lepromatous disease. The appearance of new skin lesions or inflammation in preexisting skin lesions with or without neuritis characterize type 1 reaction, whereas erythema nodosum leprosum is a multisystem disease characterized by high-grade fever, tender erythematous nodules, lymphadenopathy, neuritis, orchitis, arthritis, and eye involvement. Type 1 reaction is due to delayed-type hypersensitivity (DTH) whereas type 2 reaction is immune-complex mediated.

The pattern of joint involvement is similar in both forms, manifesting as symmetric polyarthritis or oligoarthritis, affecting hand joints commonly and mimicking classic RA [11]. Involvement of shoulders, elbows, wrists, knees, and ankles is also seen. The arthritis is usually nonerosive and either resolves over a few weeks to months or becomes chronic, till appropriate therapy is instituted. Radiological evidence of erosions can be seen [11]. A recent cross-sectional study by the Erythema Nodosum Leprosum International STudy (ENLIST) group, which included 292 patients of borderline and pure lepromatous leprosy patients, reported arthritis in 105 patients (36%), with large joint involvement being the most common [12]. Dactylitis was seen in 14% of patients in the above study.

The frequency of acute polyarthritis, chronic arthritis similar to RA, and neuropathic joint in an Indian cohort of leprosy patients was 17%, 24%, and 3%, respectively [13]. Lepra reactions were common, predominantly of type 2 reaction. Symmetric polyarthritis affecting small and large joints is common in the reactional state, compared to oligoarticular and monoarticular involvement [14]. The study by Pereira et al. found a reactional state, predominantly ENL, in 50 of 79 leprosy patients with joint involvement [7]. The joints frequently involved were wrists, proximal interphalangeal (PIP), metacarpophalangeal (MCP), knees and metatarsophalangeal (MTP), in that order. In a cohort of 44 patients with leprosy, acute-onset polyarthritis involving small and large joints was seen in 32% and oligoarticular involvement in 16% of patients [15]. Twenty-eight patients (64%) presented with ENL in the above study.

13.4.2 Chronic Arthritis in Leprosy

Chronic arthritis is also known to occur in leprosy [16]. The arthritis is insidious in onset and may manifest as long as 7 years after the onset of leprosy symptoms. There can be periods of exacerbations and remissions. Long-standing arthritis with a mean duration of 11 years involving small joints, with or without large joints was reported in one study [17]. Wrists, knees, MTP joints, MCP, and PIP joints of the hands are commonly affected. Involvement of the sacroiliac joint is also known and bilateral sacroiliitis can be a presentation [17]. Erosions can also be seen.

13.4.3 Neuropathic Arthropathy

Neuropathic arthropathy or Charcot joint due to leprosy is a known complication of long-standing disease, manifesting as a destructive joint involvement with dislocations and/or pathological fractures. Weight-bearing joints of the lower limbs are commonly affected. The exact prevalence of Charcot's arthropathy in leprosy is likely underestimated and may contribute substantially to the disability associated with leprosy in endemic countries.

13.4.4 Swollen Hands and Feet Syndrome (SHFS)

Swollen hands with or without feet involvement is a distinct entity, first described in 1980 [18]. The swelling typically extends from mid-forearm proximally to MCP joints distally and is usually pitting in nature. The pathology includes inflammation extending beyond the synovium involving the subcutaneous tissue thus differentiating it from RA in which it is limited to the joint capsule. SHFS can mimic remitting seronegative symmetrical synovitis with pitting edema (RS3PE), warranting careful evaluation for leprosy. RS3PE is a distinctive syndrome seen in isolation or associated with connective tissue diseases and malignancies. SHFS is common in leprosy, with a study including predominantly lepromatous disease reporting it in 10 out of 16 patients with rheumatic manifestations [19]. SHFS was also reported in 20% of patients in an Indian cohort [13].

13.4.5 Tenosynovitis and Enthesitis

Tenosynovitis associated with arthritis or in isolation is reported in leprosy and can be the presenting manifestation. Isolated tenosynovitis often poses a diagnostic challenge. Calcaneal enthesophytes can be seen in leprosy patients, mainly those with a lepromatous disease, compared to age- and sex-matched healthy controls [20]. Enthesitis is also seen.

The frequency of different patterns of joint involvement described in leprosy among various studies are shown in Table 13.1.

13.5 Diagnosis

The diagnosis of leprosy requires a high index of clinical suspicion, along with a detailed physical examination, especially of the palpable peripheral nerves. The presence of hypoesthetic skin rash and evidence of peripheral nerve involvement often clinches the diagnosis. The objective finding of a thickened and tender nerve trunk with hypoesthesia or rarely hyperesthesia in its distribution is almost exclusive to leprosy. A thickened great auricular nerve is often visible and suggests the diagnosis. Focal loss of hair and loss of temperature sensations may be early signs and need to be looked for. The clinical manifestations characteristic of leprosy are shown in Figs. 13.1, 13.2, 13.3, 13.4, 13.5, 13.6, 13.7, and 13.8. The examination of the musculoskeletal system would reveal arthritis, tenosynovitis, dactylitis, etc.

Table 13.1 Frequency of different patterns of joint involvement in leprosy among various studies[a]

	Wakhlu et al. (n = 29) [13]	Prasad et al. (n = 44) [15]	Sarkar et al. (n = 102) [14]	Salvi and Chopra (n = 33) [6]	Pereira et al. (n = 79) [7]
Acute polyarthritis	5 (17.2)	14 (31.8)	49 (48)	28 (84.8)	55 (69.6)[b]
Chronic arthritis akin to RA	7 (24.1)	–	–	–	–
Neuropathic arthropathy (Charcot's joint)	1 (3.4)	1 (2.2)	0	0	–
Tenosynovitis	5 (17.2)	9 (20.4)	16 (15.7)	0	–
SHFS	6 (20.7)	11 (25)	0	0	–
Lepra reaction	15 (51.7)	28 (63.6)	43 (42.1)	15 (45.4)	50 (63.2)
ENL	13 (44.8)	28 (63.6)	13 (12.7)	9 (27.2)	35 (44.3)

RA Rheumatoid arthritis, *SHFS* Swollen hands and feet syndrome, *ENL* Erythema nodosum leprosum

[a] Values are shown as numbers, *n* (%)

[b] Remaining patients had arthralgia

Fig. 13.1 Erythematous nodules over the face in a patient with erythema nodosum leprosum

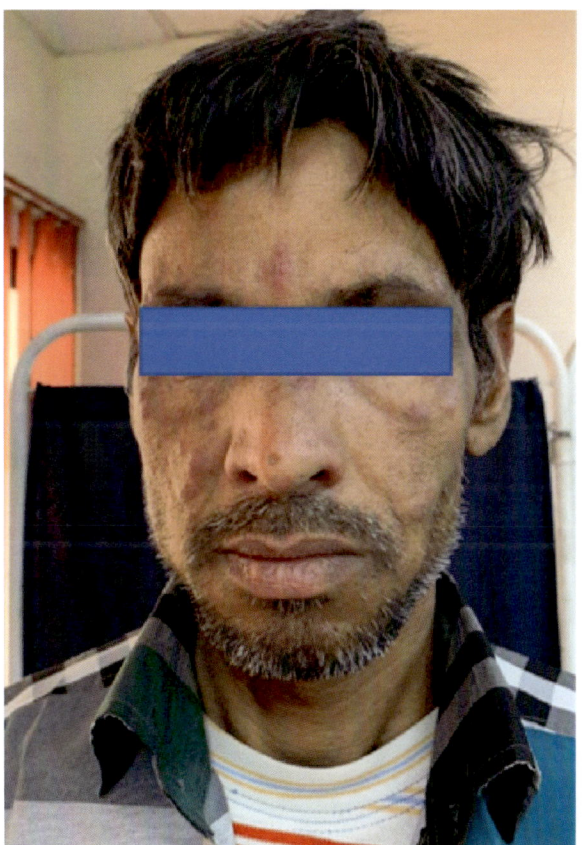

Fig. 13.2 Involvement of ear cartilage and lobule in leprosy

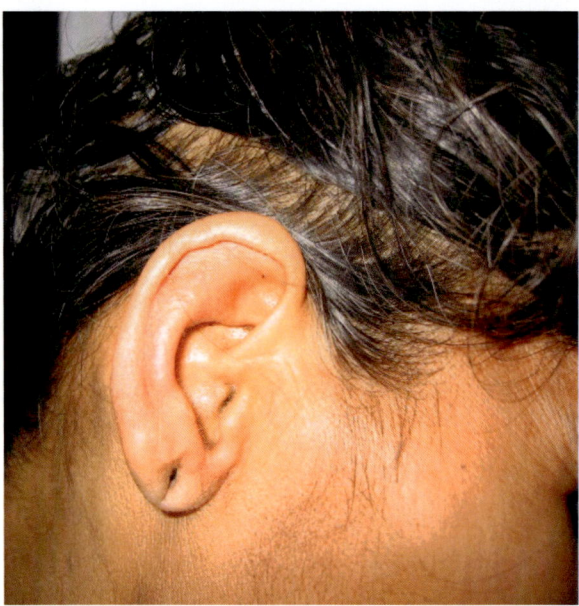

13.5.1 Laboratory

Inflammatory parameters such as ESR and CRP may be modestly elevated, especially in reactional states. The diagnosis of leprosy is mainly clinical, microbiological, and histological. Autoantibodies may be unreliable when differentiating leprosy mimicking rheumatic diseases from actual rheumatic diseases, as rheumatoid factor (RF) and antinuclear antibody (ANA) positivity can be seen in one-third of patients, with a higher frequency in lepromatous disease [21]. Antibodies against citrullinated proteins (ACPA) are less common in leprosy and if seen, are in low titers [22]. False-positive anti-neutrophil cytoplasmic antibody on immunofluorescence is also common, although antibodies against proteinase 3 and myeloperoxidase are uncommon. Demonstration of *M. leprae* in the synovial fluid of affected joints is usually difficult but can be done [4].

13.5.2 Radiology

The frequency of radiological findings in leprosy arthritis varies among studies and is more prevalent among patients with long-standing disease and those with deformities. The specific bone changes in hands and feet include honeycombing, bone cyst, thinning and irregularity of cortex, areas of bone destruction, and primary periostitis [23]. Absorption of terminal phalanges, subluxation/dislocation of joints, soft tissue, and paranasal sinus changes are common nonspecific bone findings. Besides, osteopenia is also common.

Fig. 13.3 Hyperpigmented and hypoesthetic macules over legs in leprosy

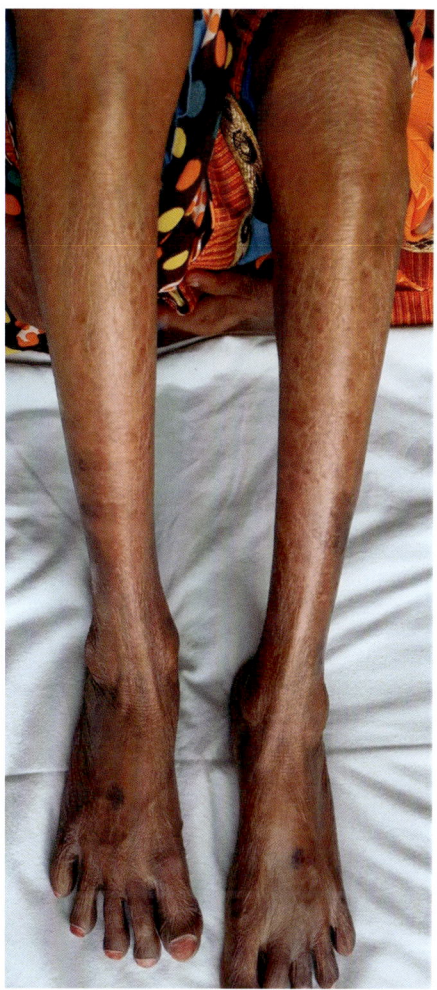

13.5.3 Histology

Slit skin smear and histopathological examination of skin or nerve biopsy specimens with appropriate stains confirm the diagnosis. A synovial biopsy may demonstrate granulomatous inflammation in patients with chronic arthritis [4].

13.6 Differential Diagnosis

Musculoskeletal manifestations in leprosy mimic various rheumatic diseases and is a diagnostic challenge to the caregivers, especially in endemic countries. Patients with indeterminate leprosy or paucibacillary disease present with one or few skin

Fig. 13.4 Erythema
nodosum in leprosy

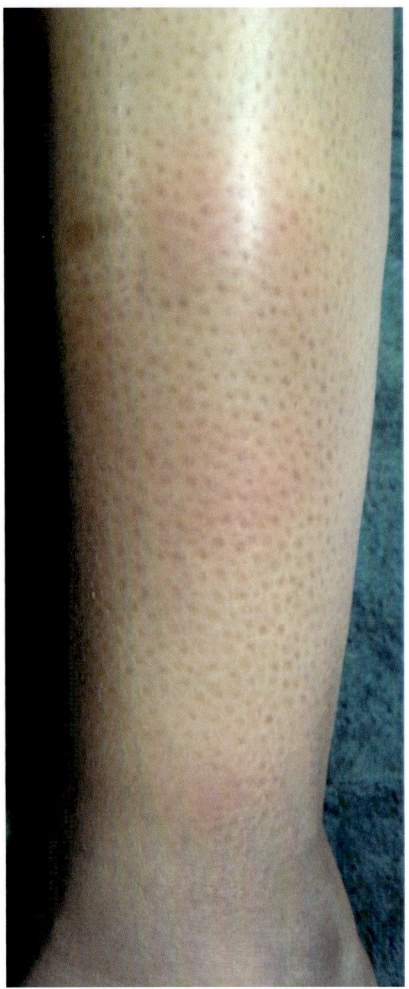

lesions and can be difficult to identify in dark-skinned people. Mild sensory symptoms or pure neuritic presentation in the absence of skin lesions tend to be overlooked. When rheumatic manifestations predominate, one tends to focus less on cutaneous and peripheral nerve examination. Arthritis, with or without tenosynovitis and dactylitis is commonly misdiagnosed as spondyloarthritis including reactive arthritis. Chronic symmetric polyarthritis often mimics RA and the diagnosis is further confounded by the presence of bone erosions and low-titer RF. The coexistence of leprosy with rheumatoid arthritis often complicates the issue and needs to be resolved for the institution of appropriate therapy. Characteristic joint involvement, erosive disease, high-titer RF/ACPA positivity, lack of response of arthritis to leprosy medicines are points favoring RA. The various rheumatic mimics of leprosy are summarized in Table 13.2.

Fig. 13.5 Thickened great auricular nerve (black arrowhead) in a patient with erythema nodosum leprosum

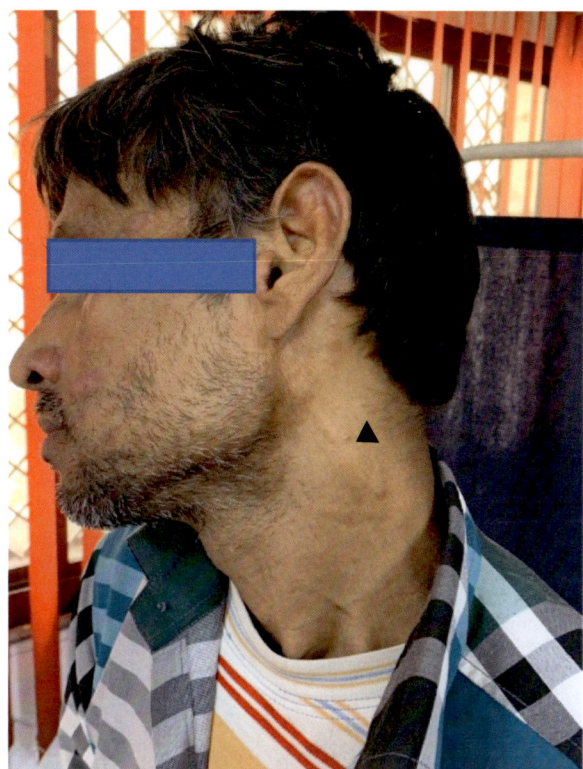

Fig. 13.6 Swollen hands with a diffuse erythematous rash over right forearm and hand in lepromatous leprosy

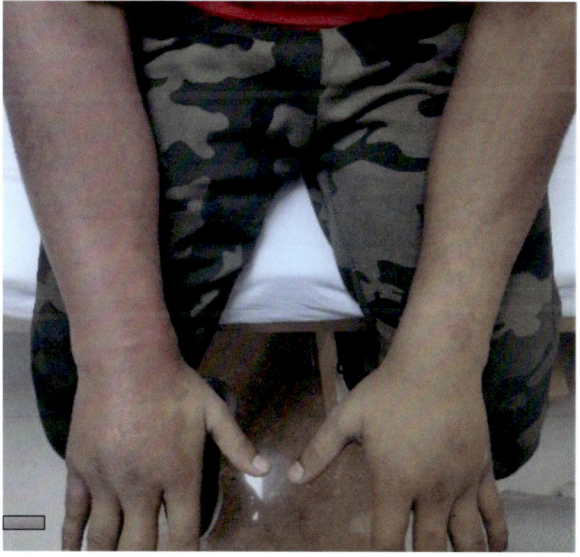

Fig. 13.7 Left second toe
dactylitis and bilateral
ankle arthritis with
hyperpigmented and
hypoesthetic macules in
leprosy

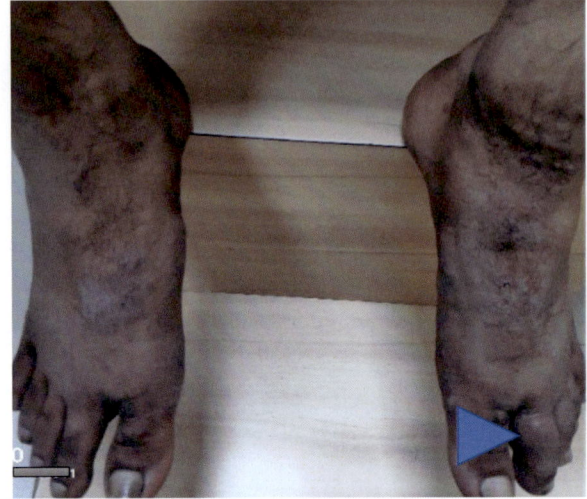

Fig. 13.8 Left ankle
arthritis with
hyperpigmented macules
in leprosy

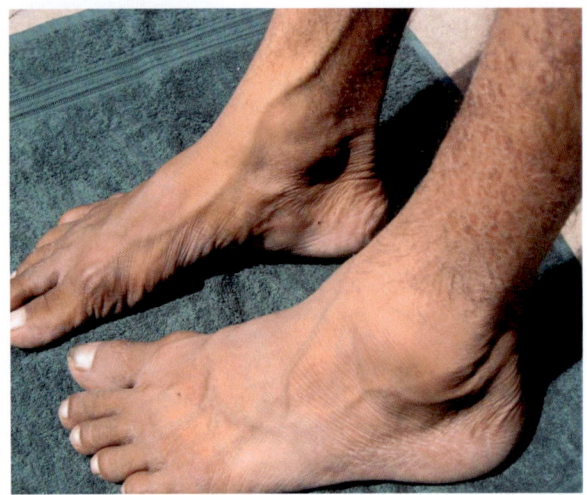

13.7 Management

13.7.1 General

Non-steroidal anti-inflammatory drugs (NSAIDs) are often the mainstay of treatment in controlling joint symptoms, including arthritis and tenosynovitis. Various
classes of NSAIDs are equally effective. Corticosteroids are indicated in patients
with lepra reactions, severe musculoskeletal manifestations, or neuritis. Reversal
reactions and ENL often necessitate high dose steroids (prednisolone equivalent to
1 mg/kg body weight per day) for a prolonged period. Steroids are always administered under the cover of multi drug therapy (MDT). Thalidomide is effective in

Table 13.2 Differential diagnosis of musculoskeletal mimics in leprosy

Clinical manifestation	Mimicked musculoskeletal conditions
Acute oligoarthritis of lower limbs	Reactive arthritis/spondyloarthritis
Symmetric polyarthritis	RA
Ankle arthritis with erythema nodosum	Sarcoidosis
Lucio phenomenon	Vasculitis, SLE
Arthritis with saddle nose and auricular chondritis	Relapsing polychondritis
SHFS	RS3PE
Destructive arthropathy	Charcot's arthropathy: Advanced osteoarthritis, diabetes mellitus, tabes dorsalis, syringomyelia, avascular necrosis

RA Rheumatoid arthritis, *SLE* Systemic lupus erythematosus, *SHFS* Swollen hands and feet syndrome, *RS3PE* Remitting symmetric seronegative synovitis with pitting edema

Table 13.3 Management of arthritis in leprosy (multi drug therapy will be required in all cases for the appropriate duration)

Clinical pattern	Treatment
Arthritis related to lepra reaction	NSAIDs and corticosteroids
Chronic arthritis	NSAIDs, corticosteroids, methotrexate
Charcot's arthropathy	Analgesics, joint stabilization
Swollen hands and feet syndrome	NSAIDs and corticosteroids
Tenosynovitis	NSAIDs and corticosteroids

NSAIDs Non-steroidal anti-inflammatory drugs

controlling ENL symptoms [9]. Supportive measures include physiotherapy, splints, braces, and occupational therapy as required. The incapacitation caused by the disease associated with personal and social stigma of the disease requires family support and counseling and should not be neglected.

13.7.2 Specific

Treatment of leprosy most often ameliorates arthritis over a period of time. Paucibacillary leprosy requires MDT including rifampicin 600 mg monthly single-dose and dapsone 100 mg daily for 6 months, whereas multibacillary disease is treated with the above two medications with the addition of clofazimine 50 mg daily and 300 mg once a month for 12 months [24]. Response to therapy with the clearing of disease should be documented. Prolonged MDT courses may also be required and relapses do occur, especially in endemic countries like India. Alternative treatment regimens are described, which are beyond the scope of this chapter. Arthritis and other rheumatic manifestations take a month or two to respond. The management of arthritis in leprosy is summarised in Table 13.3.

Leprosy neuropathy is often arduous to control, because of the potential for irreversible damage. Steroids are the cornerstone of treatment in controlling inflammation, in addition to symptomatic management and MDT. Neurolysis with surgical decompression is also successful in refractory disease.

The treatment of Charcot's arthropathy in leprosy aims to stabilize the joint with braces and splints and requires arthrodesis in advanced disease.

13.7.3 Prevention

There are no markers to predict the development of arthritis in leprosy. Preventive strategies necessarily include early diagnosis of leprosy when manifesting with arthritis, so as to institute appropriate treatment and prevent complications such as Charcot's joint. Also, recognition that leprosy is causing a rheumatologic manifestation akin to vasculitis or sarcoidosis or reactive arthritis, will prevent delay in instituting appropriate therapy.

13.8 Conclusion

Musculoskeletal manifestations are common in leprosy and at times, indistinguishable from classic rheumatic syndromes. Unless suspected, the disease tends to be misdiagnosed with poor patient outcomes. Owing to the huge burden of the disease in endemic countries, leprosy should be included in the differentials while attending patients with rheumatic manifestations. In the absence of the classical cutaneous and peripheral nerve involvement, rheumatic presentations of this disease have outfoxed even the most astute of physicians and rheumatologists.

References

1. Galhotra A, Panigrahi SK, Pal A. Leprosy—a raging persistent enigma. J Fam Med Prim Care. 2019;8:1863–6.
2. Leprosy (Hansen's disease) [Internet]. [cited 2021 Oct 29]. https://www.who.int/news-room/fact-sheets/detail/leprosy.
3. Maymone MBC, Laughter M, Venkatesh S, Dacso MM, Rao PN, Stryjewska BM, et al. Leprosy: clinical aspects and diagnostic techniques. J Am Acad Dermatol. 2020;83:1–14.
4. Chauhan S, Wakhlu A, Agarwal V. Arthritis in leprosy. Rheumatology (Oxford). 2010;49:2237–42.
5. El-Gendy H, El-Gohary RM, Shohdy KS, Ragab G. Leprosy masquerading as systemic rheumatic diseases. J Clin Rheumatol. 2016;22:264–71.
6. Salvi S, Chopra A. Leprosy in a rheumatology setting: a challenging mimic to expose. Clin Rheumatol. 2013;32:1557–63.
7. Pereira HL, Ribeiro SL, Pennini SN, Sato EI. Leprosy-related joint involvement. Clin Rheumatol. 2009;28:79–84.
8. Lele RD, Sainani GS, Sharma KD. Leprosy presenting as rheumatoid arthritis. J Assoc Physicians India. 1965;13:275–7.
9. Kamath S, Vaccaro SA, Rea TH, Ochoa MT. Recognizing and managing the immunologic reactions in leprosy. J Am Acad Dermatol. 2014;71:795–803.
10. Sehgal VN. Reactions in leprosy. Clinical aspects. Int J Dermatol. 1987;26:278–85.

11. Gibson T, Ahsan Q, Hussein K. Arthritis of leprosy. Br J Rheumatol. 1994;33:963–6.
12. Walker SL, Balagon M, Darlong J, Doni SN, Hagge DA, Halwai V, et al.; Erythema Nodosum Leprosum International STudy Group. ENLIST 1: an international multi-centre cross-sectional study of the clinical features of erythema nodosum leprosum. PLoS Negl Trop Dis. 2015;9:e0004065.
13. Wakhlu A, Sawlani KK, Himanshu D. Rheumatological manifestations of Hansen's disease. Indian J Rheumatol. 2018;13:14–9.
14. Sarkar RN, Phaujdar S, Banerjee S, Siddhanta S, Bhattacharyya K, De D, et al. Musculoskeletal involvement in leprosy. Indian J Rheumatol. 2011;6:20–4.
15. Prasad S, Misra R, Aggarwal A, Lawrence A, Haroon N, Wakhlu A, et al. Leprosy revealed in a rheumatology clinic: a case series. Int J Rheum Dis. 2013;16:129–33.
16. Atkin SL, el-Ghobarey A, Kamel M, Owen JP, Dick WC. Clinical and laboratory studies of arthritis in leprosy. Br Med J. 1989;298:1423–5.
17. Cossermelli-Messina W, Festa Neto C, Cossermelli W. Articular inflammatory manifestations in patients with different forms of leprosy. J Rheumatol. 1998;25:111–9.
18. Albert DA, Weisman MH, Kaplan R. The rheumatic manifestations of leprosy (Hansen disease). Medicine. 1980;59:442–8.
19. Paira SO, Roverano S. The rheumatic manifestations of leprosy. Clin Rheumatol. 1991;10:274–6.
20. Carpintero-Benítez P, Logroño C, Collantes-Estevez E. Enthesopathy in leprosy. J Rheumatol. 1996;23:1020–1.
21. Gupta L, Zanwar A, Wakhlu A, Agarwal V. Leprosy in the rheumatology clinic: an update on this great mimic. Int J Rheum Dis. 2016;19:941–5.
22. Dionello CF, Rosa Utiyama SR, Radominski SC, Stahlke E, Stinghen ST, de Messias-Reason IJ. Evaluation of rheumatoid factor and anti-citrullinated peptide antibodies in relation to rheumatological manifestations in patients with leprosy from Southern Brazil. Int J Rheum Dis. 2016;19:1024–31.
23. Mohammad W, Malhotra SK, Garg PK. Clinico-radiological correlation of bone changes in leprosy patients presenting with disabilities/deformities. Indian J Lepr. 2016;88:83–95.
24. Guidelines for the diagnosis, treatment and prevention of leprosy [Internet]. [cited 2021 Dec 9]. https://www.who.int/publications-detail-redirect/9789290226383.

Chikungunya Arthritis

14

J. Kennedy Amaral, Trina Pal, and Robert T. Schoen

14.1 Introduction

Chikungunya (CHIK) is caused by chikungunya vírus (CHIKV), a small (60–70 nm, 12 kb), single-stranded positive-sense RNA virus in the Alphavirus genus of the Togaviridae family [1]. CHIKV is transmitted to humans by mosquito vectors, primarily *Aedes aegypti* in tropical countries and *A. albopictus* in more temperate climates [1]. The chikungunya fever (CHIKF) illness is often biphasic, beginning with acute illness, characterized by high fever, arthralgia and arthritis, headache, maculopapular rash, and intense fatigue, commonly accompanied by anorexia, nausea, vomiting, and diarrhea [2]. The viraemic phase of CHIKF typically resolves within 5–14 days [1]. In many patients, no further disease manifestations occur, but some patients develop late-stage arthritic manifestations that persist for more than 3 months, and are referred to as chronic chikungunya arthritis (CCA) [3]. These patients develop widespread musculoskeletal pain, arthralgia, or frank arthritis, which is not only persistent but often painful and disabling [4]. The word "chikungunya" means "that which bends up" or "to become contorted" in the Makonde language, referring to the painful, prostrated appearance of affected patients [1].

CHIK has existed for at least over a century. A chikungunya-like illness was recorded in Zanzibar in 1820. At the same time, in the Western Hemisphere, a

J. K. Amaral
Department of Infectious Diseases and Tropical Medicine, Federal University of Minas Gerais, Belo Horizonte, Minas Gerais, Brazil
e-mail: kennedyamaral@ufmg.br

T. Pal · R. T. Schoen (✉)
Section of Rheumatology, Allergy, and Immunology, Yale University School of Medicine, New Haven, CT, USA
e-mail: trina.pal@yale.edu; robert.schoen@yale.edu

© The Author(s), under exclusive license to Springer Nature
Switzerland AG 2022
V. Ravindran et al. (eds.), *Rarer Arthropathies*, Rare Diseases of the Immune
System, https://doi.org/10.1007/978-3-031-05002-2_14

similar disease was described in the Caribbean and the southern United States [5]. In modern times, CHIK was an endemic, mosquito-borne illness, initially confined to East Africa. CHIKV was isolated in Tanzania in 1952–1953 [6]. CHIK reemerged as a global epidemic in Kenya in 2004 (500,000 cases) spreading to Reunion Island in the Indian Ocean in 2005 (250,000 cases), and India in 2006 (1.4 million cases) [7]. In Asia, CHIK was reported in Bangkok in 1958 but reemerged in 2005–2006 with large outbreaks in South and Southeast Asia with seroprevalence rates of 4% in Myanmar, 6% in Sri Lanka, 25% in Vietnam, 27% in the Philippines, and 27.4% in Indonesia [8, 9] (Fig. 14.1).

CHIK spread to Italy, then France, in 2007 [10]. In the Americas, CHIK was reported in the Caribbean in 2013 [11]. Since then, more than 2.9 million cases have been reported in 45 countries in North, Central, and South America [12]. Brazil alone reported almost 500,000 CHIK cases between 2014 and 2017 [13]. Between 2014 and 2015, 460,000 cases were reported in Colombia [14]. In the United States, most cases have occurred in travelers returning from endemic areas [11]. Since 1950s, when CHIK was a geographically confined, mainly East-African endemic disease, it has reemerged as a global epidemic, affecting more than 6.5 million people [12].

Countries and territories where chikungunya cases have been reported*
(as of October 30, 2020)

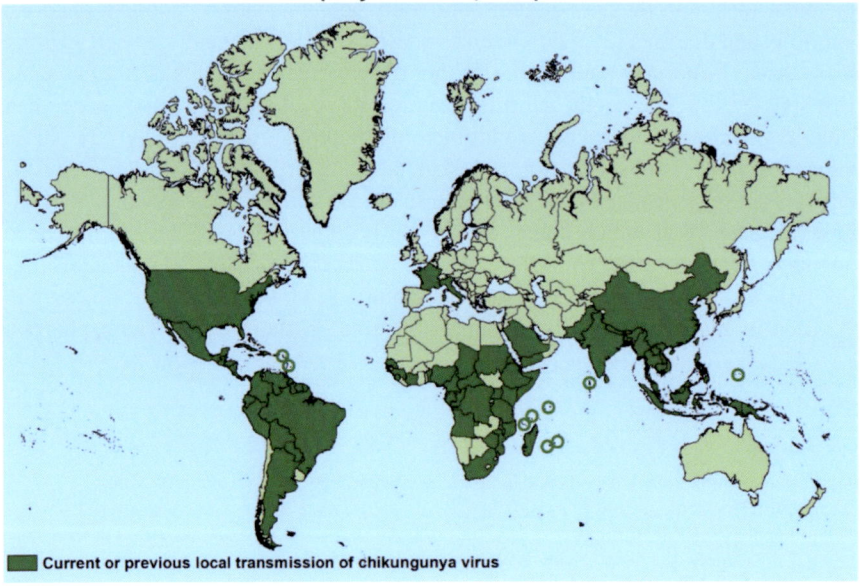

☐ Current or previous local transmission of chikungunya virus

*Does not include countries or territories where only imported cases have been documented.

Fig. 14.1 Countries and territories where chikungunya cases have been reported (as of October 30, 2020). https://www.cdc.gov/chikungunya/pdfs/Chik_World_Map_10-30-20-P.pdf, accessed 8/22/2021

14.2   Acute Chikungunya Fever

14.2.1 Clinical Features

One to 12 days (average 2–4 days) following an *Aedes* vector mosquito bite, most CHIKF patients develop high fever, arthralgia, and rash [15]. Headache, back pain, nausea, vomiting, lymphadenopathy, and abdominal pain also occur. Asymptomatic infection occurs in less than 25% of infected individuals [12]. Arthralgia and frank arthritis occur early in a symmetrical pattern, affecting large and small joints, most commonly the wrists, followed by the phalanges, shoulders, and ankles [2]. Joint pain is more distal than proximal, although axial skeleton involvement is noted in up to half of the cases [16]. The most common dermatological manifestations are generalized, maculopapular, and pruritic rash, as well as nodular, vesicular, bullous, and scaly skin lesions [15]. In one study, pigmentary changes were the most common skin finding (42%), followed by maculopapular eruptions (33%) and intertriginous aphthous ulcers (37%) [17]. CHIKF skin lesions affect the extremities, trunk, and face and tend to be transient, resolving after 2–5 days [18].

Other CHIKF manifestations include neurological complications such as encephalitis, myelitis, facial paralysis, sensorineural deafness, Guillain-Barre syndrome, and neuro-ocular disease (uveitis, retinitis, optic neuritis) [19]. Ocular symptoms such as conjunctivitis, retinitis, photophobia, conjunctival hyperemia, and retro-orbital pain are common [19]. Posterior uveitis and optic neuritis develop in some patients 1 month after disease onset [20]. Although rare, cases of heart failure, cardiac arrhythmias, acute myocardial infarction, and myocarditis have been described [21]. CHIKF is generally not life-threatening, but excess mortality is seen in CHIKF epidemics, particularly in the elderly, newborns, and immunocompromised individuals [22].

14.2.2 Management

14.2.2.1   Prevention
Environmental control measures and personal protection may limit mosquito bites and reduce CHIK infection risk [3]. CHIK vaccines are in development, including a live-attenuated, measles-vectored vaccine expressing CHIK structural proteins [23]. In 260 subjects from a non-CHIK endemic region, this vaccine, induced durable seroconversion in 86–100% of subjects after 2 doses and was well-tolerated [23]. A CHIKV particle-like vaccine is also in development [24]. In a phase 2 study of 400 CHIK-endemic Caribbean subjects who received 2 doses of this vaccine, 88% had a more than fourfold increase in baseline neutralization titers [24]. Studies on both these vaccines are ongoing.

14.2.2.2   Treatment
Antiviral therapies for the treatment of CHIKF, including traditional antiviral compounds, synthetic small molecule inhibitors of viral polymerase and other

nonstructural proteins, in silico high-throughput screening (HTS) for existing compounds with anti-CHIKV activity and drugs that target host proteins are being investigated [25]. However, none is validated thus far, so the treatment of CHIKF remains supportive care, primarily, rest, fluids, and pain management [3]. Acetaminophen, tramadol, and when needed, codeine and oxycodone are recommended. Aspirin or NSAIDs should only be used when dengue coinfection has been excluded because of the risk of bleeding complications. During acute CHIKF, when viremia is present, corticosteroids should not be used. Neuropathic pain can be managed with gabapentin and amitriptyline. It is important to maintain joint mobility [3].

Management of arthritic symptoms during the acute phase of CHIKF is also supportive. Glucocorticoids and disease-modifying anti-rheumatic drugs (DMARDs) such as those used to treat rheumatoid arthritis (RA) are generally deferred unless arthritic manifestations become chronic, because a) the majority of patients have a resolution of symptoms in several weeks and b) during the acute phase, immunosuppression should be avoided because viremia is present. It is worth noting however that the distinction between acute and CCA may be somewhat arbitrary. During a Martinique epidemic, ultrasound imaging of acute CHIKF patients (disease duration 5 ± 1 day) with arthritic symptoms demonstrated multiple patients with joint effusions and synovitis [26].

14.3 Chronic Chikungunya Arthritis

14.3.1 Clinical Features

The clinical expression of arthritis over time in CHIK infection is variable. CHIKF usually causes arthralgia. In those presenting with arthritis, it is usually mild and self-limited. In others, the illness is biphasic, with CHIKF followed by a more severe arthritic phase. In some patients, painful polyarthritis is present and unremitting from disease onset. It is useful to differentiate between acute and chronic Chikungunya arthritis (CCA), the duration watershed has been somewhat arbitrarily defined as 12 weeks [2]. There may be pathogenic and clinical differences between these stages and available evidence supports different treatment strategies [2]. During the early arthritic phase, viremia is present for at least several weeks and robust antiviral interleukin and INF-alpha responses are present [27]. Later, in CCA patients, it has not been possible to detect CHIKV in synovial fluid, [28] and the cytokine signature, including IL-6, IL-17, TNF, GM-CSF, matrix metalloproteinases, resembles other chronic inflammatory rheumatic diseases [29]. These findings suggest that early CHIK arthritis is infectious, but CCA may be a post-infectious inflammatory disorder [2].

The rate of CCA varies among CHIKF cohorts. In one Columbian study, it was 12%, [30] but in another Columbian cohort, persistent rheumatic symptoms were present at 26 weeks in 53.7%, morning stiffness in 49.5%, joint edema in 40.6%, and polyarthritis and morning stiffness combined in 38.2% [31]. Another large study reported similar rates of CCA with 57% developing post-viral polyarthralgia, 22% inflammatory polyarthritis, and 19.5% tenosynovitis [32]. CCA remits over time. In a Reunion Island study, chronic arthritis was observed in 93%, 57%, and 47% of patients at 3, 15, and 24 months, respectively [11].

Several groups have attempted to define patterns of arthritis. Javelle and colleagues evaluated 159 cases of CCA (CHIKF followed by arthritic symptoms for more than 2 years) [33]. In this study, 112 patients had "post-chikungunya chronic inflammatory rheumatism," mimicking four clinical patterns—spondyloarthropathy (33 patients), rheumatoid arthritis (40 patients), undifferentiated polyarthritis (21 patients), and there was also a fibromyalgia group [33]. Most reports describe symmetrical polyarthralgia/polyarthritis with involvement of hands and feet, as well as large joints [2]. In one report, the frequency of joints affected was—hands 57%, knees 57%, wrists 50%, ankles 46%, and shoulders 45% [34]. In another study, knees were involved in 83%, ankles in 62%, and elbows in 59% [35]. In a third of a cohort of 180 patients evaluated at 36 months, hands, wrists, ankles, and knees were commonly affected [36]. In this group, 60–80% of patients had intermittent arthritis and 20–40% were unremitting [37].

Because the pattern of joint involvement in CCA is symmetrical polyarthritis with hand and foot involvement, many have stressed clinical similarity to RA [2]. Among 173 patients with a history of CHIKF, 78.6% had persistent musculoskeletal symptoms at 27.5 months and 5% met American College of Rheumatology (ACR) 2010 criteria for RA [38]. In a study of 10 relief workers who contracted CHIKF in Haiti, 8 met ACR RA criteria [39]. These RA mimics are even more striking given the variable but increased rates of rheumatoid factor (RF) and sometimes anti-cyclic citrullinated protein (anti-CCP) antibody test positivity reported in some studies [2]. In an Indian cohort, 13 of 95 patients and 4 of 67 patients were RF and anti-CCP antibody positive, respectively, [40] Other studies have reported RF positivity between 2 and 43% [41]. None of the 8 patients in the Haitian study were positive for RF [39].

We evaluated a Brazilian cohort of 50 patients with CCA, 90% of whom were self-referred, 14.2 months after disease onset [42]. This delay in treatment was consistent with other reports [33]. Ninety-two percent of our patients were female. Thirty (60%) had arthralgia, while 20 (40%) also had frank arthritis with clinically evident synovitis. The prevalence of involvement of joints has been depicted in Fig. 14.2 [42]. Arthralgia was most common in the hands (56%), ankles (48%), and knees (44%). Arthralgia was polyarticular (>4 joints) in 76% and oligoarticular (2–4 joints) in 24%. All the 20 patients with frank arthritis had hand involvement. Other arthritis-affected joints were wrists (16 patients), ankles (12 patients), and knees (9 patients). In our cohort, 11 patients (22%) met ACR criteria for RA and 7 (14%) met ACR criteria for fibromyalgia [42]. As has been seen in other studies [34], we found that preexisting rheumatic disease predicts a more severe CCA [42]. Other risk factors for severe arthritis include female sex, age more than 45 years, diabetes, hypertension, dyslipidemia, and more severe infection at onset [43, 44].

Multiple cohorts document that CCA is associated with significant pain and disability [4, 45]. In one study, Health Assessment Questionnaire (HAQ) scores of

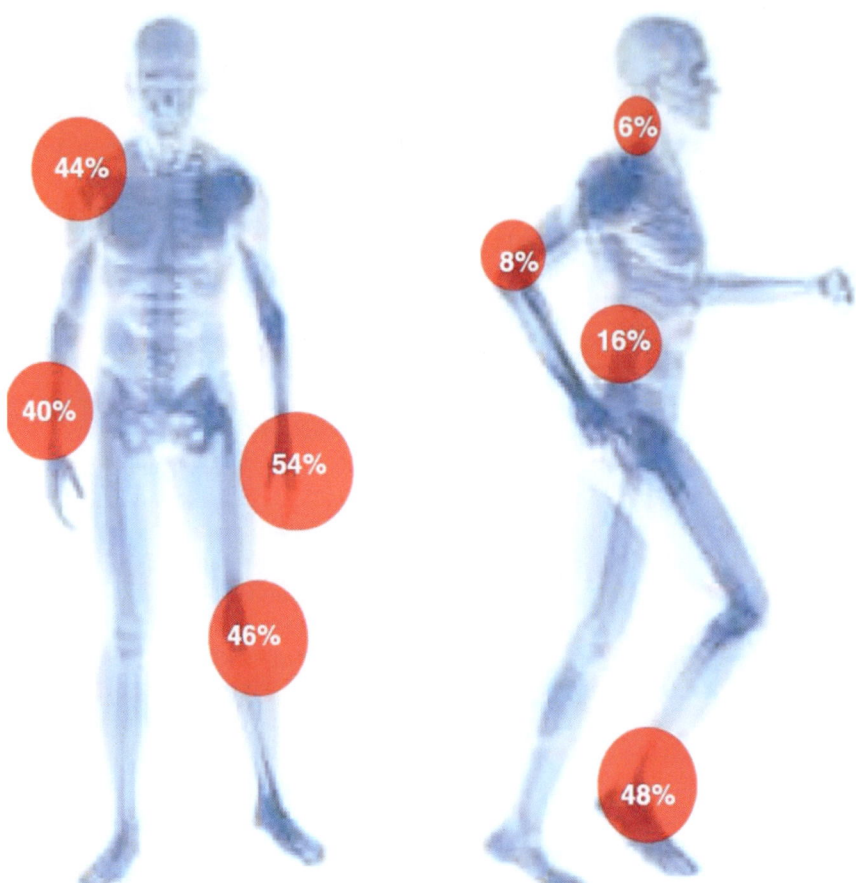

Fig. 14.2 Joints affected (arthralgia/arthritis)

2.18 ± 0.63 were present in 16 CCA patients (symptoms >3 months despite NSAIDs and hydroxychloroquine (HCQ) therapy) [45]. These HAQ scores resemble other rheumatic diseases such as RA (1.75), low back pain (1.27), knee osteoarthritis (OA) (1.29), hand OA (1.24), and fibromyalgia (1.30) [46]. We obtained similar results in 35 Brazilian CCA patients [4]. Our patients had a moderate disability and significant pain (HAC-DI = 1.0 ± 0.40; Visual Analog Pain Scale (VAS) median = 8) [4].

14.3.2 Investigations

The diagnosis of CCA is based on clinical presentation, including epidemiological risk, particularly in endemic areas or in travelers from affected regions, and laboratory confirmation [2]. During CHIKF, reverse transcription method (RT) PCR detects CHIKV up to 7 days after onset of infection [16]. Once CHIK infection is established, anti-CHIK immune responses, both IgM (at 5–10 days) and IgG (after the first week) can be detected by ELISA [16]. IgM positivity peaks at 3 weeks, persisting for up to 2–3 months. ELISA IgG responses remain positive for years [16]. At the onset, CHIK must be distinguished from other febrile, tropical infections, including other mosquito-borne infections, such as dengue. Once chronic arthritis is established, the differential diagnosis may include other inflammatory rheumatic diseases, particularly RA, OA, and fibromyalgia [2, 42].

14.3.3 Management

Chronic Chikungunya arthritis may be a postinfectious inflammatory disease [2]. If so, therapy resembles the treatment of other chronic rheumatic diseases, aimed to relieve pain, improve function and quality of life, limit structural damage, and avoid toxicity. Glucocorticoids improve symptoms in CCA and have not been associated with exacerbation of CHIKV infection in patients with chronic illness, but usage is limited by well-recognized toxicities [3]. HCQ is relatively safe and has been extensively studied, but evidence of significant benefit is lacking [3]. Sulfasalazine has also shown limited efficacy [3].

The most promising DMARD at present for CCA is MTX [47]. In an unblinded randomized trial, 72 subjects received two DMARD regimens, triple therapy with MTX (15 mg/week), sulfasalazine (SSZ) (1 g/day) and HCQ (400 mg/day) compared to HCQ monotherapy for 24 weeks [48]. Both groups received prednisolone (7.5 mg/daily), which was discontinued at 6 weeks. The primary outcome measure was DAS28-ESR good clinical response at 24 weeks. MTX triple therapy was markedly superior to HCQ monotherapy (DAS28-ESR <3.2, 82 vs 14%, respectively) (Fig. 14.3) [48]. In another study, subjects treated with SSZ and HCQ who failed to achieve good clinical response at 3 months were randomized to add MTX [45]. There was a significant improvement in the MTX treated group (MTX vs no MTX, good clinical response, 71.4 vs 12.5%, respectively) [45].

We evaluated MTX in a cohort of 48 Brazilian CCA patients, assessing pain reduction, measured by VAS, as the primary outcome measure [42]. MTX [9.2 ± 3.2 mg/week] resulted in VAS pain reduction of 4.3 (3.0) ($p < 0.0001$) and 4.4(2.6) ($p < 0.0001$), respectively (Fig. 14.4) [42]. In all these reports, MTX was well tolerated. It is reassuring that in CCA patients, it has not been possible to detect CHIKV in synovial fluid [28], and MTX does not increase CHIKV infection or replication in human synovial fibroblasts [36]. There is limited evidence defining the duration of MTX therapy, but we consider discontinuing MTX treatment at 3–6 months in CCA patients who achieve remission [3]. The response seen in one of our MTX–treated patients with CCA is illustrated in Fig. 14.5. Larger, randomized placebo-controlled trials to evaluate the safety and efficacy of MTX in CCA are needed.

There are limited reports of biologic therapy in CCA [3]. In one study of 147 CHIK arthritis patients in Martinique, most were treated with MTX, with "good

Fig. 14.3 Comparison of DMARD triple therapy to hydroxychloroquine monotherapy in chronic persistent chikungunya arthritis (Reprinted with permission from [48])

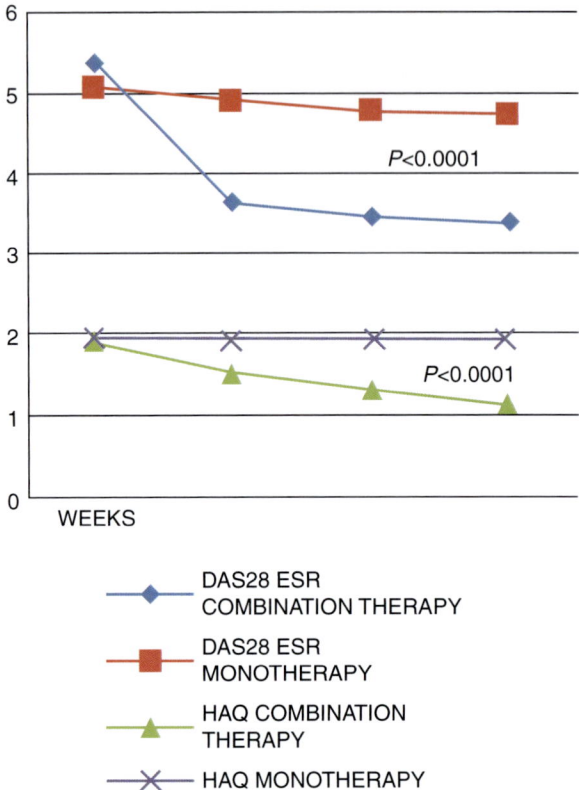

DAS28 ESR COMBINATION THERAPY

DAS28 ESR MONOTHERAPY

HAQ COMBINATION THERAPY

HAQ MONOTHERAPY

Fig. 14.4 Pain score improvement with methotrexate therapy (Reprinted with permission from [42])

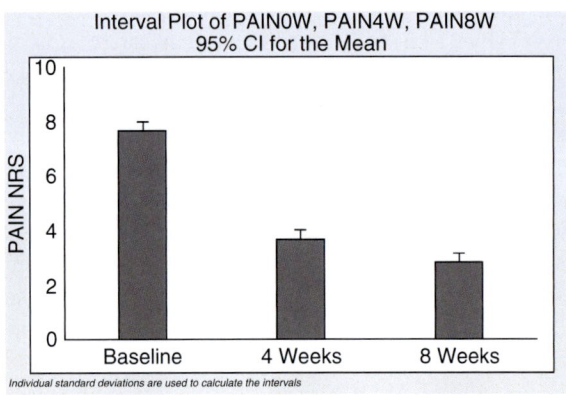

results" [49]. Twelve of these patients were treated with anti-tumor necrosis factor inhibitors "with good tolerance and efficacy" [49]. In another epidemic, 53 of 328 RA patients developed CHIKF while on biologic therapy. Their illnesses resembled other CHIKF patients during this outbreak. Biologic therapy did not appear to improve or worsen their outcomes [50].

Fig. 14.5 Hand arthritis in chronic chikungunya arthritis. A young woman with chronic chikungunya arthritis presenting 2 years after disease onset. (**a**) Prior to methotrexate therapy. (**b**) After oral methotrexate 20 mg once a week for 8 weeks (Reprinted with permission from [42])

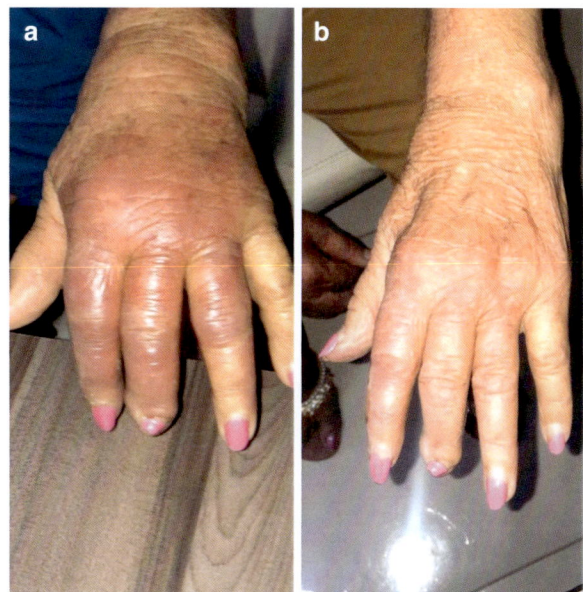

14.4 Conclusion

CHIK is an established viral infection that has spread throughout the world over the past 20 years. The early disease causes significant morbidity, pain and disability, and adverse economic impact. When CHIK becomes chronic, it causes disabling arthritis. Patients with CCA can benefit from treatment of CCA as postinfectious, inflammatory arthritis with strategies borrowed from the treatment of RA and related disorders. However, there exists a knowledge gap in prevention, vaccination, and treatment for this disease which has significant global impact.

References

1. Thiberville S, Moyen N, Dupuis-Maguiraga L, Nougairede A, Gould EA, Roques P, et al. Chikungunya fever: epidemiology, clinical syndrome, pathogenesis, and therapy. Antiviral Res. 2013;99(3):345–70. https://doi.org/10.1016/j.antiviral.2013.06.009.
2. Amaral JK, Taylor PC, Teieira MM, Morrison TE, Schoen RT. The clinical features, pathogenesis, and methotrexate therapy of chronic chikungunya arthritis. Viruses. 2019;11:289. https://doi.org/10.3390/v11030289.
3. Amaral Pereira JK, Schoen RT. Management of chikungunya arthritis. Clin Rheumatol. 2017;36:2179–86.
4. Amaral JK, Bilsborrow JB, Schoen RT. Brief report: the disability of chronic chikungunya arthritis. Clin Rheumatol. 2019;38(7):2011–4. https://doi.org/10.1007/s10067-019-04529-x.
5. Robinson MC. An epidemic of virus disease in Southern Province, Tanganyika territory, in 1952-53. I. Clinical features. Trans R Soc Trop Med Hyg. 1955;49:28–32.

6. Nsoesie EO, Kraemer MU, Golding N, Pigott DM, Brady OJ, Moyes CL, et al. Global distribution and environmental suitability for chikungunya virus, 1952 to 2015. Euro Surveill. 2016;21(20).
7. Wahid B, Ali A, Rafique S, Idrees M. Global expansion of chikungunya virus: mapping the 64-year history. Int J Infect Dis. 2017;58:69–76.
8. Ngwe TM, Inoue S, Thant KZ, Talemaittoga N, Aryati A, Dimaano EM, et al. Retrospective seroepidemiological study of chikungunya infection in South Asia, Southeast Asia, and the Pacific region. Epidemol Infect. 2016;144(11):2268–75.
9. Centers for Disease Control and Prevention. Countries and territories where chikungunya cases have been reported (as of October 30, 2020). https://www.cdc.gov/chikungunya/pdfs/Chik_World_Map_10-30-20-P.pdf. Accessed 22 Aug 2021.
10. Devaux CA. Emerging and re-emerging viruses: a global challenge illustrated by chikungunya virus outbreaks. World J Virol. 2012;1(1):11. https://doi.org/10.5501/wjv.v1.i1.11.
11. Yactayo S, Staples JE, Millot V, Cibrelus L, Ramon-Pardo P. Epidemiology of chikungunya in the Americas. J Infect Dis. 2016;214:S441–5.
12. Morrison TE. Reemergence of chikungunya virus. J Virol. 2014;88(20):11644–7. https://doi.org/10.1128/jvi.01432-14.
13. Amaral JK, Schoen RT. Chikungunya in Brazil: rheumatologists on the front line. J Rheumatol. 2018;45(10):1491–2. https://doi.org/10.3899/jrheum.171237.
14. Villero-Wolf Y, Mattar S, Puerta-González A, Arrieta G, Muskus C, Hoyos R, Pinzon H, Peláez-Carvajal D. Genomic epidemiology of chikungunya virus in Colombia reveals genetic variability of strains and multiple geographic introductions in outbreak. 2014. Sci Rep. 2019;9(1):9970. https://doi.org/10.1038/s41598-019-45981-8.
15. Staples J, Breiman R, Powers A. Chikungunya fever: an epidemiological review of a re-emerging infectious disease. Clin Infect Dis. 2009;49(56):942–8. https://doi.org/10.1086/605496.
16. Pathak H, Mohan MC, Ravindran V. Chikungunya arthritis. Clin Med (Lond). 2019;19(5):381–5.
17. Inamadar AC, Palit A, Sampagavi VV, Raghunath S, Deshmukh NS. Cutaneous manifestations of chikungunya fever: observations made during a recent outbreak in South India. Int J Dermatol. 2008;47:154–9. https://doi.org/10.1111/j.1365-4632.2008.03478.x.
18. Robin S, Ramful D, Zettor J, Benhamou L, Jaffar-Bandjee MC, Riviere JP, et al. Severe bullous skin lesions associated with chikungunya virus infection in small infants. Eur J Pediatr. 2010;169:67–72.
19. Mehta R, Gerardin P, de Brito C, Soares CN, Ferreira M, Solomon T. The neurological complications of chikungunya virus: a systematic review. Rev Med Virol. 2018;28(3):e1978. https://doi.org/10.1002/rmv.1978.
20. Venkatesh A, Patel R, Goyal S, Rajaratnam T, Sharma A, Hossain P. Ocular manifestations of emerging viral diseases. Eye (Lond). 2021;35(4):1117–39. https://doi.org/10.1038/s41433-020-01376-y.
21. Obeyesekere I, Hermon Y. Arbovirus heart disease: myocarditis and cardiomyopathy following dengue and chikungunya fever-a follow-up study. Am Heart J. 1973;85(2):186–94.
22. Mavalankar D, Shastri P, Bandyopadhyay T, Parmar J, Ramani KV. Increased mortality rate associated with chikungunya epidemic, Ahmedabad, India. Emerg Infect Dis. 2008;14:412–5. https://doi.org/10.3201/eid1403.070720.
23. Reisinger EC, Tschismarov R, Beubler E, Wiedermann U, Firbas C, Loebermann M, et al. Immunogenicity, safety and tolerability of the measles-vectored chikungunya virus vaccine MV-CHIK: a double blind, randomized, placebo controlled and active controlled phase 2 trial. Lancet. 2019;392:2718–27.
24. Chen GL, Coates EDE, Plummer SH, Carter CA, Berkowitz N, Conan-Cibotti M, et al. Effect of a chikungunya virus-like particle vaccine on safety and tolerability outcomes: a randomized clinical trial. JAMA. 2020;323(14):1369–77.
25. Powers AM. Vaccine and therapeutic options to control chikungunya virus. Clin Microbiol Rev. 2017;31:e00104–16.
26. Blettery M, Brunier L, Banydeen R, Derancourt C, de Brant M. Management of acute-stage chikungunya disease: contribution of ultrasound joint examination. Int J Infect Dis. 2019;84:1–4.

27. Ng LF, Chow A, Sun Y, Kwek DJ, Lim P, Dimatatac F, et al. IL-1beta, IL-6, and RANTES as biomarkers of chikungunya severity. PLoS One. 2009;4(1):e4261. https://doi.org/10.1371/journal.pone.0004261.
28. Chang AY, Martins KA, Encinales L, Reid SP, Acuna M, Encinales C, et al. Chikungunya arthritis mechanisms in the Americas. Arthritis Rheumatol. 2018;70:585–93.
29. Chow A, Her Z, Ong EK, Chen J, Dimastatac F, Kwek DJ, et al. Persistent arthritis induced by chikungunya virus infection is associated with interleukin-6 and granulocyte macrophage colony stimulating factor. J Infect Dis. 2010;203(20):149–57.
30. Chang AY, Encinales L, Porras A, Pacheco N, Reid SP, Martins KA, Simon GL. Frequency of chronic joint pain following chikungunya virus infection. Arthritis Rheumatol. 2018;70: 578–84.
31. Rodriguez-Morales AJ, Gil-Restrepo AF, Ramirez-Jaramillo V, Montoya-Arias CP, Acevedo-Mendoza WF, Bedoya-Arias JE, et al. Post-chikungunya chronic inflammatory rheumatism: results from a retrospective follow up study of 283 adult and child cases in La Virginia, Risaralda, Colombia. F1000Res. 2016;5:360.
32. Mathew AJ, Goyal V, George E, Thekkemuriyil DV, Jayakumar B, Chopra A. Rheumatic-musculoskeletal pain and disorders in a naïve group of individuals 15 months following a chikungunya viral epidemic in South India: a population based observational study. Int J Clin Pract. 2011;65(12):1306–12.
33. Javelle E, Ribera A, Degasne I, Gauzere B, Marimoutou C, Simon F. Specific management of post-chikungunya rheumatic disorders: a retrospective study of 159 cases in Reunion Island from 2006-2012. PLoS Negl Trop Dis. 2015;9(3):e0003603. https://doi.org/10.1371/journal.pntd.000360.
34. Kennedy AC, Fleming J, Solomon L. Chikungunya viral arthropathy: a clinical description. J Rheumatol. 1980;7(2):231–6.
35. Borgherini G, Poubeau P, Jossaume A, Gouix A, Cotte L, Michault A, et al. Persistent arthralgia associated with chikungunya virus: a study of 88 adult patients on Reunion Island. Clin Infect Dis. 2008;47(4):469–75.
36. Bedoui Y, Giry C, Jaffar-Bandjee M, Guiraud P, Gasque P. Immunomodulatory drug methotrexate used to treat patients with chronic inflammatory rheumatisms post-chikungunya does not impair the synovial antiviral and bone repair processes. PLoS Negl Trop Dis. 2018;12:e0006634.
37. Schilte C, Staikovsky F, Couderc T, Madec Y, Carpentier F, Kassab S, et al. Correction: chikungunya virus-associated long-term arthralgia: a 36-month prospective, longitudinal study. PLoS Negl Trop Dis. 2013;7(3):e2137. https://doi.org/10.1371/annotation/850ee20f-2641-46ac-b0c6ef4ae79b6de6.
38. Essackjee K, Goorah S, Ramchurn SK, Cheeneebash J, Walker-Bone K. Prevalence of and risk factors for chronic arthralgia and rheumatoid-like polyarthritis more than 2 years after infection with chikungunya virus. Postgrad Med J. 2013;89(1054):440–7.
39. Miner JJ, Aw Yeang HK, Fox JM, Taffner S, Malkova ZO, Oh ST, et al. Brief report: chikungunya viral arthritis in the United States: a mimic of seronegative rheumatoid arthritis. Arthritis Rheumatol. 2015;67(5):1214–20.
40. Chopra A, Anuradha V, Lagoo-Joshi V, Kunjir V, Salvi S, Saluja MA. Chikungunya virus aches and pain: emerging challenge. Arthritis Rheumatol. 2008;58:2921–2.
41. Horcada ML, Diaz-Calderon C, Garrido L. Chikungunya fever. Rheumatic manifestations of an emerging disease in Europe. Rheumatol Clin. 2015;11:161–4.
42. Amaral JK, Bingham COL, Schoen RT. Successful methotrexate treatment of chronic chikungunya arthritis. J Clin Rheumatol. 2020;26(3):119–24.
43. Gerardin P, Fianu A, Michault A, Mussard C, Boussaid K, Rollot O, et al. Predictors of chikungunya rheumatism: a prognostic survey ancillary to the TELECHIK cohort study. Arthritis Res Ther. 2013;15:R9.
44. Yaseen HM, Simon F, Deparis X, Marimoutou C. Identification of initial severity determinants to predict arthritis after chikungunya infection in a cohort of French gendarmes. BMC Musculoskelet Disord. 2014;15:249.

45. Ganu MA, Ganu AS. Post-chikungunya chronic arthritis—our experience with DMARDs over two year follow up. J Assoc Physicians India. 2011;59:83–6.
46. Carmona L. The burden of musculoskeletal diseases in the general population of Spain: results from a national survey. Ann Rheum Dis. 2001;60(11):1040–5. https://doi.org/10.1136/ard.60.11.1040.
47. Amaral JK, Sutaria R, Schoen RT. Treatment of chronic chikungunya arthritis with methotrexate: a systematic review. Arthritis Care Res (Hoboken). 2018;70(10):1501–8.
48. Ravindran V, Alias G. Efficacy of combination DMARD therapy in chronic persistent chikungunya arthritis: a 24-week randomized controlled open label study. Clin Rheumatol. 2017;36:1335–40.
49. Blettery M, Brunier L, Polomat K, Moinet F, Deligny C, Arfi S, Jean-Baptiste G, De Brandt M. Brief report: management of chronic post-chikungunya rheumatic disease: the Martinican experience. Arthritis Rheumatol. 2016;68(11):2817–24.
50. Rosario V, Munoz-Louis R, Valdez T, Adames S, Medrano J, Paulino I, et al. Chikungunya infection in the general population and in patients with rheumatoid arthritis on biological therapy. Clin Rheumatol. 2015;34(7):1285–7.

Brucella Arthritis

Yojana Gokhale

15.1 Introduction

Osteoarticular brucellosis is the most frequent complication of brucellosis, a worldwide zoonosis. Due to severe rheumatism associated with this febrile illness or due to osteoarticular complications of the disease, these patients can present to the clinicians, during acute as well as chronic phases of the disease. The sacroiliac joint is the commonest joint involved and acute unilateral sacroiliitis should make one consider a diagnosis of brucellosis. Due to marked predilection for reticuloendothelial cells, the spine is often involved and brucella spondylitis was the commonest complication of untreated brucellosis in the pre-antibiotic era. Clinicians, therefore should be well versed with clinical and radiological features of brucellosis as well as its laboratory diagnosis [1, 2].

15.2 Epidemiology

Brucellosis is a common zoonotic disease with worldwide distribution. Cattle (sheep, goats, pigs, bison, buffalo, camels, dogs, horses, reindeer, and yaks) are the major source of infection. Recently, the infection has also been identified in marine mammals, dolphins, and seals, which may be an emerging hazard to persons occupationally exposed to these. Transmission of brucellosis to humans occurs through consumption of unpasteurized milk and milk products (soft cheese) and contact with infected animal products (raw meat). Brucellosis is an occupational hazard to farmers, people working in the cattle industry, wool industry, meat packers, laboratory technicians, and veterinarians. The organism can enter the human body through skin contact (breached as well as intact skin), gut,

Y. Gokhale (✉)
Lokmanya Tilak Municipal Medical College, Mumbai, India

© The Author(s), under exclusive license to Springer Nature
Switzerland AG 2022
V. Ravindran et al. (eds.), *Rarer Arthropathies*, Rare Diseases of the Immune
System, https://doi.org/10.1007/978-3-031-05002-2_15

respiratory passage, and conjunctiva. In cattle, it is a sexually transmitted disease. Thus, a single infected bison can infect the whole herd. Human to human transmission through contact or sex is extremely rare. Tourism or commerce related travel to endemic areas and consumption of ethnic food can lead to transmission of brucellosis. Only 17 countries in the world have been declared brucella free by the World Health Organization. It is an important economic problem and a serious health hazard in the Middle-east countries, the Mediterranean region, the Indian subcontinent, Mexico, and South-Central America. The disease is transmitted to man by consumption of contaminated milk or milk products or contact with infected cattle. Infection can also be acquired during foreign travel or consumption of soft Mexican cheese. The organisms enter the human body through skin, conjunctiva, gut, or respiratory mucosa [1].

15.3 Microbiology

Brucellae are gram-negative aerobic, cocco-bacilli. They are fastidious organisms, have a long incubation period (4–6 weeks), and grow well on Castaneda biphasic (solid and liquid) medium. There are many subtypes, four of which commonly cause human infection; namely, *B. melitensis* (sheep, goat, camel), *B. abortus* (cow, buffalo, camel, horses), *B. suis* (pigs), and *B. cannis* (dogs). *B. melitensisis* is the most virulent. Brucellae are killed by boiling or pasteurization of milk but survive in biological material for long periods at low temperatures. The infected animal should be culled to protect the herd. As this is not done for the economic concerns and the infected animal keeps spreading the infection to man through infected milk and also to the rest of the herd. Uninfected cattle and newborns should be vaccinated to prevent the disease from spreading. In cattle, it causes recurrent abortion [1].

15.4 Pathogenesis

Exposure to brucellosis generates both humoral and cell-mediated immune responses. Antibodies promote clearance of extracellular brucellae. Polymorphonuclear cells engulf the organism. These intracellular organisms can establish persistent intracellular infection. Initial replication of brucellae takes place within the cells of the lymph nodes draining the point of entry. Subsequent hematogenous spread may result in chronic localizing infection at almost any site, although the reticuloendothelial system, musculoskeletal, and the genitourinary system are most frequently involved. Local tissue response may include abscess or granuloma formation with or without necrosis and caseation. IgM antibodies appear by 1 week of acquiring the infection and persist for 9–12 months. The IgG antibodies appear by 4 weeks and persist beyond 18–24 months. Blocking antibodies appear in over 50% of patients by 3–6 months of acquiring the infection. They are responsible for the false-negative standard "Tube Agglutination Test" (TAT) [3]. *B. cannis* does not share cell membrane antigen with other Brucella species, the one used in TAT. Thus, in those infected with *B. cannis* standard TAT is negative [4]. The incubation period is highly variable (5 days to 6 months) and averages 2–4 weeks.

15.5 Clinical Features

Brucellosis is a febrile illness (hence, it is also referred to as Malta fever, Mediterranean fever, undulant fever and typhomalaria) which during the acute phase is often mistaken for other febrile illnesses that are endemic locally, e.g., malaria, typhoid, and during the chronic phase for tuberculosis. This is because manifestations of brucellosis are nonspecific. History of exposure to domesticated animals or consumption of unpasteurized milk or milk products is elicited in 70–80% of cases. Often brucellosis is not considered as a cause of the fever by the treating physician and the patient may be labeled as a case of pyrexia of unknown origin (PUO). The history of consumption of unpasteurized milk or milk products, contact with cattle, travel to endemic countries (Middle-eastern countries, Spain, Indian subcontinent), consumption of ethnic food, camel rides, and occupations such as abattoirs, farmers, and working in the leather industry should be elicited.

The fever is accompanied by sweats which may be drenching. Malaise, myalgia, arthralgia, backache, and weight loss are common associated symptoms. The patients may look well even at height of fever. Later fever appears only on exertion and subsides on rest. Most patients get night sweats. During the acute phase, there may be enlargement of the lymph nodes, liver, and/or spleen. There may be relapses and the acute phase is followed by a protracted convalescence with some form of severe rheumatism. Invasion of the central nervous system occurs in about 5–7% of the cases with *B. melitensis* infection. Brucella meningitis is lymphocytic meningitis, which can be mistaken for tubercular meningitis. It also produces similar complications such as hydrocephalus. *Brucella* endocarditis occurs in less than 2% of cases but accounts for the majority of deaths [1, 2, 4].

Bone and joint involvement is the most frequent complication of brucellosis and may present in the following ways [5]:

- Backache due to spondylitis/sacroiliitis
- Arthritis
- Pyrexia of unknown origin
- Osteomyelitis
- Bursitis and tenosynovitis

15.6 Bone and Joint Brucellosis

Osteoarticular involvement was recognized as early as 1861 by Martson. The frequency of bone and joint involvement in brucellosis ranges from 2 to 85% as reported by different authors. It is most frequently related to *B. melitensisis* followed by *B. suis* and then *B. Abortus*. They may occur at any age. Arthralgia and arthritis due to brucellosis are more common in childhood than in older age groups, whereas brucella spondylitis is more common in adults than in children. While extra-spinal osteomyelitis is extremely rare, bursitis and tenosynovitis are occasionally seen. The more frequent involvements have been described below [1, 5].

15.6.1 Brucella Spondylitis [3, 6]

It occurred in 50% of the patients with brucellosis in the pre-antibiotic era. The most common site of affection is the lumbar spine (L4), but the dorsal, as well as the cervical spine, may be involved. Multiple vertebral sites may also be involved. The lesion generally starts at the superior endplate of the fourth lumbar vertebra producing an erosion that may heal by sclerosis producing what is known as "Pedro Pons' sign" (Fig. 15.1) on the lateral radiograph. The lesion may spread to involve the entire vertebra or even the adjacent vertebra. There may be a collapse of the vertebra (Fig. 15.2) radiologically mimicking tuberculous spondylitis. Paravertebral, epidural, as well as psoas abscesses [7] may develop.

Patients with Brucella spondylitis present with low back pain, with gradual or sudden onset, radiating to the leg(s), resembling prolapsed intervertebral disc. The pain is aggravated by walking and relieved by rest. The patient may become bedridden due to severe pain. The affected vertebral spine is usually tender. There is a paraspinal muscle spasm. The straight leg raising test may be positive. Deformities and neurological deficits are rare as compared to the tuberculous spine, but they do occur in the setting of a delayed diagnosis [6]. History of febrile illness in 3–6 months preceding the onset of back pain is elicited in most patients [6].

There are no characteristic features of Brucella spondylitis as such. A history of animal contact, consumption of raw milk or milk products, visiting endemic countries, and febrile illness in a patient with back pain should arouse suspicion of

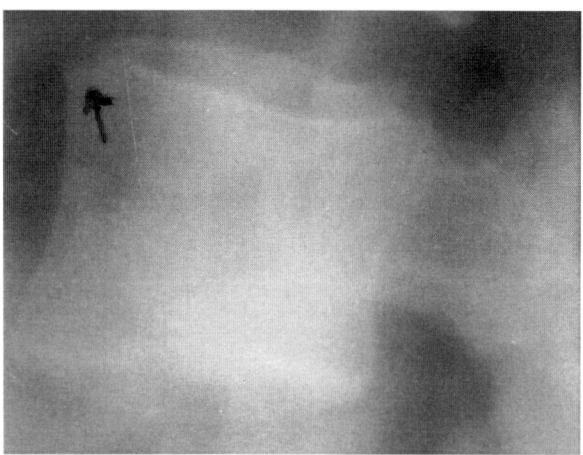

Fig. 15.1 Pedro Pons' sign, erosion at anterior superior angle of L4

Fig. 15.2 Brucella spondylitis, X-ray showing L5 collapse

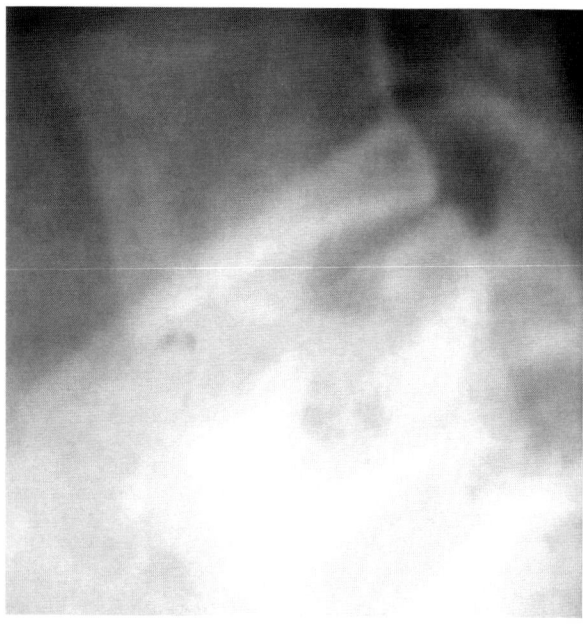

brucella spondylitis. Bacteriological studies or blood cultures are the gold standards but the yield is poor in spondylitis, especially in afebrile patients. Hence, one must rely on serological tests. IgM and IgG antibodies to Brucella can be detected in the patients' serum by ELISA. It is highly sensitive and specific. For the TAT, titers more than 1:80 or above may be considered positive. The TAT may be falsely negative due to blocking antibodies after 3–6 months of acquiring the infection. PCR-based assays for Brucella are reported to be very specific and sensitive. Blood culture by classical Castaneda method takes 4–6 weeks to grow brucella. With continuous-monitoring blood culture systems such as BACTEC, in 5–7 days Brucellae can be cultured in nearly 70% of patients [7, 8].

Very early in the disease and up to 3 months, the plain radiographs may be normal. Scintigraphy using Tm99 is particularly useful in such cases. It shows increased tracer uptake at affected vertebral sites and/or the sacroiliac joint (Fig. 15.3). Later, in the radiographs, the earliest lesion seen is an area of bone destruction at the disco-vertebral junction. This may have a rim of sclerosis. An anterior osteophyte resembling that due to degenerative spondylitis of the lumbar spine is a common finding due to an old healed lesion. In advanced cases, there is vertebral body collapse and decreased intervertebral disc space (Fig. 15.4). Paravertebral soft tissue may be seen. An MRI scan in early lesion depicts areas of low signal intensity at the superior endplate in T1 images, they become hyperintense in T2 images. Such lesions may be seen at multiple vertebral levels (Fig. 15.5a, b). Para spinal, epidural, or psoas abscesses may be seen [2]. The MRI lesions usually resolve completely on prompt initiation of treatment (Fig. 15.5a, b—pretreatment and Fig. 15.5c, d—posttreatment).

Fig. 15.3 Bone scan: increased uptake in the right sacroiliac joint

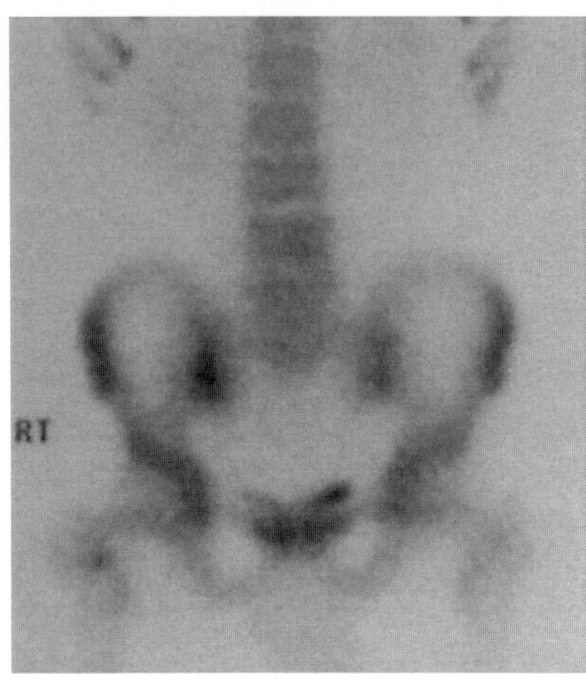

Fig. 15.4 Brucella spondylitis, X-ray showing L4–5 discitis

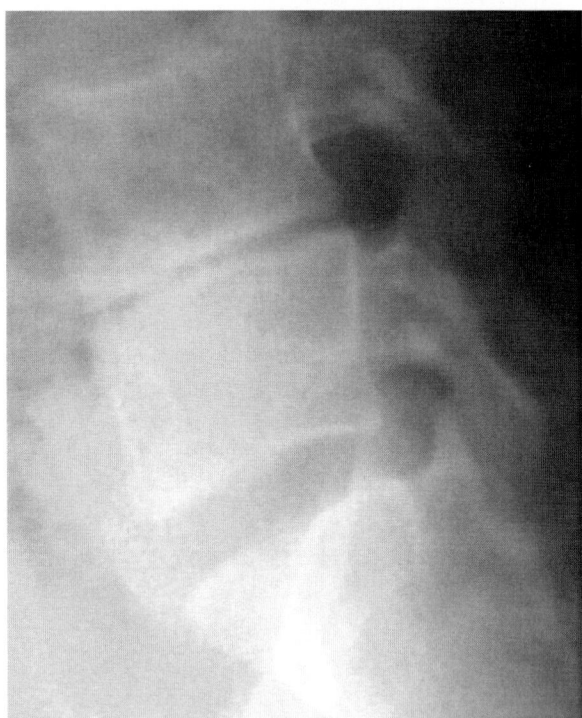

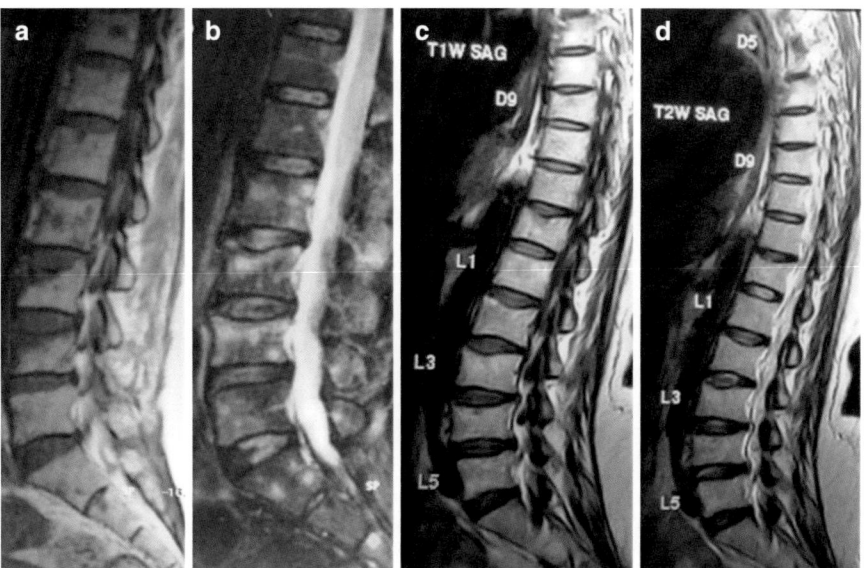

Fig. 15.5 MRI spine, Brucella Spondylitis: (**a**) T1 image showing hypointense marrow signals, (**b**) T2 image showing hyperintense marrow signals. The patient was extensively investigated for myeloma, lymphoreticular malignancy, and metastasis in a cancer hospital. Her serological test for brucellosis was strongly positive and there was an excellent clinical response to anti-brucella therapy, along with improvement in MRI (**c**, **d**)

15.6.2 Brucella Sacroiliitis

The sacroiliac joint is the most common joint involved in patients with brucella arthritis. It is reported in 13–52% of patients with brucellosis. Acute sacroiliitis due to brucellosis occurs in the early febrile stage of infection. It presents as unilateral pain over the sacroiliac joint, fever with chills, and sweats. The sacroiliac maneuvers are very painful, as also the hip movements and straight leg raising (SLR). It lasts for a few weeks to then resolve spontaneously. All acute unilateral sacroiliitis should be investigated for brucellosis. In a few cases, the opposite sacroiliac joint may subsequently get affected. Sacroiliitis may be associated with lumbar spondylitis with low back pain mimicking ankylosing spondylitis [6, 9, 10].

15.6.2.1 Differential Diagnosis of Brucella Spondylitis and Sacroiliitis

Spinal tuberculosis: Clinically as well as radiologically, spinal tuberculosis can mimic Brucella spondylitis. Brucellosis has a predilection for the lumbar spine whereas tuberculosis more often affects the dorsal spine. Spinal deformities are common in tuberculosis. Positive Brucella serology is useful in making the diagnosis of brucella spondylitis. Brucellae can rarely be grown from the surgical specimen, whereas in the tuberculous spine, often Mycobacteria can be cultured.

Prolapsed intervertebral disc: Patients with Brucella spondylitis experience low back pain radiating to the leg and SLR can be positive. The radiograph may be normal in early brucella spondylitis. An abnormal bone scan and positive Brucella serology can aid the diagnosis.

Degenerative lumbar spondylosis: Anterior osteophytes in the elderly patients' radiographs may mimic old Brucella spondylitis. Such changes on lateral radiographs are common in elderly patients in endemic areas.

Ankylosing spondylitis: Sacroiliitis and osteophytes due to healed superior end-plate lesions may mimic ankylosing spondylitis.

Malignancy or metastatic deposits: Back pain, abnormal tracer uptake in bones and the spine on bone scan and abnormal marrow signals on the MRI may be mistaken for malignancies such as myeloma or secondaries.

15.6.3 Brucella Arthritis

Reported incidence of Brucella arthritis is 10–100% (occurs during acute brucellosis). Arthralgia is reported in over 80% patients of with Brucellosis. Arthritis may be mono-arthritis, usually affecting the large joints or migratory polyarthritis. Arthritis is common in children whereas spondylitis is common in adults (Fig. 15.6a–d). Brucella arthritis has no unique distinguishable features. Onset may be sudden and severe or mild and gradual. Arthritis may last for days to months (until the disease is active). It responds well to anti-Brucella treatment. The synovial fluid may grow Brucella. The radiographs may be normal in early cases. Bone scans show increased tracer uptake. Septic and destructive arthritis of one joint may occur due to Brucellosis. If there is a delay in diagnosis destructive changes and radiological abnormalities, such as joint space narrowing or bony ankylosis occur. Brucella arthritis is easily diagnosed in countries where brucellosis is endemic. It is more common in children than adults. There are reports of tenosynovitis, bursitis, and osteomyelitis due to brucellosis [3–5].

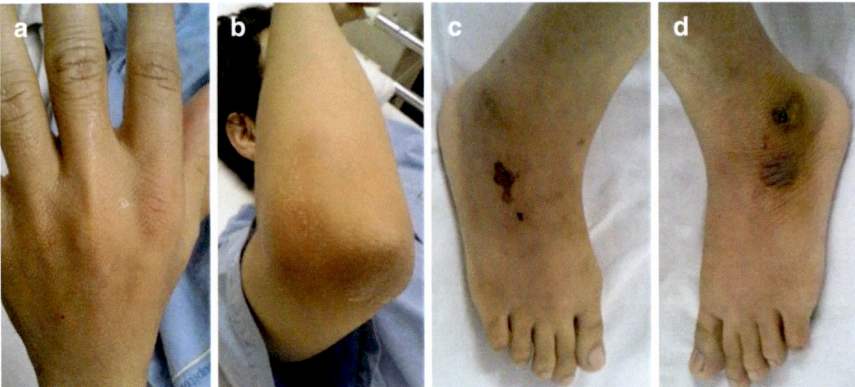

Fig. 15.6 (**a–d**) Arthritis of the left second and third metacarpophalangeal joint, right elbow, feet. (**c, d**) necrotic purpura on both feet in a 30-year-old male

15.6.4 Brucellosis Presenting as Pyrexia of Unknown Origin (PUO)

From various parts of the world, Brucellosis has been reported as a cause of PUO in proportions ranging from 0.8% of PUO cases from Kashmir in India [11], 1.8% from Turkey [12], 5.2% from Nigeria [13] using the TAT for screening, to 27% from CMC Vellore in India [14], and 59% from Kuwait [15] with the use of ELISA test for screening. This variation is due to false-negative TAT by 3–6 months and different prevalence of the disease in different parts of the world.

15.7 Involvement of Other Systems in Brucellosis [16]

Respiratory: Symptoms like cough, pleuritic pain, and hemoptysis are reported in brucellosis but are generally mild. Chest radiographs may show infiltrates and pleural effusion (Fig. 15.7).

Neurological: Chronic lymphocytic meningitis, myelitis, radiculoneuropathy, and depression.

Genitourinary: Epididymo-orchitis is a frequent complication.

Cardiovascular: Involvement can be in the form of infective endocarditis (more so in countries with rheumatic valvular heart disease) or pericardial effusion. Cardiovascular involvement is reported in 2% of patients.

Dermatological: Cutaneous manifestations may be encountered as erythema, papules, petechiae, purpura (Fig. 15.6c, d) urticaria, impetigo, eczematous rash, erythema nodosum (during the acute phase), subcutaneous abscess, and cutaneous vasculitis. Skin involvement is reported in 5–10% of cases.

Fig. 15.7 HRCT chest—bilateral pleural and pericardial effusion

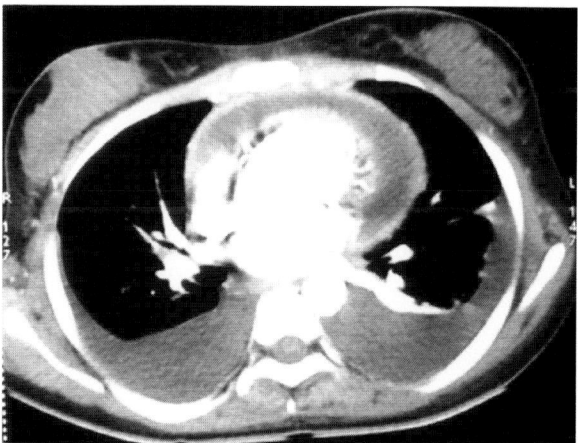

15.8   Treatment of Osteoarticular Brucellosis

The general principles of management are,

1. Always use combination therapy (2–3 drugs)
2. The duration of therapy should be 6–12 weeks or more.
3. Paraspinal abscesses do respond to the medical line of treatment. Therefore, surgery should be reserved for patients with neurological deficits or relapses due to abscesses.

Drugs used in the management are Doxycycline 100 mg twice a day, Rifampicin 900 mg daily, Ciprofloxacin 500 mg twice a day, Co-trimoxazole 10 mg/kg of trimethoprim (i.e., 3 tablets twice a day), and parenteral Streptomycin 1 g daily for 3 weeks. Ceftriaxone is also effective against brucellae and is used for the treatment of Brucella endocarditis [1, 2].

Relapse is known to occur in 20% of the cases. One can document the rising titers of antibodies. Treatment of each relapse is similar to that of the first episode.

15.9   Conclusion

Brucellosis is a common zoonosis with worldwide distribution. Osteoarticular complications are common in Brucellosis, spondylitis being the commonest. Very few countries have eradicated animal brucellosis. Due to increasing international travel, physicians and rheumatologists around the world may come across cases of brucellosis as pyrexia of unknown origin (PUO), arthralgia, arthritis, back pain, lymphocytic meningitis, epididymo-orchitis or a bone scan or spinal MRI of a patient with Brucellosis being mistaken for metastasis. Though with conventional methods culture time for brucellae is 4–6 weeks, with continuous-monitoring blood culture systems such as BACTEC it has been reduced to 5–7 days. Serological tests such as ELISA are also highly sensitive and specific. Brucellosis can be cured when treated with a combination of appropriate antibiotics for several weeks.

References

1. Unuvar GK, Kilic AU, Doganay M. Current therapeutic strategy in osteoarticular brucellosis. North Clin Istanb. 2019;6(4):415–20. Published 2019 Oct 24. https://doi.org/10.14744/nci.2019.05658.
2. Esmaeilnejad-Ganji SM, Esmaeilnejad-Ganji SMR. Osteoarticular manifestations of human brucellosis: a review. World J Orthop. 2019;10(2):54–62.
3. Ariza J, Pellicer T, Pallarés R, Fos A, Gudiol F. Specific antibody profile in human brucellosis. Clin Infect Dis. 1992;14:131–40.
4. Madkour MM. Madkour's brucellosis. Berlin: Springer; 2001.
5. Khateeb MI, Araj GF, Majeed SA, Lulu AR. Brucella arthritis: a study of 96 cases in Kuwait. Ann Rheum Dis. 1990;49(12):994–8. https://doi.org/10.1136/ard.49.12.994.

6. Gokhale YA, Ambardekar AG, Bhasin A, Patil M, Tillu A, Kamath J, et al. Brucella spondylitis and sacroilitis in the general population in Mumbai. J Assoc Physicians India. 2003;51:659–66.
7. Maleknejad P, Hashemi FB, Fatollahzadeh S Jafari B, Peeri Dogaheh H. Direct urease test and acridine orange staining on BACTEC blood culture for rapid presumptive diagnosis of brucellosis. Iran J Public Health. 2005;34:52–5.
8. Yagupsky P, Paled N, Press J. Use of BACTEC 9240 blood culture system for detection of Brucella melitensis in synovial fluid. J Clin Microbiol. 2001;39:738–9.
9. Pascual E. Brucella arthritis. In: Isenberg DA, Madison PJ, Woo P, Klars D, Breedveld FC, editors. Oxford text book of rheumatology. Oxford: Oxford University Press; 2004. p. 937–44.
10. Gokhale YA, Bichile LS, Gogate A, Tillu AV, Zamre. Brucella spondylitis: an important treatable cause of low backache. J Assoc Physicians India. 1999;47:384–8.
11. Kadri SM, Rukhsana A, Laharwal MA, Tanvir M. Seroprevalence of brucellosis in Kashmir (India) among patients with pyrexia of unknown origin. J Indian Med Assoc. 2000;98:170–1.
12. Ciftçi E, Ince E, Dogru U. Pyrexia of unknown origin in children: a review of 102 patients from Turkey. Ann Trop Paediatr. 2003;23:259–6.
13. Baba MM, Sarkindared SE, Brisibe F. Serological evidence of brucellosis among predisposed patients with pyrexia of unknown origin in the north eastern Nigeria. Cent Eur J Public Health. 2001;9:158–61.
14. Mathai E, Singhal A, Verghese S, D'Lima D, Mathai D, Ganesh A, Thomas K, Moses P. Evaluation of an ELISA for the diagnosis of brucellosis. Indian J Med Res. 1996;103:323–4.
15. Al-Fadhli M, Al-Hilali N, Al-Humoud H. Is brucellosis a common infectious cause of pyrexia of unknown origin in Kuwait? Kuwait Med J. 2008;40(2):127–9.
16. Mantur BG, Amarnath SK, Shinde RS. Review of clinical and laboratory features of human brucellosis. Indian J Med Microbiol. 2007;25:188–202.

Hypertrophic Osteoarthropathy

16

Kok Ooi Kong and Gervais Khin-Lin Wansaicheong

16.1 Introduction

Hypertrophic osteoarthropathy (HOA) has been referred to as osteoarthropatia hypertrophica, Pierre Marie syndrome, Bamberger syndrome, Pierre Marie-Bamberger syndrome, Mankowsky syndrome, and Hagner syndrome. It is characterized by a combination of clinical findings, including symmetrical, severe disabling arthralgia and arthritis, digital clubbing (or acropachy), and periostosis of tubular bones mainly due to fibrovascular proliferation. Digital clubbing is one of the oldest clinical signs in medicine. Its original recognition has been attributed to Hippocrates (circa 450 BCE) [1]. Pierre Marie [2] and Eugen von Bamberger [3] first described this syndrome in 1890 and 1891, respectively. Marie coined the term hypertrophic pulmonary osteoarthropathy (HPOA), referring to the more prevalent association with pulmonary diseases such as lung carcinoma, cystic fibrosis, or pulmonary tuberculosis. For this reason, secondary HOA is also referred to as Pierre Marie-Bamberger syndrome. Subsequently, as the sites of primary disease were recognized to be in areas other than the lungs, this

K. O. Kong (✉)
Department of Rheumatology, Allergy and Immunology, Tan Tock Seng Hospital, Singapore, Singapore

Lee Kong Chian School of Medicine, Nanyang Technological University of Singapore, Singapore, Singapore

Yong Loo Lin School of Medicine, National University of Singapore, Singapore, Singapore
e-mail: Kok_Ooi_Kong@ttsh.com.sg

G. K.-L. Wansaicheong
Lee Kong Chian School of Medicine, Nanyang Technological University of Singapore, Singapore, Singapore

Department of Diagnostic Radiology, Tan Tock Seng Hospital, Singapore, Singapore
e-mail: Gervais_Wansaicheong@ttsh.com.sg

© The Author(s), under exclusive license to Springer Nature Switzerland AG 2022
V. Ravindran et al. (eds.), *Rarer Arthropathies*, Rare Diseases of the Immune System, https://doi.org/10.1007/978-3-031-05002-2_16

designation was changed to HOA. Paleopathologic studies have demonstrated changes consistent with HOA in human skeletal remains from different ancient civilizations [4]. There are no systematic studies on the prevalence of digital clubbing in either the general population or hospital inpatients. It is accepted that HOA does not have racial or sexual predominance, except for primary HOA, with a typical age of presentation of 55–75 years, unless in association with congenital cyanotic heart disease.

16.2   Etiology

There are two forms of HOA, primary and secondary. Primary HOA, pachydermoperiostosis, also known as Touraine-Solente-Golé syndrome, or Friedreich-Erb-Arnold syndrome, is a rare autosomal dominant heritable genetic mutation with a variable expression that results in similar clinical manifestations, although it tends to have more generalized cutaneous thickening and soft tissue findings [5]. A third of these patients will have a close relative with the same disease. It has a male: female ratio of 9:1. They also have skin overgrowth which roughens the facial features and may reach the extreme of cutis verticis gyrata. There may be also glandular dysfunction, manifested as hyperhidrosis, seborrhoea, or acne. Other abnormalities that have been described in primary HOA include cranial suture defects, males with female escutcheon, and hypertrophic gastropathy.

Ninety-five to 97% of reported cases of HOA are however of secondary origin. The causes of secondary HOA are broadly divided into generalized, with symmetrical involvement of multiple bones and localized disease. Most of the generalized diseases are of pulmonary origin and a large majority of reported HOA is associated with malignancy as a paraneoplastic syndrome. Pulmonary malignancies, including primary metastatic lung cancer and intrathoracic lymphoma, account for 80% of cases of secondary HOA. Non-small cell lung cancer (NSCLC), particularly adenocarcinoma, is the most common cause of secondary HOA; while small cell carcinoma is the least frequent histopathologic type of lung cancer-associated with HOA. Although lower in absolute incidence, a higher percentage of pleural tumors result in HOA (22% of solitary fibrous tumors of pleura compared to 5% of NSCLC) [6, 7]. The other diseases of extrapulmonary origin can cause generalized secondary HOA, including a wide variety of cardiopulmonary, gastrointestinal [8], endocrine, hematologic, rheumatologic, and inflammatory conditions as shown in Table 16.1.

Forms of HOA localized to one or two limbs are rarely seen [9]. These often occur as a result of a prominent endothelial injury of that particular limb, such as in cases of arterial aneurysms, endothelial infections, or infection of arterial graft. Such patients present with painful swelling of the affected limb associated with radiographic periostosis, often without clubbing. Hemiplegia is another consideration when clubbing is localized [10]. Localized HOA limited only to the cyanotic limbs can also be found in patients with patent ductus arteriosus complicated by pulmonary hypertension.

Table 16.1 Causes of hypertrophic osteoarthropathy

Primary	Idiopathic
	Pachydermoperiostosis
Secondary	
Generalized	Pleuro-Pulmonary
	Bronchogenic carcinoma
	Pulmonary metastases, especially osteosarcoma
	Mesothelioma
	Pulmonary lymphoma
	Solitary fibrous tumor of pleura, pleural fibroma
	Cystic fibrosis
	Pulmonary tuberculosis
	Chronic lung infections
	Lung abscess
	Bronchiectasis
	Idiopathic pulmonary fibrosis
	Pulmonary arteriovenous malformation
	Sarcoidosis
	Lung transplant
	Cardiac
	Congenital cyanotic heart disease
	Atrial myxoma
	Infective endocarditis
	Right to left shunt
	Gastrointestinal
	Polyposis
	Inflammatory bowel disease
	Coeliac disease
	Whipple disease
	Gastrointestinal lymphoma
	Malignancy, e.g., gastric, pancreatic, oesophageal carcinoma
	Achalasia
	Laxative use
	Hepatobiliary
	Liver Cirrhosis including Cryptogenic cirrhosis
	Wilson disease
	Biliary atresia
	Primary biliary cirrhosis
	Primary sclerosing cholangitis
	Hepatopulmonary syndrome
	Rheumatologic condition
	Rheumatoid arthritis
	Ankylosing spondylitis
	Systemic lupus erythematosus
	Antiphospholipid syndrome
	Polyarteritis nodosa

(continued)

Table 16.1 (continued)

		Takayasu's disease
		Familial Mediterranean fever
		Miscellaneous
		Thymoma
		POEMS syndrome
		Myelofibrosis
		Hematological malignancy
		Other malignancies, e.g., nasopharyngeal carcinoma, renal cell carcinoma, breast phyllodes tumor, melanoma, thyroid cancer, osteosarcoma, ovarian, and adrenal malignancies
Localized		Patent ductus arteriosus
		Aneurysms
		Infected arteritis or vascular graft
		Hemiplegia

16.3 Clinical Features

In most cases, digital clubbing is the first manifestation, and as the syndrome progresses, periostosis becomes evident. Affected patients can present at any point in a continuum of symptom complexes, from asymptomatic to a classic triad of clubbing, periostosis/periostitis, and synovial effusions. Regardless of the etiology, clubbing is the most common manifestation of this syndrome, and periostitis is the hallmark of HOA.

Classically, patients complain of a deep-seated burning sensation of digits in early stages to the excruciating pain of lower extremity long bones, aggravated in a dependent position in later stages. Bone and joint pain often mislead to a diagnosis of inflammatory arthritis. Symptoms of primary organ dysfunction often provide diagnostic cues, including cyanosis, new-onset cough, hemoptysis, weight loss, exophthalmos, myxoedema, stigmata of the chronic liver, or biliary disease.

Physical examination often reveals the characteristic findings. Digital clubbing with a unique bulbous deformity or a "drumstick" appearance of the nailbeds, where edema and increased soft tissue produce rocking of the nailbed [11], is identifiable by a meticulous digital examination. Convex nail (Fig. 16.1) with shiny overlying skin and loss of normal crease renders the characteristic appearance to both fingers and toes. However, toes are more difficult to appreciate due to the normal splaying of toe tips. Several methods [12, 13] have been proposed for diagnosing clubbing but their interobserver variabilities are significant (Fig. 16.2). They include:

(a) Lovibond angle or profile sign (angle between the skin proximal to the cuticle and proximal take-off of the nail) exceeding 180°,
(b) Hyponychial angle (angle between the skin proximal to the cuticle and distal nail) exceeding 192°,

Fig. 16.1 Magnified view of the left index finger and middle finger. This shows clubbing with a phalangeal depth ratio of more than one in the index finger

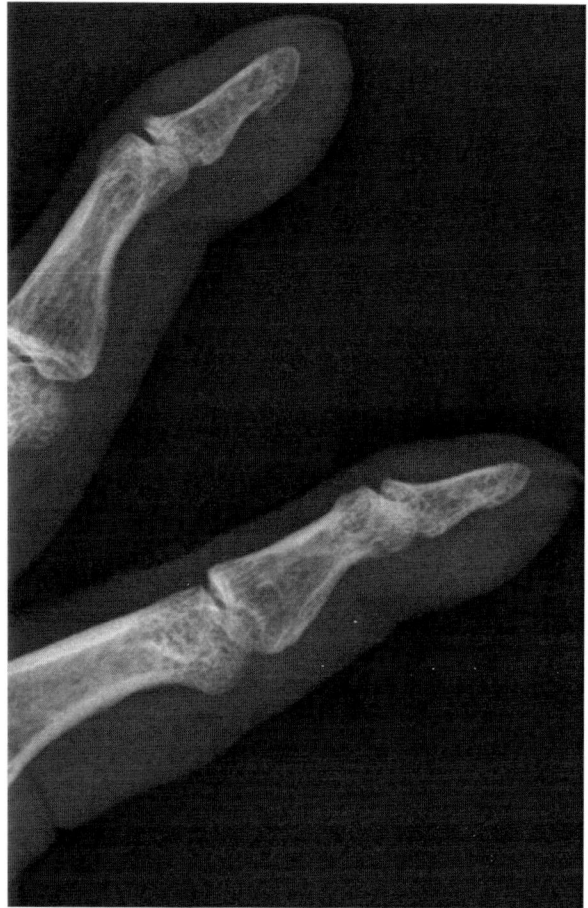

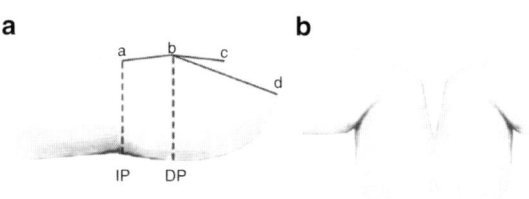

Fig. 16.2 Methods to diagnose digital clubbing during physical examination. (**a**) (1) hyponychia angle (abc), (2) profile angle (abd), (3) phalangeal depth ratio (depth at interphalangeal [IP] level: depth at distal phalangeal [DP] level), and iv) digital index (perimeter at IP level and nailbed [DP] level); (**b**) Schamroth sign

(c) Phalangeal depth ratio (ratio between the depths measured at the distal phalangeal level and interphalangeal level) greater than 1,

(d) The Schamroth sign (or Schamroth window test), which is defined as the loss of the diamond-shaped window between two juxtaposed nailbeds, and

(e) The digital index, which is computed by adding the nailbed-to-distal interphalangeal ratios of all the digits in the hands after obtaining the ratio of the digit perimeter at the nailbed to the digit perimeter at the distal interphalangeal joint of each digit, greater than 10.

In primary HOA, skin hypertrophy with coarse facial features and cylindrical soft tissue swelling of the soft tissues of the legs (elephant legs) are the typical features besides clubbing. The thickening of long bones may be evident in nonmuscular locations such as ankles and wrists. Tenderness may be elicited on palpation of the area affected by periostitis. Swelling of small joints due to effusion may be found in the joints adjacent to the site of periostosis/periostitis. Joint involvement, typically symmetrical with sizeable joint effusion due to sympathetic response to adjacent periostosis, are more commonly found in the knee and wrists. Arthrocentesis yields a non/pauci-inflammatory fluid with less than 500/mm^3 leucocytes and a tendency to clot spontaneously [14]. As opposed to inflammatory arthritis, both the joint and the adjacent bones are symptomatic. The range of motion of the affected joint is often slightly decreased only. Rarely does HOA presents without clubbing and features of primary organ dysfunction. In these cases, refractory symmetrical bone and joint pain with noninflammatory effusion in the adjacent joints presents a diagnostic challenge to clinicians.

16.4 Investigations

Clinical diagnosis is often challenging as the symptoms at presentation can be very similar to connective tissue diseases, although the rheumatoid factor is often negative. However, there are reports of HOA associated with lung malignancy being associated with positive antinuclear, anti-Sm and anti-neutrophil cytoplasmic antibodies serology. There are no specific serological markers for HOA but indirect evidence of increased bone formation by elevated circulating markers such as bone alkaline phosphatase, osteocalcin, or amino-terminal propeptide of type 1 procollagen may be seen. However, these markers do not have a diagnostic role in routine clinical practice.

Imaging is the mainstay of diagnosis. Symmetrical periostosis, as smooth periosteal reaction in the absence of cortical destruction or fracture, is the hallmark of HOA (Fig. 16.3). It typically starts in the shafts of tubular bones (diaphysis), though in primary HOA, epiphysis may also be involved. With progression, metaphysis is also involved. There is an initial monolayer circumferential widening without transformation of bone shape (Figs. 16.4 and 16.5), followed by multilayered, laminated (Figs. 16.6 and 16.7), centripetal thickening with an irregular appearance in advanced stages (Fig. 16.8a and b). Typical HOA shows preservation of joint space;

Fig. 16.3 Proximal left
tibia and fibula. This shows
a subtle periosteal reaction
(monolayer) along the
lateral aspect of the
diaphysis of the fibula

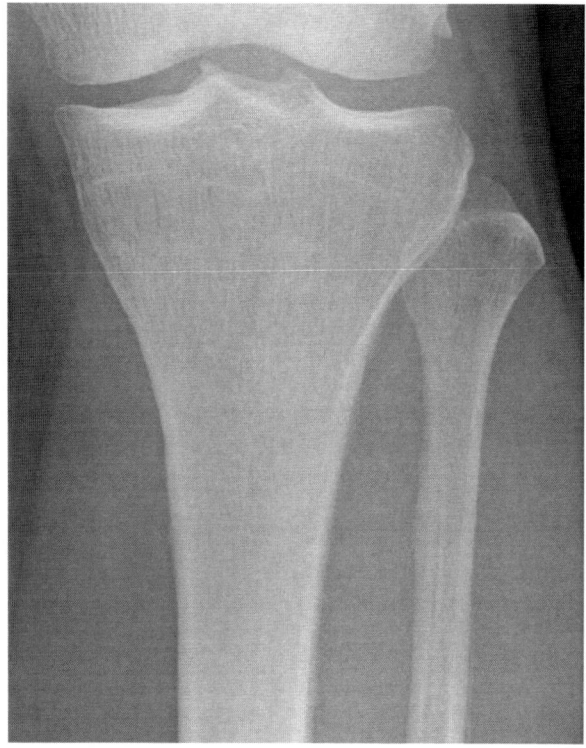

erosions or para-articular osteopenia are absent. Tibia, fibula, radius, and ulna are most commonly affected, followed by phalanges [15]. Primary and secondary HOA feature similar changes [16]. Identification of periostosis/periostitis on radiography should alert the treating physician to consider malignancy, osteomyelitis, or drug-related (prostaglandins, fluoride, voriconazole, vitamin A) periostitis. Thyroid acropachy may have radiological signs of multifocal periosteal reactions. Chronic venous insufficiency typically shows a solid undulating reaction separated from the cortex. Rarely, Camurati Engelmann disease or progressive diaphyseal dysplasia, an autosomal dominant condition with overactive TGFβ1 as a result of its mutated TGFB1 gene, may also have radiographic features of multifocal periostosis.

Long-standing clubbing can cause osseous resorption at terminal phalanges. Also, tuft overgrowth is seen in malignancy-associated HOA, first in toes and then in fingers. Such findings can be seen if the radiographs of the affected hands and/or feet are carefully reviewed.

Bone scintigraphy with technetium 99m (99m-Tc) methylene diphosphonate (MDP) is the most sensitive test showing periosteal involvement and is considered the gold standard. Early suspicion based on radiographs should prompt a bone scan along with a search for primary etiology with thoracic imaging [17]. Characteristic finding, known as the "double stripe" or "tramline" sign (Fig. 16.9), describes symmetrical enhanced linear tracer uptake along cortical margins of tubular bones in the

Fig. 16.4 Right wrist. This shows a subtle periosteal reaction (monolayer) along the dorsal aspect of the metaphysis of the radius

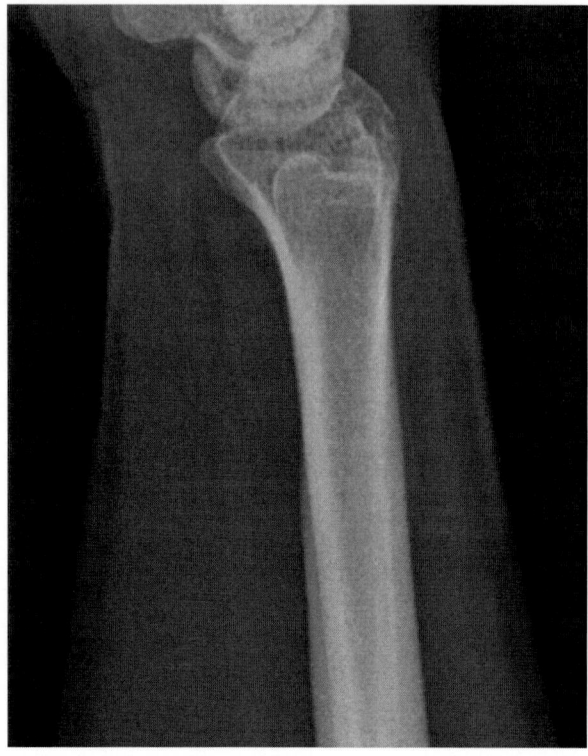

bone scan. It often reveals the involvement of the shafts and ends of tibiae, femurs, and radii, especially around the knees, ankles, and wrists. Differential diagnoses include (a) normal variant, where lateral cortices of the tibiae often appear with asymmetric linear uptake; (b) shin splints, which have very similar findings but are limited to the tibia; and (c) chronic venous insufficiency. Digital clubbing also results in prominent tracer uptake. These findings may resolve after successful treatment of the underlying etiology giving the bone scan an immense utility in monitoring the treatment response.

Magnetic resonance imaging usually shows a low to intermediate signal intensity on T1 and T2 weighted images, highlighting periosteal elevation and reaction [10]. It also helps in identifying synovial effusions. However, MRI does not have a significant role in the diagnosis and management of HOA. Findings of HOA are mostly incidental findings in imaging for unrelated conditions.

There are reports of HOA diagnosis based on PET scan findings of irregular bilateral periosteal new bone formation with increased fluorodeoxyglucose (FDG) uptake. For the same reason, there is a possibility of misdiagnosis of metastatic disease based on FDG avidity [18]. PET scan, in particular PET-CT, may be used to identify the site of the primary malignancy that results in secondary HOA. Often, HOA is noted incidentally on the PET-CT done to search for the metastases.

Fig. 16.5 Left ankle. This shows a definite periosteal reaction (monolayer) along the medial aspect of the metaphysis of the tibia

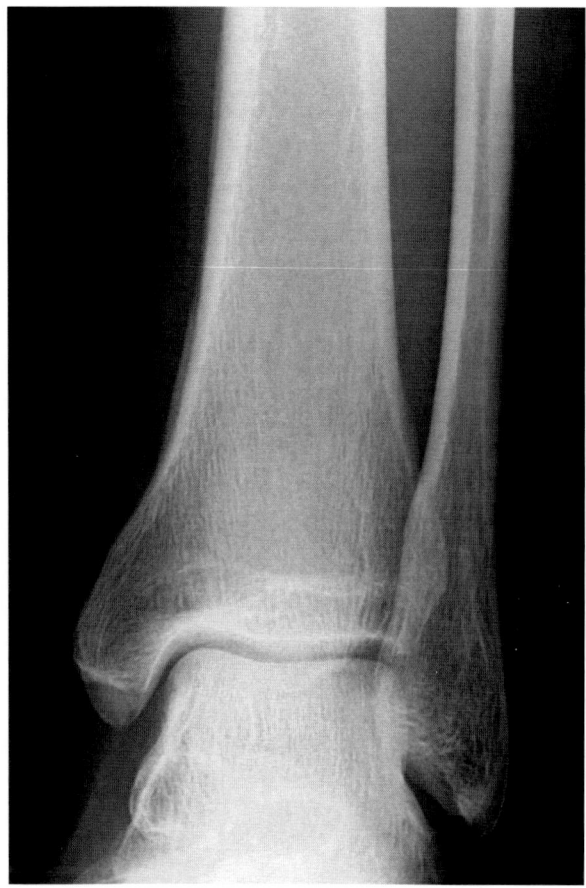

Secondary HOA should be actively entertained in the differential of bone and joint pain and new-onset clubbing in a patient with known malignancy, chronic lung disease, liver disease, or cyanotic heart disease. A new diagnosis of HOA based on clubbing, periostitis, and arthropathy should always trigger a search for a primary cause.

16.5 Pathophysiology

There is now evidence to support the contention that clubbing and HOA represent different stages of the same disease process [19]. Although several hypotheses have been proposed, the exact pathophysiologic mechanism in HOA is unknown, as it is challenging to offer good theories to explain the pathophysiologic process that leads to the same manifestations from such diverse etiologies.

Fig. 16.6 Left shin. This
shows a periosteal reaction
(lamellated or
multilayered) along the
medial aspect of the
diaphysis of the tibia

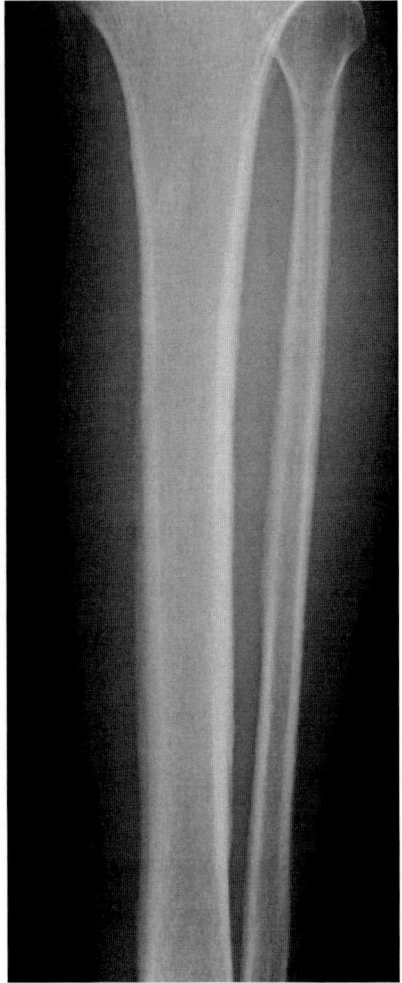

The etiopathogenesis of secondary HOA has mainly been attributed to either a neurogenic or vascular pathway triggered by circulating growth factors. The vascular pathway can be classified into two subtypes:

1. hypersecretion of vasoactive agents by the tumor itself or hypoxemia, and
2. the mechanical release of vasoactive agents in systemic circulation due to arteriovenous shunting within the pulmonary circulation.

In the neurogenic pathway, the affected organs with vagal innervation trigger a neural reflex which results in vasodilatation and increases blood circulation to the extremities, leading to clinical manifestations. Chemical and surgical vagotomy have achieved symptom suppression with varying levels of success [20].

Fig. 16.7 Right wrist. This shows a periosteal reaction (lamellated or multilayered) along the metaphysis and diaphysis of the radius and ulna

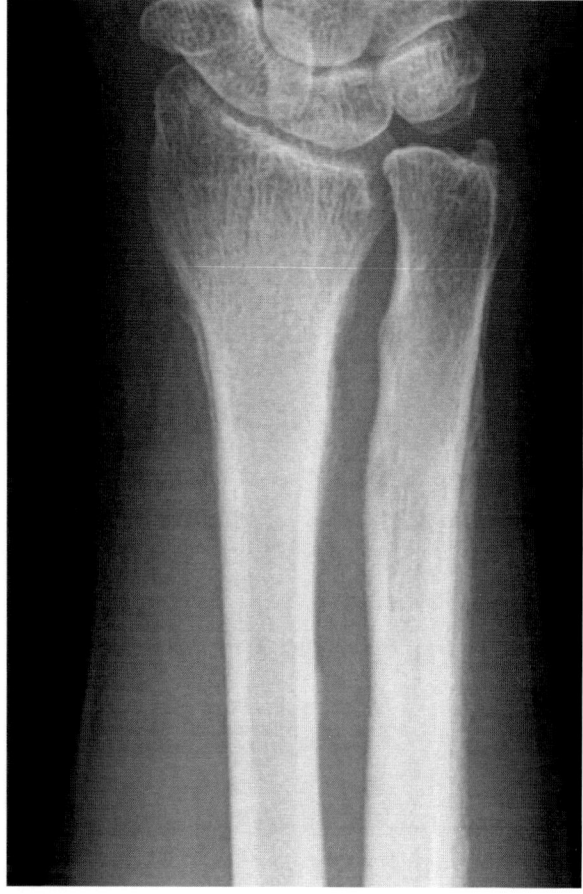

In the vascular pathway, a hypoxemia-driven surge of circulating growth factors, like platelet-derived growth factor (PDGF), vascular endothelial growth factor (VEGF), or prostaglandin E2 (PGE2) have been suggested to incite the triad of changes in HOA, i.e., clubbing, effusion of small joints, and periostosis of tubular bones [21]. Studies have demonstrated overexpression of PDGF and VEGF in HOA patients compared to healthy subjects. The functions of PDGF include stimulating endothelial and smooth muscle proliferation, increasing vascular permeability, and causing neutrophil chemotaxis. VEGF, which is derived from platelets, stimulates angiogenesis. Newly formed immature vessel walls tend to be more permeable. At the tissue level, VEGF induces vasodilatation, vascular hyperplasia, interstitial edema, and collagen deposition. The bulbous deformity of the digits is the result of excessive collagen deposition and interstitial edema. Connective tissue proliferation in the outer margin of bones elevates the periosteum and deposits the osteogenic matrix underneath. VEGF has a direct stimulatory effect on osteoblasts and osteoclasts. Paraneoplastic hypersecretion of VEGF by bronchogenic carcinoma and

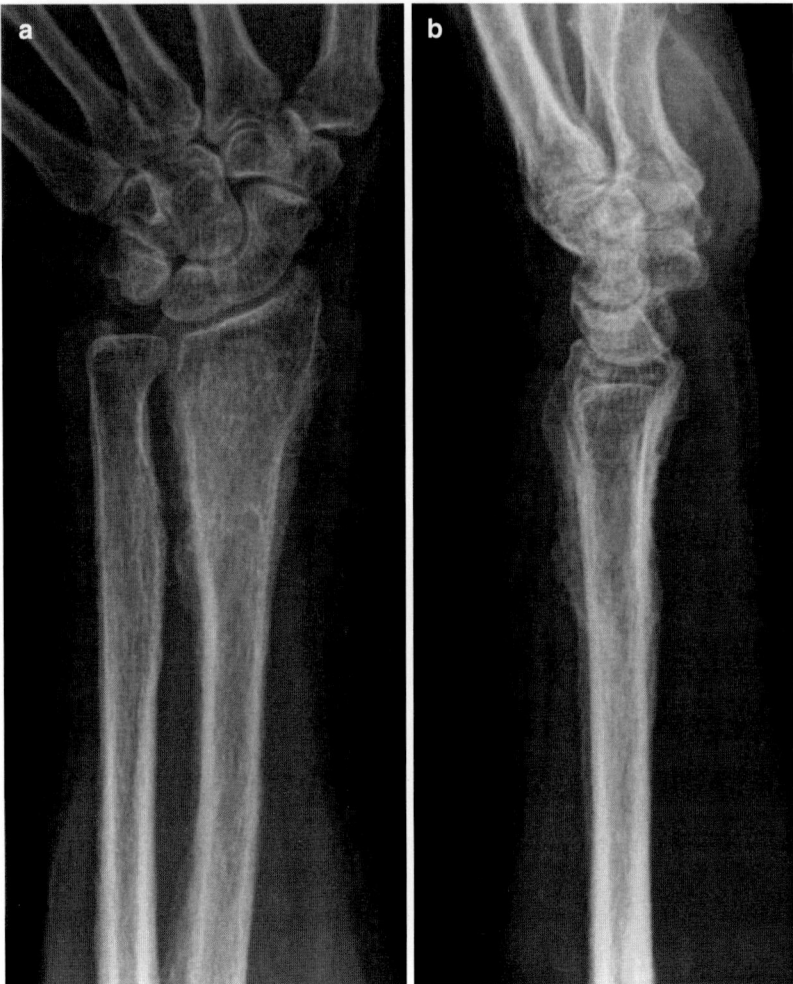

Fig. 16.8 (**a**) Left wrist (AP view). This shows a periosteal reaction (irregular) along the metaphysis and diaphysis of the radius and ulna. (**b**) Left wrist (Lat view). This shows a periosteal reaction (irregular) along the metaphysis and diaphysis of the radius and ulna

pleural fibrous tumor results in a similar surge of their function. When concurrent with malignancies, removal of primary tumors results in a decline of these levels and thus the periostitis/periostosis.

In the presence of pathological intracardiac or intrapulmonary shunt, the megakaryocytes bypass fragmentation in the pulmonary circulation and enter into systemic circulation instead [22]. This is evidenced by patients with patent ductus arteriosus complicated by pulmonary hypertension in whom the acropachy is limited to the cyanotic limbs. The release of PDGF from entrapped platelet fragments at the capillary level promotes hypervascularization and fibroblast activity. Patients

Fig. 16.9 Bone scan
shows classic tramline or
double stripe uptake in the
distal femurs and distal
tibiae bilaterally

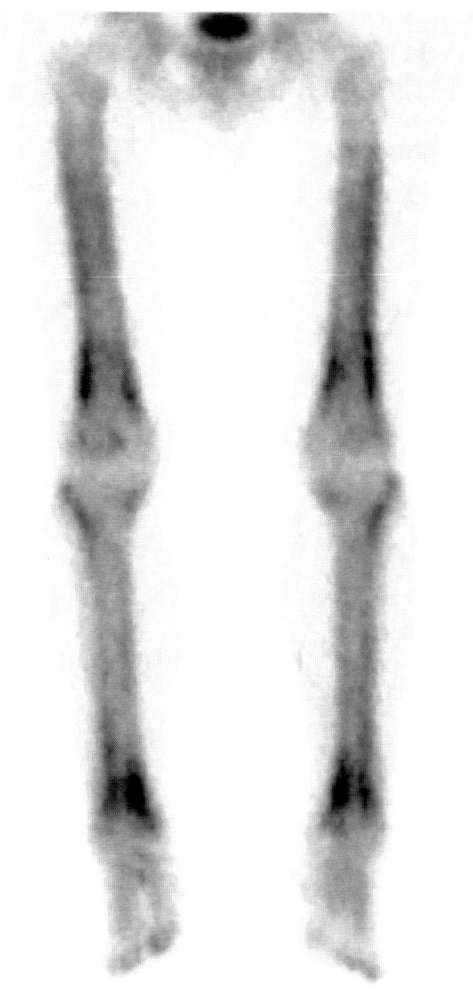

with congenital cyanotic heart diseases of myriad forms have a common histological feature of pleomorphic giant macrothrombocytes with aberrant volume distribution curves. There is also glomerular enlargement with entrapped megakaryocytic nuclei, as well as a high circulating level of von Willebrand factor antigen. Structural damage to vessel integrity is confirmed on electron microscopy, showing the presence of Weibel–Palade bodies, prominences of Golgi complexes, activated endothelia, duplicated capillary basement membranes, and perivascular lymphocytic infiltrate. Synovial cell proliferation is minimal in the adjacent joints, with prominent arterial wall thickening and intravascular deposition of electron-dense material. These findings suggest the activation of platelets and endothelial cells as the primary histologic mechanisms with subsequent release of growth factors as a secondary step, leading to the common clinical manifestations.

Genomic studies of primary HOA support the role of PGE2 in pathogenesis. Families with primary HOA carry homozygous and compound heterozygous mutations in the 15-hydroxyprostaglandin dehydrogenase [NAD+] encoding gene (HPGD) [23] and solute carrier organic anion transporter family member 2A1 (SLCO2A1) [24]. The encoded enzyme is critical for platelet degradation. There is a resultant high circulating level of PGE2 and its metabolites (PGEM). PGE2 is presumed to have an indirect role in secondary HOA through facilitating VEGF expression in bones and joints. Five infants were reported to have developed limb pain and swelling associated with periostitis after chronic infusion of PGE for congenital ductal-dependent heart disease [25].

A somewhat different but well-demonstrated pathology is seen in vascular graft infection-associated HOA, where the bacteria adherent to graft releases certain endotoxins and vasoactive agents. However, the pathogenesis is not well studied, though endothelial activation is suggested [26].

16.6   Management

A multidisciplinary team consisting of specialists (internist, rheumatologist, oncologist, cardiologist, pulmonologist, palliative medicine specialist, etc.), speciality nurses, and pharmacists is best positioned to manage patients with HOA. Most patients will require some degree of reassurance concerning the occurrence of HOA. They will need to be educated on the need for further investigations to identify the underlying cause. Compliance with a thorough evaluation is crucial for accurate diagnosis. Patient's understanding of the secondary nature of this disease will help with treatment compliance and eventually improve outcomes.

Treatment strategy can be broadly classified as treating the underlying etiology and symptomatic relief. Treatment of primary etiology where definitive treatment is targeted at curing the underlying cause [27], including surgical resection, definitive chemotherapy or radiofrequency ablation for primary malignancy, antimicrobial therapy as in pulmonary tuberculosis, lung transplantation in cystic fibrosis, treatment of liver disease with liver graft or orthoptic liver transplantation, surgical correction of cyanotic heart disease, and surgical removal of prosthetic graft coupled with systemic antibiotic therapy.

Symptomatic relief can be challenging when the primary etiology cannot be cured or treated. Considering the advanced stage of the underlying disease, the extent of symptoms in this subset of patients may be severe. The involvement of a palliative medicine specialist may be beneficial [28]. At times, the use of palliative radiation therapy may be useful in symptom control. Other modalities include non-steroidal anti-inflammatory drugs (NSAIDs), bisphosphonates, octreotide, vagotomy, adrenergic blockade, and VEGF inhibitors, which may be considered.

Following the publication of a case series of five infants with arthritis and periostitis following PGE2 infusion for patent ductus arteriosus [25], several reports showing a robust response of HOA symptoms to NSAIDs [29], e.g., indomethacin and ketorolac, and cycloxygenase-2 inhibitors have been published. In contrast, opioid analgesics were not found to be nearly as effective.

Case reports have shown that intravenous pamidronate and zoledronic acid provide symptomatic relief of HOA in bronchogenic and metastatic breast carcinoma and cyanotic congenital heart disease [30, 31]. Therapeutic response was noted in terms of symptom alleviation and the radiographic resolution of periostitis in the bone scans. The mechanism of action of the bisphosphonates traces them to a proven inhibition of circulating VEGF levels in plasma.

Octreotide has a well-demonstrated role in inhibiting endothelial proliferation through VEGF as well as inhibiting nociceptive neurons. It has been used with some success in treating HOA at a daily dose of 200 mcg [32, 33].

A combination regimen of adrenergic antagonists with propranolol and phenoxybenzamine was reported to have achieved symptomatic relief in HOA associated with small cell carcinoma lung. The treatment response was objectively measured by improvement in the thermographic index and the functional ability, including ring size and grip strength [34].

In the 1950s and 1960s, ipsilateral vagus nerve dissection was reported to relieve the symptom of HOA in inoperable primary lung malignancy cases. It was not a preferred modality due to its invasiveness and increasing popularity of the humoral theory of pathogenesis. However, the approach was revisited in 2006 by Ooi et al. in a patient with inoperable lung malignancy where HOA symptom control was successfully achieved by truncal vagotomy using video-assisted thoracoscopic surgery (VATS) [35].

VEGF circulating levels and tissue expression are enhanced in almost all HOA cases, irrespective of the etiology. Specific VEGF inhibitors are hypothesized to be able to achieve symptom suppression in HOA. Therapeutic trials of combining bevacizumab with conventional chemotherapy regimens in non-small cell lung cancer are underway. Isolated case reports from Japan suggest reducing periostitis in advanced lung malignancy with erlotinib, an epidermal growth factor receptor tyrosine kinase inhibitor [36]. Certain anticancer chemotherapies that target fibroblastic growth factors may also be useful.

The outcomes for patients with HOA depend on the underlying cause. Cases associated with a malignancy usually have a poor outcome, despite treatment. HOA may remit completely with only symptomatic treatment and specific curative treatment of the underlying cause. Recurrence of symptoms may herald a recurrence or exacerbation of the underlying condition. Secondary HOA does not add to the mortality or morbidity of the associated disease. The only complication that may occur is osteoarthritis in cases with long-standing HOA.

16.7 Conclusion

Despite being an ancient condition, understanding of the pathogenesis of HOA is still limited, even though recent research has identified potential mechanisms and the role of significant vasoactive agents, such as VEGF and PGE2. Further research is needed to confirm the findings and associations. Targeted therapy, such as anti-VEGF agents, may then be developed based on the improved understanding of the pathogenesis. With the improvement in early detection of lung cancer, advances in early surgical correction of cyanotic heart diseases, and improved public health practices that reduce the incidences of pyogenic lung diseases, HOA is becoming rarer. It is always prudent to consider HOA in cases with oligoarthritis and start a search for underlying pathology as this is often associated with malignant disease.

References

1. Hippocrates. The book of prognostics: the genuine works of Hippocrates, 9th ed. London: Sydenham Society; 1849.
2. Marie P. De l'osteo-arthropathie Hypertrophiante Pneumique. Rév Med. 1890;10:1–36.
3. Bamberger E. ÜberKnochenver€änderungen bei chronischen Lungen und Herzkrankheiten. Z Klin Med. 1891;18:193–217.
4. Martinez-Lavin M, Mansilla J, Pineda C, Pijoan C, Ochoa P. Evidence of hypertrophic osteoarthropathy in human skeletal remains from pre-Hispanic Mesoamerica. Ann Intern Med. 1994;120(3):238–41.
5. Martinez-Lavin M. Miscellaneous non-inflammatory musculoskeletal conditions. Pachydermoperiostosis. Best Pract Res Clin Rheumatol. 2011;25(5):727–34.
6. Davis MC, Sherry V. Hypertrophic osteoarthropathy as a clinical manifestation of lung cancer. Clin J Oncol Nurs. 2011;15(5):561–3.
7. Ito T, Goto K, Yoh K, Niho S, Ohmatsu H, Kubota K, et al. Hypertrophic pulmonary osteoarthropathy as a paraneoplastic manifestation of lung cancer. J Thorac Oncol. 2010;5(7):976–80.
8. Ede K, McCurdy D, Garcia-Lloret M. Hypertrophic osteoarthropathy in the hepatopulmonary syndrome. J Clin Rheumatol. 2008;14(4):230–3.
9. Martinez-Lavin M. Hypertrophic osteoarthropathy. Best Pract Res Clin Rheumatol. 2020;34(3):101507.
10. Yap FY, Skalski MR, Patel DB, Schein AJ, White EA, Tomasian A, et al. Hypertrophic osteoarthropathy: clinical and imaging features. Radiographics. 2017;37(1):157–95.
11. Vazquez-Abad D, Pineda C, Martinez-Lavin M. Digital clubbing: a numerical assessment of the deformity. J Rheumatol. 1989;16(4):518–20.
12. Gibb C, Smith PJ, Miller R. Clubbing. Br J Hosp Med (Lond). 2013;74(11):C170–2.
13. Myers KA, Farquhar DR. The rational clinical examination. Does this patient have clubbing? JAMA. 2001;286(3):341–7.
14. Schumacher HR Jr. Articular manifestations of hypertrophic pulmonary osteoarthropathy in bronchogenic carcinoma. Arthritis Rheum. 1976;19(3):629–36.
15. Morgan B, Coakley F, Finlay DB, Belton I. Hypertrophic osteoarthropathy in staging skeletal scintigraphy for lung cancer. Clin Radiol. 1996;51(10):694–7.
16. Pineda C, Fonseca C, Martinez-Lavin M. The spectrum of soft tissue and skeletal abnormalities of hypertrophic osteoarthropathy. J Rheumatol. 1990;17(5):626–32.
17. Mohan HK, Groves AM, Clarke SE. Detection of finger clubbing and primary lung tumor on Tc-99 MDP bone scintigraphy in a patient with a scaphoid fracture. Clin Nucl Med. 2004;29(7):450–1.
18. Aparici CM, Bains S. Hypertrophic osteoarthropathy seen with NaF18 PET/CT bone imaging. Clin Nucl Med. 2011;36(10):928–9.
19. Martinez-Lavin M. Digital clubbing and hypertrophic osteoarthropathy: a unifying hypothesis. J Rheumatol. 1987;14(1):6–8.
20. Treasure T. Hypertrophic pulmonary osteoarthropathy and the vagus nerve: an historical note. J R Soc Med. 2006;99(8):388–90.

21. Kozak KR, Milne GL, Morrow JD, Cuiffo BP. Hypertrophic osteoarthropathy pathogenesis: a case highlighting the potential role for cyclo-oxygenase-2-derived prostaglandin E2. Nat Clin Pract Rheumatol. 2006;2(8):452–6; quiz following 6.
22. Dickinson CJ, Martin JF. Megakaryocytes and platelet clumps as the cause of finger clubbing. Lancet. 1987;2(8573):1434–5.
23. Uppal S, Diggle CP, Carr IM, Fishwick CW, Ahmed M, Ibrahim GH, et al. Mutations in 15-hydroxyprostaglandin dehydrogenase cause primary hypertrophic osteoarthropathy. Nat Genet. 2008;40(6):789–93.
24. Zhang Z, Zhang C, Zhang Z. Primary hypertrophic osteoarthropathy: an update. Front Med. 2013;7(1):60–4.
25. Letts M, Pang E, Simons J. Prostaglandin-induced neonatal periostitis. J Pediatr Orthop. 1994;14(6):809–13.
26. Alonso-Bartolomé P, Martínez-Taboada VM, Pina T, Blanco R, Rodriguez-Valverde V. Hypertrophic osteoarthropathy secondary to vascular prosthesis infection: report of 3 cases and review of the literature. Medicine (Baltimore). 2006;85(3):191.
27. Nguyen S, Hojjati M. Review of current therapies for secondary hypertrophic pulmonary osteoarthropathy. Clin Rheumatol. 2011;30(1):7–13.
28. Pourmorteza M, Baumrucker SJ, Al-Sheyyab A, Da Silva MA. Hypertrophic pulmonary Osteoarthropathy: a rare but treatable condition in palliative medicine. J Pain Symptom Manag. 2015;50(2):263–7.
29. Shakya P, Pokhrel KN, Mlunde LB, Tan S, Ota E, Niizeki H. Effectiveness of non-steroidal anti-inflammatory drugs among patients with primary hypertrophic osteoarthropathy: a systematic review. J Dermatol Sci. 2018;90(1):21–6.
30. Amital H, Applbaum YH, Vasiliev L, Rubinow A. Hypertrophic pulmonary osteoarthropathy: control of pain and symptoms with pamidronate. Clin Rheumatol. 2004;23(4):330–2.
31. Jayakar BA, Abelson AG, Yao Q. Treatment of hypertrophic osteoarthropathy with zoledronic acid: case report and review of the literature. Semin Arthritis Rheum. 2011;41(2):291–6.
32. Angel-Moreno Maroto A, Martinez-Quintana E, Suarez-Castellano L, Perez-Arellano JL. Painful hypertrophic osteoarthropathy successfully treated with octreotide. The pathogenetic role of vascular endothelial growth factor (VEGF). Rheumatology (Oxford). 2005;44(10):1326–7.
33. Birch E, Jenkins D, Noble S. Treatment of painful hypertrophic osteoarthropathy associated with non-small cell lung cancer with octreotide: a case report and review of the literature. BMJ Support Palliat Care. 2011;1(2):189–92.
34. Reardon G, Collins AJ, Bacon PA. The effect of adrenergic blockade in hypertrophic pulmonary osteoarthropathy (HPOA). Postgrad Med J. 1976;52(605):170–3.
35. Ooi A, Saad RA, Moorjani N, Amer KM. Effective symptomatic relief of hypertrophic pulmonary osteoarthropathy by video-assisted thoracic surgery truncal vagotomy. Ann Thorac Surg. 2007;83(2):684–5.
36. Kikuchi R, Itoh M, Tamamushi M, Nakamura H, Aoshiba K. Hypertrophic Osteoarthropathy secondary to lung cancer: beneficial effect of anti-vascular endothelial growth factor antibody. J Clin Rheumatol. 2017;23(1):47–50.

Carcinomatous Polyarthritis

17

Jasmin Raja and Rafi Raja

17.1 Introduction

Malignancy is known to cause a wide variety of systemic conditions, including rheumatological conditions with various musculoskeletal manifestations. There can be three types of associations between malignancies and rheumatological conditions. Firstly, a direct triggering of a new-onset rheumatological condition by a tumor or its metastasis. Secondly, the development of cancer within a temporal interval of up to 20 years in individuals with established rheumatic disease. The third group of patients have paraneoplastic syndromes, where the rheumatological manifestations have a temporal relationship with malignancy which becomes clinically evident within months to a few years.

Paraneoplastic syndromes are rare and occur in the presence of an apparent or occult malignancy, but are not due to the direct effects of the tumor mass or its metastasis. Approximately 7–10% of paraneoplastic syndromes have rheumatological manifestations [1]. The clinical picture in such paraneoplastic syndromes can mimic rheumatic diseases as the selective influence of a tumor can affect various parts of the musculoskeletal system including the synovium, periosteum, muscles, fascia, subcutaneous connective tissue, vessels, and bones. Some examples of such paraneoplastic syndromes are carcinomatous polyarthritis, inflammatory myositis, scleroderma, fasciitis, and vasculitis [1–5].

J. Raja (✉)
Division of Rheumatology, Department and Faculty of Medicine, University of Malaya,
Kuala Lumpur, Malaysia
e-mail: rjasmin@ummc.edu.my

R. Raja
Rheumatology and Immunology Department, Christchurch Hospital,
Christchurch, New Zealand

© The Author(s), under exclusive license to Springer Nature
Switzerland AG 2022
V. Ravindran et al. (eds.), *Rarer Arthropathies*, Rare Diseases of the Immune
System, https://doi.org/10.1007/978-3-031-05002-2_17

Carcinomatous polyarthritis (CP) is defined as the presence of inflammatory arthritis in association with malignancy, but it is not due to direct invasion by the tumor or due to metastasis. Its exact prevalence is unknown, but on all counts, it is a rare clinical entity with a variable presentation. The early identification of CP becomes crucial given the underlying malignancy and the need for early and effective treatment. This review focuses on CP, the possible pathological mechanisms involved, its various presentations, clues to suspecting underlying cancer, and the treatment.

17.2 Pathophysiology

The exact pathophysiology of paraneoplastic rheumatic syndromes is unknown. Possible tumor-secreted mediators involved in the immune mechanisms are various hormones, peptides, antibodies, cytotoxic lymphocytes, and autocrine and paracrine mediators [2, 6, 7]. The interplay between malignancy and rheumatological conditions is mostly attributed to the abnormalities in cell-mediated and humoral immunity. There are a few hypotheses that have been proposed as underlying mechanisms for the immunological alteration that accounts for the coexistence of cancer and CP.

Circulating immune complexes (CIC) and cytokines are thought to play a role in the pathogenesis of CP [8]. The presence of autoantibodies such as rheumatoid factor or antinuclear antibody (ANA) and perhaps the appearance of the synovial biopsy may provide a clue regarding this immune trigger. One study found elevated levels of a platelet-activating factor, thought to be CIC that disappeared with tumor resection and resolution of symptoms [9]. It has been suggested that platelet aggregation may be an indicator of circulating immune complexes in vivo [10]. Serum sIL-2R level, which is one of the markers for immune activation also decreased in the case of gastric adenocarcinoma when the manifestation resolved [11]. In the case of ovarian malignancy, partial regression of arthritis in response to chemotherapy, taken together with the serum biomarkers CA125 and HE4, suggests the possible role of CIC [12]. However, this circumstantial evidence of circulating immune complexes involved could not be substantiated. In a published report, immune complexes failed to be demonstrated in immunofluorescent studies of the synovium in a patient with CP secondary to spindle cell carcinoma of the lung [8].

Another proposed underlying mechanism is apoptosis of neoplastic cells which is responsible for cross-immune reactions between tumor antigens and synovium. This mechanism was demonstrated in a case where the pattern of the T cell antigen-receptor γ gene from T lymphocytes infiltrating the renal cell carcinoma and the synovial tissue from the Baker's cyst that was removed before the diagnosis of renal cell carcinoma was analyzed [13]. It revealed the presence of monoclonal T cells in both types of tissue. This suggests that lymphocytes directed against the tumor can cross-react with synovial antigens to trigger CP.

The demonstration of autoantibodies to nuclear proteins and to a wide array of tissue-associated antigens in the sera of patients with paraneoplastic rheumatic syndromes also supports this hypothesis [14]. Cases of CP with positive anti-CCP antibodies theoretically have been linked to this. Peptidyl arginine deiminase (PAD) enzymes convert target peptides from apoptotic cells to citrullinated peptides (e.g., anti-CCP antibodies) in inflammatory arthritis. Synovial tissues from patients with rheumatoid arthritis (RA) and with other arthropathies were studied and it was found that the presence of antibody formation, not citrullinated proteins, in the inflamed synovium is more specific to RA and is likely a result of an abnormal humoral response to these proteins [15]. Whether anti-CCP antibodies are involved in the pathogenesis of joint inflammation or are a by-product of synovial inflammation secondary to a specific humoral response is unknown. Anti-CCPs are formed against citrullinated peptides, and could also result from the antigenic stimulation by citrullinated peptides due to overexpression of PAD14 enzymes in neoplastic tissues [16]. The complete understanding of the role of these antibodies as mediators of CP remains elusive and further studies are required to confirm their role.

17.3 Clinical Features (Table 17.1)

Carcinomatous polyarthritis occurs relatively late, at a mean age of 50 years [18, 19]. The elderly are the most often affected, and present with new-onset arthritis [2]. The age of onset of RA on the other hand is between 30 and 55 years; however, as this incidence increases with increasing age, the distinction between RA and CP becomes particularly challenging in older populations. Moreover, elderly onset RA represents a poorer prognostic subset of the disease, adding to the diagnostic confusion [20]. Unlike female preponderance in RA, available evidence suggests that males have a higher predilection to CP [2, 18, 19].

Table 17.1 Key clinical features of carcinomatous polyarthritis [17]

Traditional characteristics of CP	New characteristics of CP
Close temporal relationship (12 months) between onset of arthritis and malignancy	Average time between arthritis and malignancy diagnosis as early as 3–6 months
Late age at onset	Age >50
Asymmetric joint involvement	Polyarthritis (symmetrical or asymmetrical)
Explosive or abrupt onset	–
Predominance of lower extremity involvement with sparing of wrists and small joints of hands	Joint involvement of upper and lower extremities, mimicking RA
Absence of rheumatoid factor (RF)	Absence or presence of RF or/and anti-CCP
Absence of rheumatoid nodules	–
No family history of rheumatic disease	–
Absence of characteristic radiologic features of RA	Erosions may be present, but rare
Nonspecific histopathologic appearance of synovial lining	–

17.3.1 When to Suspect Carcinomatous Polyarthritis?

Carcinomatous polyarthritis by definition (Table 17.2) must occur during the course of an identified malignant disease or precede clinical evidence of malignancy [1, 22]. Symptoms of CP should not be the direct consequence of tumor invasion or compression. A close temporal relationship or interval between the onset of arthritis and the diagnosis of the associated tumor often does not exceed 2 years. In most instances, arthritis precedes the development of malignancy by 8–12 months or as little as 3 months [18, 23]. Gur et al. found that 5.8% of the leukemia patients who presented with arthritis were seen for arthritis an average of 3.2 months before the diagnosis of their leukemia [24]. Malignancy was diagnosed after articular symptoms in 88.5%, while in 11.5% it was diagnosed at the time of their rheumatic presentation [18].

17.3.2 Common Patterns of Presentation

Historically, CP has been characterized by asymmetric joint involvement, a predilection for lower extremity joints, and sparing of the wrists and hands [25]. Presentations such as symmetrical polyarthritis involving wrists, metacarpophalangeal, and proximal interphalangeal joints of both hands that resemble RA (Fig. 17.1), are seen in up to 85% of the cases [18, 19, 27, 28]. In a study of 18

Table 17.2 Criteria for carcinomatous polyarthritis [1, 21]

1. Arthritis should occur during the course of an identified malignant disease or precede clinical evidence of a malignancy
2. Symptoms of arthritis should not be attributable to a direct tumor invasion
3. Symptoms of arthritis improve with treatment of the underlying malignancy

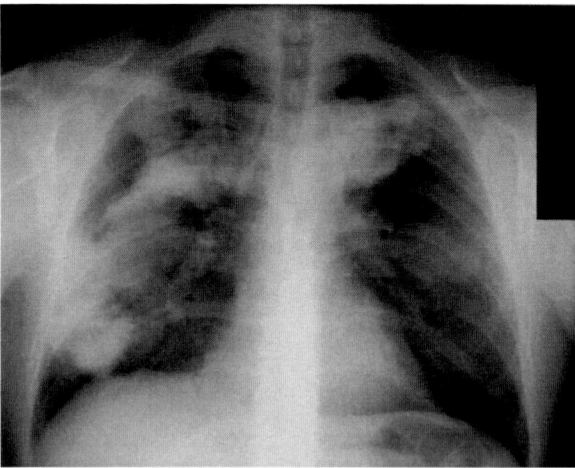

Fig. 17.1 Chest X-ray showing multiple bilateral lung nodules in a man presenting with polyarthritis, who was later diagnosed to have lymphomatoid granulomatosis. His rheumatoid factor and anti-CCP levels were significantly elevated during the initial presentation (Adapted with permission from [26])

patients, 8 presented with the typical joint involvement pattern of RA [29]. In another series of 26 patients with CP diagnosed within 2 years of the discovery of malignancy, four met the American College of Rheumatology (ACR) criteria for RA [23]. The differentiation of CP from RA is quite challenging given that the patients may fulfill ACR criteria for RA, but clinical awareness and suspicion of CP should always remain, given the certain clues for neoplasia and atypical features of arthritis presentation.

Other various patterns of presentation are asymmetrical polyarthritis, monoarthritis, oligoarthritis, and migratory inflammation of the joints [2, 18, 19, 27]. In a case series differentiating paraneoplastic arthritis from early rheumatoid arthritis, patients with oligoarthritis were significantly higher in the former and those with symmetrical polyarthritis were significantly higher in the latter group [19]. Bilateral sacroiliitis with asymmetrical large joint arthritis, a clinical scenario for diagnosis of axial spondyloarthropathy was also reported in hematological malignancies, where these patients were not responding to regular NSAIDs [30].

The onset of CP is abrupt or explosive and can be debilitating [28]. Arthritis in CP may also have a gradual onset over weeks to months, making CP difficult to differentiate from RA [17]. Patients describe their painful joint swellings as sudden and severe, painful during rest or at night, and early morning stiffness of joints lasting at least for an hour. Physical examination of the joints involved shows tender synovitis or soft tissue swelling, limited range of motion of affected joint, usually with no deformities. The presence of long bone pain or tenderness is suggestive of hypertrophic osteoarthropathy rather than CP. Patients with CP do not have rheumatoid nodules [18, 25].

17.3.3 Risk Factors and Extra-Articular Features Suggestive of Carcinomatous Polyarthritis

A comprehensive history and physical examination are pivotal in distinguishing CP from other more common causes of inflammatory arthritis, with careful attention to social and family history to detect any possible risk factors for malignancy. The presence of a family history of malignancy or certain risk factors such as smoking should increase the suspicion for the development of malignancy. The percentage of smokers among CP patients was higher among those with solid tumors (75%) [18]. A family history of RA is generally not found in patients with CP [18, 25].

Extra-articular features and presentations that are consistent with an underlying neoplasm should prompt relevant clinical assessments. Patients with CP may have a general state of deterioration accompanied by constitutional symptoms such as malaise, lethargy, fever, and significant loss of weight which may be there at presentation or develop gradually thereafter [18, 25]. A detailed physical examination is crucial to look for signs of malignancy, for example, a palpable mass in cases of solid tumor and cervical lymphadenopathy or hepatosplenomegaly in cases of hematological malignancies.

17.3.4 Types of Malignancies Commonly Associated with Carcinomatous Polyarthritis

Carcinomatous polyarthritis has been reported in a variety of solid tumors including those of lungs, breast, kidneys, ovaries, thyroid glands, and the gastrointestinal system [12, 13, 17, 18, 21, 27, 31, 32]. Most frequently occurring solid tumors are adenocarcinomas of the lungs and breast [2, 18, 21]. RA-like arthritis was detected in 16% of cases of paraneoplastic syndromes in patients with lung cancer [31].

Carcinomatous polyarthritis has been reported less commonly in hematological malignancies compared to solid tumors [2]. In the two case series reported by Morel and Kisacik, around 10% of paraneoplastic arthritis were due to lymphomas [18, 19]. As such, leukemias have a higher prevalence of CP than other hematological malignancies. In this context, the diagnosis of hematological malignancies was observed to be more delayed than that of solid tumors [18].

17.3.5 Differential Diagnosis

Clinicians must be able to exclude other common causes of inflammatory arthritis. Differential diagnosis of migratory polyarthritis or oligoarthritis is broad and includes rheumatoid arthritis, crystal arthropathy, spondyloarthropathies, connective tissue disorders, and infectious causes. In comparison, paraneoplastic syndromes such as CP contribute to less common etiologies.

17.4   Investigations

There are no definitive diagnostic tests for CP hence most investigations are performed to exclude other diseases. Inflammatory markers, i.e., erythrocyte sedimentation rate and C-reactive protein levels are usually elevated when the arthritis is active [17–19, 27]. Previously proposed features of CP included negative serological tests for rheumatoid factor and anti-CCP [25]. However, in up to 50% of cases, seropositive polyarthritis (Fig. 17.1) can be the presenting feature in CP [17–19, 21, 23, 27]. The presence of rheumatoid factor in such cases can be partially explained by the incidental rheumatoid factor positivity in 10–20% of patients with underlying malignancies. Cases of malignancies with positivity for anti-CCP have also been reported, which can be misleading and may lead to an incorrect diagnosis of RA [17, 19, 21, 26, 33]. The presence of a significant titer of ANA is also seen in about 20% of cases [2, 18, 27].

Another common useful investigation is joint arthrocentesis with synovial fluid analysis to exclude the presence of crystals and infection. The synovial fluid generally shows nonspecific inflammatory changes with moderately raised leukocyte or neutrophil counts [1, 18, 21, 26, 27]. Synovial tissue histology shows nonspecific synovitis [13, 33]. Radiographic studies are generally unremarkable with the absence of erosions and joint space narrowing except for age-related changes [27]. Erosive disease in CP has been described in only a few cases in the literature [23, 34].

The clues in hematological investigations and imaging studies are important as they often precede other clinical manifestations of neoplasms that aid the diagnosis of an underlying malignancy. Anemia is a common concurrent feature seen in CP [17, 25]. There may be bi-cytopenia seen in cases of leukemia. Lactate dehydrogenase is a useful marker for the differentiation of malignant hematological diseases and helps differentiate these from solid tumors and early rheumatoid arthritis [19]. Other investigations such as tumor markers, CT scan, FDG-PET scan imaging, and a biopsy of the suspicious mass or bone marrow are also warranted.

17.5 Management

One of the important clues pointing towards CP is poor response to NSAIDs or glucocorticoids [21, 27, 28]. Some patients may have a transient response to the glucocorticoids given either intra-articular, parenterally or orally [17, 21, 26, 32]. NSAIDs were efficacious in 45% and glucocorticoids in 91%, though sustained remission was not achieved [18]. DMARDs were shown not to be efficient to improve symptoms in CP [18, 19]. Poor response to methotrexate, sulfasalazine, and hydroxychloroquine has been reported [17, 18, 28, 32]. Conversely, the use of glucocorticoids, DMARDs and rituximab to treat arthritis can lead to a minimal or partial response in lymphomas, leading to temporary resolution of the symptoms [35].

One of the main criteria for CP is improvement and resolution in arthritis symptoms following treatment of the underlying malignancy, for example, surgical resection of the tumor or following chemotherapy [1]. The paraneoplastic synovitis and constitutional symptoms improve with regression of the associated malignancy [12, 18, 21, 32, 36]. In a survival study of patients with CP, the cure of malignancy resulted in complete resolution of CP in 76% of patients [18]. Patients with solid tumors had significantly higher rates of resolution of articular symptoms as compared to patients with hematological malignancies [18]. Return of arthritis can herald tumor recurrence [37]. In most cases however a tumor relapse or metastasis of the primary malignancy is not accompanied by the recurrence of arthritis [18, 36]. Arthritis symptoms did not recur in 75% of patients with tumor relapse [18].

17.6 Conclusion

Paraneoplasia provides an interesting relationship between malignancy and rheumatological manifestations such as CP, which are complex and not yet completely understood. The differential diagnosis of CP is broad and it may mimic RA. Despite CP being rare, several of its classical features should prompt suspicion in facilitating the early diagnosis and timely treatment. A comprehensive detailed evaluation is required to diagnose and then work towards the cure of underlying malignancy, which often results in the resolution of symptoms.

References

1. Fam AG. Paraneoplastic rheumatic syndromes. Baillieres Best Pract Res Clin Rheumatol. 2000;14(3):515–33.
2. Manger B, Schett G. Paraneoplastic syndromes in rheumatology. Nat Rev Rheumatol. 2014;10(11):662–70.
3. Sendur OF. Paraneoplastic rheumatic disorders. Turk J Rheumatol. 2012;27(1):18–23.
4. Calabro JJ. Cancer and arthritis. Arthritis Rheum. 1967;10(6):553–67.
5. Racanelli V, Prete M, Minoia C, Favoino E, Perosa F. Rheumatic disorders as paraneoplastic syndromes. Autoimmun Rev. 2008;7(5):352–8.
6. Azar L, Khasnis A. Paraneoplastic rheumatologic syndromes. Curr Opin Rheumatol. 2013;25(1):44–9.
7. Shah AA, Casciola-Rosen L, Rosen A. Review: cancer-induced autoimmunity in the rheumatic diseases. Arthritis Rheumatol. 2015;67(2):317–26.
8. Bradley JD, Pinals RS. Carcinoma polyarthritis: role of immune complexes in pathogenesis. J Rheumatol. 1983;10:826–8.
9. Bennett RM, Ginsberg MH, Thompsen S. Carcinomatous polyarthritis: the presenting symptom of an ovarian tumor and association with a platelet activating factor. Arthritis Rheum. 1976;19:953–8.
10. Myllyla G, Vaheri A, Pentinnen K. Detection and characterization of immune complexes by the platelet aggregation test. Clin Exp Immunol. 1971;8:399–408.
11. Ochi K, Horiuchi Y, Seki M, Nishi K, Nozaki H, Yabe H. Polyarthritis and posterior interosseous nerve palsy associated with gastric carcinoma. Rheumatol Int. 2012;32(8):2557–9.
12. Gatti A, Plotti F, Montera R, Terranova C, Nardone CDC, et al. Paraneoplastic arthritis in advanced ovarian cancer and its correlation with CA125 and HE4 levels: a case report. Ann Case Rep. 2021;6:608.
13. Schultz H, Krenn V, Tony HP. Oligoarthritis mediated by tumor-specific T lymphocytes in renal-cell carcinoma. N Engl J Med. 1999;341(4):290–1.
14. Abu-Shakra M, Buskila D, Ehrenfeld M, Conrad K, Shoenfeld Y. Cancer and autoimmunity: autoimmune and rheumatic features in patients with malignancies. Ann Rheum Dis. 2001;60(5):433–41.
15. Vossenaar ER, Smeets TJ, Kraan MC, Raats JM, van Venrooij WJ, Tak PP. The presence of citrullinated proteins is not specific for rheumatoid synovial tissue. Arthritis Rheum. 2004;50(11):3485–94.
16. Chang X, Han J, Pang L, Zhao Y, Yang Y, Shen Z. Increased PADI4 expression in blood and tissues of patients with malignant tumors. BMC Cancer. 2009;9:40.
17. Silvério-António M, Parlato F, Martins P, Khmelinskii N, Braz S, Fonseca JE, Polido-Pereira J. Gastric adenocarcinoma presenting as a rheumatoid factor and anti-cyclic citrullinated protein antibody-positive polyarthritis: a case report and review of literature. Front Med (Lausanne). 2021;8:627004.
18. Morel J, Deschamps V, Toussirot E, Pertuiset E, Sordet C, Kieffer P, Berthelot JM, Champagne H, Mariette X, Combe B. Characteristics and survival of 26 patients with paraneoplastic arthritis. Ann Rheum Dis. 2008;67(2):244–7.
19. Kisacik B, Onat AM, Kasifoglu T, Pehlivan Y, Pamuk ON, Dalkilic E, et al. Diagnostic dilemma of paraneoplastic arthritis: case series. Int J Rheum Dis. 2014;17(6):640–5.
20. Yazici Y, Paget SA. Elderly-onset rheumatoid arthritis. Rheum Dis Clin North Am. 2000;26:517–26.

21. Watson GA, O'Neill L, Law R, McCarthy G, Veale D. Migrating polyarthritis as a feature of occult malignancy: 2 case reports and a review of the literature. Case Rep Oncol Med. 2015;2015:934039.
22. Lansbury J. Collagen disease complicating malignancy. Ann Rheum Dis. 1953;12(4):301–5.
23. Sheon RP, Kirsner AB, Tangsintanapas P, Samad F, Garg ML, Finkel RI. Malignancy in rheumatic disease: interrelationships. J Am Geriatr Soc. 1977;25(1):20–7.
24. Gur H, Koren V, Ehrenfeld M, Ben-Bassat I, Sidi Y. Rheumatic manifestations preceding adult acute leukemia: characteristics and implication in course and prognosis. Acta Haematol. 1999;101(1):1–6.
25. Stummvoll GH, Aringer M, Machold KP, Smolen JS, Raderer M. Cancer polyarthritis resembling rheumatoid arthritis as a first sign of hidden neoplasms. Report of two cases and review of the literature. Scand J Rheumatol. 2001;30:40–4.
26. Raja R, Lamont D, Yung A, Solanki K. A can of red herrings. Int J Rheum Dis. 2010;13(3):e46–50.
27. Zupancic M, Annamalai A, Brenneman J, Ranatunga S. Migratory polyarthritis as a paraneoplastic syndrome. J Gen Intern Med. 2008;23(12):2136–9.
28. Mok CC, Kwan YK. Rheumatoid-like polyarthritis as a presenting feature of metastatic carcinoma: a case presentation and review of the literature. Clin Rheumatol. 2003;22(4–5):353–4.
29. Caldwell DS. Carcinoma polyarthritis manifestations and differential diagnosis. Med Grand Rounds. 1982;1:378–85.
30. Mondal S, Sinha D, Ete T, Goswami R, Bardhan J, Ghosh A. A foe incognito: paraneoplastic sacroiliitis. J Med Cases. 2016;7(8):341–3.
31. Syniachenko O, Iermolaieva M, Stepko P, Verzilov S, Potapov Y. Paraneoplastic rheumatoid-like arthritis associated with lung cancer. Pain Joints Spine. 2020;10(1):51–6.
32. Pathak H, Lonsdale R, Dhatariya K, Mukhtyar C. Carcinomatous polyarthritis as a presenting manifestation of papillary carcinoma of thyroid gland. Indian J Rheumatol. 2016;11:164–6.
33. Mackenzie AH, Scherbel AL. Connective tissue syndromes associated with carcinoma. Geriatrics. 1963;18:745–53.
34. Handy CE, Robles G, Haque U, Houston B. T cell ALL presenting as seropositive rheumatoid arthritis: case report and review of the literature on seropositive paraneoplastic arthritis. Clin Rheumatol. 2015;34(9):1647–50.
35. Bahat G, Kamali S, Saka B, Erten N, Karan MA, Tascioglu C. Paraneoplastic arthritis may mimic rheumatoid arthritis with symmetrical and upper extremity predilecting presentation. J Clin Rheumatol. 2009;15(6):319–20.
36. Yamashita H, Ueda Y, Ozaki T, Tsuchiya H, Takahashi Y, Kaneko H, Kano T, Mimori A. Characteristics of 10 patients with paraneoplastic rheumatologic musculoskeletal manifestations. Mod Rheumatol. 2014;24(3):492–8.
37. Eggelmeijer F, MacFarlane J. Polyarthritis as the presenting symptom of the occurrence and recurrence of a laryngeal carcinoma. Ann Rheum Dis. 1992;51:556–7.

Arthritis Associated with Immune Checkpoint Inhibitors

18

Noha Abdel-Wahab ⓘ and Maria E. Suarez-Almazor ⓘ

18.1 Introduction

Cancer treatment has been transformed with the development and approval of immune checkpoint inhibitors (ICI). Several ICIs have been approved for the treatment of cancer, providing remarkable survival benefits in both metastatic and adjuvant settings. Immune checkpoint inhibitors are monoclonal antibodies that target the regulatory immune checkpoints which inhibit T cell activation [1]. Thus, ICIs take the brakes off of the immune system enhancing the host's antitumor immune response. The approved ICIs are: (1) ipilimumab, and tremelimumab, which are antibodies against cytotoxic T lymphocyte-associated protein 4 (CTLA-4); (2) nivolumab, pembrolizumab, cemiplimab-rwlc, dostarlimab-gxly, and camrelizumab, which are antibodies against programmed death receptor-1 (PD-1); and (3) atezolizumab, durvalumab, and avelumab, which are antibodies against programmed death-ligand 1 (PD-L1). The use of combination therapy including 2 ICI with

N. Abdel-Wahab
Section of Rheumatology and Clinical Immunology, The University of Texas MD Anderson Cancer Center, Houston, TX, USA

Department of Melanoma Medical Oncology, The University of Texas MD Anderson Cancer Center, Houston, TX, USA

Department of Rheumatology and Rehabilitation, Assiut University Faculty of Medicine, Assiut University Hospitals, Assiut, Egypt
e-mail: nahassan@mdanderson.org

M. E. Suarez-Almazor (✉)
Section of Rheumatology and Clinical Immunology, The University of Texas MD Anderson Cancer Center, Houston, TX, USA

Department of Health Services Research, The University of Texas MD Anderson Cancer Center, Houston, TX, USA
e-mail: msalmazor@mdanderson.org

© The Author(s), under exclusive license to Springer Nature Switzerland AG 2022
V. Ravindran et al. (eds.), *Rarer Arthropathies*, Rare Diseases of the Immune System, https://doi.org/10.1007/978-3-031-05002-2_18

different mechanisms of action is becoming more common to address tumor resistance to treatment with a single agent.

Though effective in eliciting antitumor responses, ICIs often result in severe and occasionally fatal off-target inflammatory and autoimmune effects owing to unpredictable immune system activation against host organs [2]. While many of these immune-related adverse events (irAEs) are transient and resolve rapidly with immunosuppressive therapies and ICI discontinuation, some, especially, endocrinopathies, neurologic, and rheumatologic syndromes can have long-lasting effects and sequelae, significantly impacting patients' function and activities of daily living (ADL).

18.2 Epidemiology

Arthralgia can occur in up to approximately 40% of patients receiving ICI. Definite arthritis with synovitis is less frequent and has been reported in up to 9% of patients treated with ICI. However, the true incidence and severity of arthritis-irAE are still undetermined as most studies are retrospective case series [3]. Arthritis-irAE seems to be underreported in oncology trials that use the Common Terminology Criteria for Adverse Events (CTCAE). The CTCAE version 5.0 defines arthritis as grade II if it limits instrumental ADL, which from a rheumatology perspective is considered sufficient for treatment as musculoskeletal functional limitations severely affect the quality of life. However, many trials report primarily irAE grades III–V, and arthritis may have been initially underreported. Prospective longitudinal studies including denominators with all patients treated with ICI are necessary to accurately estimate the true incidence rate, severity, and outcome of arthritis-irAE.

18.3 Risk Factors

Arthritis-irAE occurs more frequently in patients receiving combination ICI therapy. A higher proportion of irAEs, in general, have been reported in Caucasians compared to African Americans; however, no racial association with arthritis-irAE was identified [4]. Although the female gender was found in one study to be an independent risk factor for irAE, it does not seem to be a risk factor for developing arthritis-irAE. Age has varied widely at presentation and does not appear to be independently associated with developing arthritis-irAE. Of note, body mass index ≥ 25 kg/m^2 was recently identified as a risk factor for irAE, including arthritis and other rheumatologic irAEs, in patients receiving anti-CTLA-4 or anti-PD-1/PD-L1 monotherapies, or ICI combination therapies [5]. As for cancer types, rheumatologic irAEs and arthritis-irAE may occur more frequently in patients with melanoma and genitourinary cancer receiving ICI [4]. Treatment with ICI combination therapy, glucocorticoid use within 1 year before ICI initiation, and history of preexisting autoimmune diseases are also associated with rheumatologic irAEs and arthritis-irAE [4]. Notably, patients with preexisting inflammatory arthritis (rheumatoid, psoriatic, and spondyloarthritis) can experience arthritis flares upon ICI initiation, and this risk is higher among patients with active symptoms and in those who discontinued immunosuppressant therapy at ICI initiation. Moreover, the presence of autoantibodies including antinuclear antibodies (ANA), rheumatoid factor (RF), antithyroglobulin, and antithyroid peroxidase before ICI initiation have been identified as risk factors for developing irAEs, in general, although these results were not specific to rheumatologic irAEs or arthritis-irAE [6]. Some patients with arthritis-irAE were found to have preexisting anti-citric citrullinated peptide (anti-CCP) antibodies, suggesting that a pre-RA status can manifest clinically after ICI initiation. So far, no new autoantibodies have been identified in association with de novo arthritis-irAE.

18.4 Pathogenesis

Our understanding of the pathogenic mechanisms of irAEs, including arthritis-irAE, is still limited. Several mechanisms have been proposed [7]: (1) breach of self-tolerance and enhanced preexisting autoimmunity result from generalized immune activation induced by ICIs. In arthritis-irAE, immunoprofiling of the synovial fluid showed expanded $CD38^{hi}$ CD8 T cells and Th17 cells; (2) release of cytokines and chemokines from immune cells causing damage in tissues with an anatomic predisposition. Indeed, circulating cytokines such as the colony-stimulating factors (G-CSF and GM-CSF), chemokines (fractalkine), growth factors (FGF-2), interferons (IFNα2 and IFNγ), and interleukins (IL12p70, IL1α, IL1β, IL1RA, IL2, IL6, IL13, and IL-17) have been linked to irAEs development [6]. In arthritis-irAE, the successful use of antitumor necrosis factor (anti-TNF) and anti-IL-6 receptor (anti-IL-6R) antibodies for arthritis management suggest a role of these cytokines in pathogenesis [8, 9]; (3) cross-antigen reactivity against tumor-specific antigens and self-antigens released from healthy tissues located within and around the tumor milieu; (4) off-target effect of ICI therapy leading to damage in nonhematopoietic cells that express the target ligand; (5) genetic predisposition must play a role in irAEs susceptibility. Germline genetic features identified through small pilot studies suggested shared biological pathways between irAEs development and autoimmune diseases [6]. Of note, carriers with interferon-gamma (IFNG)—1616T > C single nucleotide polymorphism homozygous variant were found to have an increased risk for rheumatologic irAEs, and the presence of human leukocyte antigen (HLA) DRB1 shared epitope alleles (a known risk factor for rheumatoid arthritis) was found to be higher in patients with arthritis-irAE compared with healthy controls; and (6) apart from the usual factors, gut microbiota, primarily Bacteroides intestinalis were associated with irAEs development in ICI combination therapy-treated patients [6].

18.5 Clinical Features

Arthritis-irAE can present anytime after initiation of ICI therapy; immediately after receiving the first dose or as a late adverse event (AE) occurring 44 months post-treatment, and it may persist even after ICI discontinuation. Some patients may initially present with arthralgia, with or without joint stiffness, but develop overt synovitis over time. Most patients developing arthritis-irAE have an undifferentiated clinical presentation that does not always fulfill diagnostic criteria for primary autoimmune inflammatory arthritis. We describe below the most common patterns (Table 18.1):

Undifferentiated inflammatory arthritis: Patients may present with oligoarthritis or polyarthritis of large joints such as knees, ankles, or wrists, which can be symmetric or asymmetric in distribution [10]. Sometimes patients present with monoarthritis. These patients are negative for RF and anti-CCP, although some may be ANA positive. They generally have normal radiographs at presentation; however, they can have persistent inflammation resulting in erosive disease [11, 12].

Table 18.1 Clinical phenotypes of immune checkpoint inhibitor-induced inflammatory arthritis

Clinical pattern	Presentation
Undifferentiated inflammatory arthritis	– Oligoarthritis or polyarthritis of large joints (symmetric or asymmetric in distribution) – Monoarthritis has been reported – Negative RF and/or anti-CCP antibodies – ANA may be positive
Rheumatoid arthritis-like	– Symmetrical polyarthritis involving small joints of the hands and wrists – Positive RF and/or anti-CCP antibodies
Seronegative spondyloarthropathy-like	– Oligo/polyarthritis and axial disease or enthesopathy – Psoriatic arthritis with/without skin changes – Reactive arthritis – Negative HLA-B27
Polymyalgia rheumatica-like	– Morning stiffness and pain of shoulders and hips – Elevated ESR and CRP – Negative RF and anti-CCP antibodies – Concomitant arthritis has been reported – Concomitant giant cell arteritis has been reported
Remitting seronegative symmetrical synovitis with pitting edema	– ESR and CRP may be elevated – Negative autoantibodies
Tenosynovitis	– ANA may be positive

RF Rheumatoid factor, *anti-CCP* Anti-citric citrullinated peptide, *ANA* Antinuclear antibodies, *HLA-B27* Human Leukocyte Antigen B-27, *ESR* Erythrocyte sedimentation rate, *CRP* C-reactive protein

Rheumatoid arthritis (RA)-like: Patients may present with symmetrical polyarthritis predominantly involving small joints of the hands and wrists, along with positive RF and/or anti-CCP antibodies in their sera, fulfilling the 2010 American College of Rheumatology (ACR)/European League Against Rheumatism (EULAR) diagnostic criteria for rheumatoid arthritis (RA) [10]. While not commonly reported, this pattern is potentially erosive and may lead to permanent joint damage.

Seronegative spondyloarthropathy (SPA)-like: In addition to oligo/polyarthritis, some patients present with axial disease (inflammatory back pain or cervical pain) and enthesopathy (pain/tenderness in connective tissues between bones and tendons or ligaments such as the heel or iliac crest) [12]. The facet, costovertebral, and sacroiliac joints are involved [12, 13], but unlike primary spondyloarthritis, the few reported patients tested negative for Human Leukocyte Antigen (HLA)-B27 alleles. Moreover, ***psoriatic arthritis with and without skin changes*** also presents following ICI initiation; all reported patients were seronegative and none had a prior history of psoriasis [10]. The triad of ***reactive arthritis*** (arthritis, conjunctivitis, and sterile urethritis) has been observed in some patients, especially after receiving ICI combination therapy [10, 12].

Polymyalgia rheumatica (PMR)-like: Some patients present with morning stiffness and pain of both shoulders and hips, with elevated inflammatory markers, such as erythrocyte sedimentation rate (ESR) and C-reactive protein (CRP), and negative RF and anti-CCP antibodies, fulfilling the 2012 EULAR/ACR classification criteria for polymyalgia rheumatica (PMR) [14]. In these patients, joint swelling is not typical, but some develop effusions in shoulders/hips, subdeltoid bursitis, or biceps tenosynovitis, which can be seen by ultrasound or MRI.

PMR/arthritis overlap: Some patients have atypical PMR features with inflammatory arthritis involving other joints most commonly the knees, followed by the small joints of the hands and elbows. A few patients have been reported presenting with normal inflammatory markers. Patients with PMR have normal muscle strength and creatine kinase (CK) levels within normal limits. Unlike primary PMR, patients with PMR-irAE may require higher doses of glucocorticoids, exceeding 20 mg daily of prednisone.

Concomitant ***giant cell arteritis*** (GCA) has been occasionally reported, with patients presenting with jaw claudication, temporal headache, scalp tenderness, and vision loss.

Remitting seronegative symmetrical synovitis with pitting edema has been reported following ICI therapy, while all reported patients had elevated ESR and CRP and were negative for autoantibodies [10, 15].

Tenosynovitis: Some patients develop tenosynovitis in the hands, forearms, shoulders, and/or knees. Tenosynovitis may occur either alone or associated with arthritis. A few patients were found to be ANA positive [16].

Further studies are required to understand why patients present with such different clinical patterns. For some presentations such as RA-like, or psoriatic arthritis, it is possible that patients may have a preexisting subclinical disease or predisposing genotypes, and that therapy with ICI triggers the subsequent clinical disease. Some patients who developed RA-like arthritis were found to have RF and/or anti-CCP antibodies in serum before they received ICI [6]. Some patients with cutaneous psoriasis also developed psoriatic arthritis after ICI treatment. One study has reported variations in clinical presentation and outcomes in patients receiving anti-PD1 alone compared to those receiving ICI combination [12]. Patients receiving single-agent anti-PD1 were more likely to develop arthritis-irAE as the only toxicity, presenting with small joints arthritis. On the other hand, those who received ICI combination were more likely to develop multiple other irAEs and to present with knee arthritis [12]. Persistence of arthritis-irAE after ICI discontinuation was reported in more than 50% of the patients in this cohort [17] and was associated with having received ICI combination, and with a longer duration of ICI treatment.

18.6   Diagnosis

The ACR generally recommends five measures for RA disease activity including (1) clinical disease activity index (CDAI); (2) simple disease activity index (SDAI); (3) disease activity score-28-ESR (DAS28 ESR); (4) disease activity score-28-CRP (DAS-28 CRP), and routine assessment of patient index data 3 (RAPID 3) and three measures for RA functional assessment including (1) health assessment questionnaire-II (HAQ-II); (2) patient activity scale II (PAS II); and patient-reported outcomes measurement information system short form—physical function 10a (PROMIS PF10a) for use in clinical practice. While few of these measures have been utilized for evaluating patients with arthritis-irAE, they still need to be validated in this setting.

Laboratory testing should include: (1) ESR and CRP, which are typically elevated in patients with active inflammatory symptoms although not seen in all patients with arthritis-irAE; (2) ANA, RF, and anti-CCP, most patients predominantly those with undifferentiated arthritis are typically negative; (3) HLA-B27 primarily in patients presented with seronegative spondyloarthropathy-like arthritis; (4) Muscle enzymes in patients presenting with PMR-like arthritis, though are typically normal; (5) Joint aspiration and synovial fluid analysis, which typically reveals inflammation with neutrophilic predominance; and (6) hepatitis B and C, human immunodeficiency virus (HIV), and tuberculosis primarily if patients will require immunosuppressive therapies as this may result in reactivation of latent infection. Of note, several biomarkers (blood-based, immunogenetic, and microbial) were suggested as predictors for irAEs development, including endocrine toxicities, colitis, dermatitis, and pneumonitis [6]. However, predictive biomarkers for arthritis-irAE have not been suggested yet. Future studies with a prospective standardized collection of biospecimens (blood and synovial fluid) are important to identify predictive biomarkers for arthritis-irAE.

Imaging can be employed to confirm diagnosis early on and to exclude other possible causes of arthritis. Plain radiography of the affected joints can detect joint erosions and joint space narrowing. Whereas ultrasound and magnetic resonance (MRI) images can detect synovitis, inflammatory signals, tendinitis, enthesopathy, and erosions [11]. Importantly, in patients presenting with PMR-like along with features suggestive of GCA, urgent ophthalmological exam and temporal artery biopsy should be considered due to the known risk of permanent blindness with this type of vasculitis. Also, MRI, electromyography, or muscle biopsy may be considered to exclude muscle inflammation or myopathy in case of diagnostic uncertainty. Close monitoring is required for patients with arthritis-irAE with periodic clinical evaluations including joint examination and serial testing of inflammatory markers (ESR and/or CRP) every 4–6 weeks to monitor the therapeutic response until symptoms improve. Imaging should also be repeated to follow up for structural damage.

18.7   Differential Diagnosis

At presentation, clinicians typically confirm that symptoms started after initiation of ICI and exclude other conditions that may cause similar symptoms including preexisting autoimmune disease, osteoarthritis, or crystal arthritis as few patients have been reported with worsening or recurrent symptoms following ICI initiation. Paraneoplastic arthritis should also be excluded especially if symptoms started around the time of cancer diagnosis. Additionally, metastatic disease within the adjacent bone or joint structures, and septic arthritis should be excluded primarily in patients with monoarthritis.

18.8   Management

The guidelines for the management of irAEs have been published by several key oncology and rheumatology societies, based on the severity of presentation as per CTCAE grades [8, 9]. For arthritis-irAE, a prompt rheumatology consult is recommended if there is joint pain for more than 4 weeks, joint swelling, arthritis ≥ grade 2, or unable to taper corticosteroids to <10 mg/day within 4 weeks, and to identify signs of joint damage early on. Afterward, an assessment should be made for the need for arthrocentesis/intra-articular corticosteroid injection, and initiation/optimal dosing of disease-modifying anti-rheumatic drugs (DMARDs). The decision to initiate ICI therapy in patients with preexisting inflammatory arthritis requires a rheumatology-oncology multidisciplinary approach to carefully weigh the benefit/risk ratio while considering the severity of the underlying autoimmune disease, the prognosis of cancer, alternative therapies, and patients' preferences. For these patients, it is important to keep their baseline immunosuppressive regimen at the lowest efficient dose before ICI initiation as these patients are at high risk of arthritis flare after therapy initiation. Generally, the existing guidelines define three treatment escalations for arthritis-irAE, which are summarized in Table 18.2 [8, 9].

Mild arthritis-irAE (grade 1 per CTCAE): Patients with mild arthritis with no functional impact on their ADL are managed with acetaminophen or non-steroidal anti-inflammatory drugs (NSAIDs) if there is no contraindication, and/or intra-articular corticosteroid injection. Continuation of ICI therapy is recommended. However, if arthritis does not improve within 4 weeks, treatment should be escalated to the next step.

Table 18.2 Current guidelines for the management of checkpoint inhibitor-induced inflammatory arthritis

Clinical pattern	Presentation
Mild arthritis-irAE (grade 1 per CTCAE)	– Acetaminophen or NSAIDs if no contraindication – Intra-articular corticosteroid injection – Continue ICI therapy – Escalate treatment to next step if no improvement of arthritis within 4 weeks
Moderate arthritis-irAE (grade 2 per CTCAE)	– Oral prednisone 10–20 mg/day or equivalent – Intra-articular corticosteroid injection – Consider holding ICI therapy – Taper corticosteroid within 4–6 weeks if arthritis improved – Escalate treatment to next step and initiate DMARDs if no improvement of arthritis within 4 weeks or if unable to taper corticosteroids to below 10 mg/day within 6–8 weeks
Severe arthritis-irAE (grade 3 and 4 per CTCAE)	– Oral prednisone 0.5–1 mg/kg/day – Taper corticosteroid within 4–6 weeks if arthritis improved – Escalate treatment to next step and initiate DMARDs if no improvement or worsening of arthritis within 2 weeks Cs-DMARDs (methotrexate, hydroxychloroquine, sulfasalazine, or leflunomide alone or in combination) b-DMARDs (anti-TNF or anti-IL-6R)

CTCAE Common Terminology Criteria for Adverse Events, *NSAIDs* Non-steroidal anti-inflammatory drugs, *ICI* immune checkpoint inhibitor, *DMARDs* Disease-modifying anti-rheumatic drugs, *cs-DMARDs* Conventional synthetic DMARDs, *b-DMARDs* biological DMARDs, *anti-TNF* Antitumor necrosis factor, *anti-IL-6R* Anti-IL-6 receptor

Moderate arthritis-irAE (grade 2 per CTCAE): Patients with moderate arthritis with functionally impacted ADL, but not interfering with self-care are managed with 10–20 mg/day of oral prednisone or equivalent for 4 weeks, and intra-articular corticosteroid injection if ≤ 2 large joints are involved. ICI therapy should be placed on temporary hold. If arthritis improves, oral prednisone should be tapered slowly over 4–6 weeks, and ICI therapy should be resumed when prednisone is ≤ 10 mg/ day. However, if arthritis does not improve within 4 weeks, or if unable to taper prednisone to ≤ 10 mg/day after 6–8 weeks, treatment should be escalated to the next step and initiation of DMARDs is recommended.

Severe arthritis-irAE (grade 3 and 4 per CTCAE): Patients with severe arthritis impacting self-care and ADL are managed with 0.5–1 mg/kg/day of oral prednisone or equivalent. ICI therapy should be placed on temporary hold. If arthritis improves, oral prednisone should be tapered slowly over 4–6 weeks, and treatment with ICI should be resumed when prednisone is ≤ 10 mg/day. However, if arthritis does not improve within 2 weeks or if worsening of symptoms is noted, initiation of conventional synthetic DMARDs (cs-DMARDs) is recommended; methotrexate, hydroxy-chloroquine, sulfasalazine, or leflunomide (alone or in combination) are the most common at doses used to treat RA. In case of severe or refractory arthritis, the use of certain biological DMARDs (b-DMARDs) such as anti-TNF or anti-IL-6R anti-bodies is recommended. One should keep in mind that persistent inflammation, as well as treatment with corticosteroids (prednisone of ≥ 2.5 mg/day or equivalent for ≥ 3 months), increase the risk of osteoporosis, and therefore patients with arthritis-irAE should be encouraged to maintain a healthy lifestyle with adequate nutrition and weight-bearing exercises and may require pharmacological therapy [18]. While on DMARDs, these patients also need close monitoring of neutrophil and platelet counts, serum lipids, liver transaminases, and serum creatinine. If arthritis improves to grade 1, ICI therapy should be resumed but should be discontinued permanently if there is no improvement after 4–6 weeks of treatment.

Finally, it is worth mentioning that the occurrence of irAEs has been suggested as a surrogate for effective antitumor immune response; patients with any grade irAEs were found to have higher objective response rate, disease control rate, and overall survival, and those with grade 2 or higher irAEs or multiple irAEs had better progression-free survival and overall survival [19]. Similarly, patients who develop rheumatic and musculoskeletal irAEs per se were found to have better tumor response [20]. Therefore, future studies should focus on investigating how we can effectively manage irAEs without hindering the antitumor immune response to ICI therapy. While published guidelines endorse corticosteroids as first-line therapy for irAEs, targeted therapies could be safer and preferable to corticosteroids especially for arthritis-irAE, which may likely require prolonged therapy. Studies from melanoma and non-small cell lung cancer patients treated with ICIs have shown that the use of prednisone ≥10 mg/day led to detrimental cancer outcomes and worsen survival [21, 22]. Also, the timing of treatment initiation was found to affect the response to ICI therapy; patients treated with corticosteroids within the first 2 months after ICI initiation had shorter progression-free survival and overall survival as compared to those who received corticosteroids later [23]. With regard to corticosteroid-sparing agents, one study showed that the use of cs-DMARDs or b-DMARDs for arthritis-irAE did not impact the tumor response to ICI [17]. However, another study showed that the use of hydroxychloroquine led to decreasing the efficacy of anti-PD-1 agents [24]. Players in the autoimmune pathways can be targeted, such as TNF-alpha, but, given its role in antitumor immunity, concerns remain regarding the safety of prolonged anti-TNF therapy and its impact on survival [25]. On the other hand, anti-IL-6R antibody shows promising results for irAE management; a recent systematic review of the literature provided data on 91 patients, where the use of tocilizumab resulted in clinical benefit and none of them were reported with tumor progression [26]. Another study that combined translational, preclinical, and clinical analyses, identified that targeting IL-6 could be an effective approach for irAE management while maintaining and possibly boosting tumor immunity [27]. However, anti-IL-6R antibody might not be suitable for patients who also had colitis-irAE or preexisting inflammatory bowel disease due to the potential risk of intestinal perforation, although isolated case reports have not shown complications in these patients [28, 29]. To date, there is only one published case reporting the use of tofacitinib; JAK inhibitor, for treatment of arthritis-irAE in a patient with metastatic lung adenocarcinoma who achieved remission of arthritis and cancer [30]. However, the FDA has recently announced a black box warning on tofacitinib use due to concerns about the increasing risk of serious cardiovascular adverse events, thrombosis, cancer, and death. To our knowledge, 15 clinical trials are currently investigating the use of therapies for prevention and management of irAEs in patients receiving ICI therapy (Table 18.3).

Table 18.3 Current clinical trials investigating targeted therapies for the management of immune-related adverse events

Clinical trials	Trial ID	Status
Tocilizumab, ipilimumab, and nivolumab for the treatment of advanced melanoma, non-small cell lung cancer, or urothelial carcinoma	NCT04940299	Recruiting
Study of rituximab or tocilizumab for patients with steroid-dependent immune-related adverse events (irAEs)	NCT04375228	Recruiting
Checkpoint inhibitor-induced colitis and arthritis—Immunomodulation with IL-6 blockade and exploration of disease mechanisms (COLAR)	NCT03601611	Completed
A phase II study of the Interleukin-6 receptor inhibitor tocilizumab in combination with Ipilimumab and Nivolumab in patients with Unresectable stage III or stage IV melanoma	NCT03999749	Recruiting
TNF-inhibitor as immune checkpoint inhibitor for advanced MELanoma	NCT03293784	Active, not recruiting
Infliximab or Vedolizumab in treating immune checkpoint inhibitor-related colitis in patients with genitourinary cancer or melanoma	NCT04407247	Recruiting
Role of gut microbiome and fecal transplant on medication-induced GI complications in patients with cancer	NCT03819296	Recruiting
Ipilimumab, Nivolumab, tocilizumab, and radiation in pretreated patients with advanced pancreatic cancer	NCT04258150	Terminated (primary endpoint was not met)
Atezolizumab with or without tocilizumab in treating men with prostate cancer before radical prostatectomy	NCT03821246	Recruiting
A study evaluating the efficacy and safety of multiple immunotherapy-based treatment combinations in patients with advanced liver cancers (Morpheus-liver)	NCT04524871	Recruiting
A study evaluating the efficacy and safety of multiple immunotherapy-based treatment combinations in patients with metastatic or inoperable locally advanced triple-negative breast cancer	NCT03424005	Recruiting
Study evaluating the efficacy and safety of multiple immunotherapy-based treatments and combinations in patients with urothelial carcinoma (MORPHEUS-UC)	NCT03869190	Recruiting
Tofacitinib for the Treatment of Refractory Immune-related Colitis From Checkpoint Inhibitor Therapy- TRICK Study	NCT04768504	Recruiting
Treatment Efficacy of Corticosteroids, Mycophenolate Mofetil and Tacrolimus in Patients With Immune Related Hepatitis (IHEP)	NCT04810156	Not yet recruiting
Fecal Microbiota Transplantation in Treating Immune-Checkpoint Inhibitor Induced-Diarrhea or Colitis in Genitourinary Cancer Patients	NCT04038619	Recruiting

18.9 Conclusion

Immune checkpoint inhibition has transformed cancer treatment. However, ICIs often result in off-target inflammatory and autoimmune effects. The chances of irAEs are higher in those with preexisting autoantibodies and rheumatic diseases.

Thus, the decision to initiate ICIs in such patients should be taken in consultation with a rheumatologist. Treatment of arthritis irAEs involves temporary withdrawal of the ICI and the administration of NSAIDs, glucocorticoids, and/or DMARDs depending upon the severity of the irAE. Rare cases may however require permanent discontinuation of ICI therapy.

Acknowledgments We thank Dr. Sirisha Yadugiri, the Senior Technical Writer in the Department of Melanoma Medical Oncology at The University of Texas MD Anderson Cancer Center for editorial support.

References

1. Wei SC, Duffy CR, Allison JP. Fundamental mechanisms of immune checkpoint blockade therapy. Cancer Discov. 2018;8(9):1069–86.
2. Abdel-Wahab N, Shah M, Suarez-Almazor ME. Adverse events associated with immune checkpoint blockade in patients with cancer: a systematic review of case reports. PLoS One. 2016;11(7):e0160221.
3. Abdel-Wahab N, Suarez-Almazor ME. Frequency and distribution of various rheumatic disorders associated with checkpoint inhibitor therapy. Rheumatology (Oxford, England). 2019;58(Suppl 7):vii40–8.
4. Cunningham-Bussel A, Wang J, Prisco LC, Martin LW, Vanni KMM, Zaccardelli A, et al. Predictors of rheumatic immune-related adverse events and de novo inflammatory arthritis after immune checkpoint inhibitor treatment for cancer. Arthritis Rheumatol. 2022;74(3):527–40. https://doi.org/10.1002/art.41949. Epub ahead of print.
5. Guzman-Prado Y, Ben Shimol J, Samson O. Body mass index and immune-related adverse events in patients on immune checkpoint inhibitor therapies: a systematic review and meta-analysis. Cancer Immunol Immunother. 2021;70(1):89–100.
6. Hommes JW, Verheijden RJ, Suijkerbuijk KPM, Hamann D. Biomarkers of checkpoint inhibitor induced immune-related adverse events—a comprehensive review. Front Oncol. 2021;10:585311.
7. Esfahani K, Elkrief A, Calabrese C, Lapointe R, Hudson M, Routy B, et al. Moving towards personalized treatments of immune-related adverse events. Nat Rev Clin Oncol. 2020;17(8):504–15.
8. Haanen J, Carbonnel F, Robert C, Kerr KM, Peters S, Larkin J, et al. Management of toxicities from immunotherapy: ESMO clinical practice guidelines for diagnosis, treatment and follow-up. Ann Oncol. 2018;29(Suppl 4):iv264–6.
9. Schneider BJ, Naidoo J, Santomasso BD, Lacchetti C, Adkins S, Anadkat M, et al. Management of immune-related adverse events in patients treated with immune checkpoint inhibitor therapy: ASCO guideline update. J Clin Oncol. 2021;39(36):4073–126. https://doi.org/10.1200/JCO.21.01440. Epub ahead of print.
10. Pundole X, Abdel-Wahab N, Suarez-Almazor ME. Arthritis risk with immune checkpoint inhibitor therapy for cancer. Curr Opin Rheumatol. 2019;31(3):293–9.
11. Albayda J, Dein E, Shah AA, Bingham CO 3rd, Cappelli L. Sonographic findings in inflammatory arthritis secondary to immune checkpoint inhibition: a case series. ACR Open Rheumatol. 2019;1(5):303–7.
12. Cappelli LC, Brahmer JR, Forde PM, Le DT, Lipson EJ, Naidoo J, et al. Clinical presentation of immune checkpoint inhibitor-induced inflammatory arthritis differs by immunotherapy regimen. Semin Arthritis Rheum. 2018;48(3):553–7.
13. Feist J, Murray A, Skapenko A, Schulze-Koops H. A rare side effect of checkpoint inhibitor therapy-nivolumab-induced axial polyarthritis of the facet and costovertebral joints. Arthritis Rheumatol. 2019;71(11):1823.
14. Calabrese C, Cappelli LC, Kostine M, Kirchner E, Braaten T, Calabrese L. Polymyalgia rheumatica-like syndrome from checkpoint inhibitor therapy: case series and systematic review of the literature. RMD Open. 2019;5(1):e000906.

15. Yamamoto S, Fujita S, Mukai T, Sawachika H, Morita Y. Paraneoplastic remitting seronegative symmetrical synovitis with pitting edema syndrome should be treated with low-dose predniso-lone during pembrolizumab therapy. Intern Med. 2020;59(4):597–8.
16. Murakami S, Nagano T, Nakata K, Onishi A, Umezawa K, Katsurada N, et al. Tenosynovitis induced by an immune checkpoint inhibitor: a case report and literature review. Intern Med. 2019;58(19):2839–43.
17. Braaten TJ, Brahmer JR, Forde PM, Le D, Lipson EJ, Naidoo J, et al. Immune checkpoint inhibitor-induced inflammatory arthritis persists after immunotherapy cessation. Ann Rheum Dis. 2020;79(3):332–8.
18. Kobza AO, Herman D, Papaioannou A, Lau AN, Adachi JD. Understanding and managing corticosteroid-induced osteoporosis. Open Access Rheumatol. 2021;13:177–90.
19. Bai R, Li L, Chen X, Chen N, Song W, Zhang Y, et al. Correlation of peripheral blood param-eters and immune-related adverse events with the efficacy of immune checkpoint inhibitors. J Oncol. 2021;2021:9935076.
20. Adda L, Batteux B, Saidak Z, Poulet C, Arnault JP, Chauffert B, et al. Rheumatic and musculo-skeletal disorders induced by immune checkpoint inhibitors: consequences on overall survival. Joint Bone Spine. 2021;88(4):105168.
21. Arbour KC, Mezquita L, Long N, Rizvi H, Auclin E, Ni A, et al. Impact of baseline steroids on efficacy of programmed cell death-1 and programmed death-ligand 1 blockade in patients with non-small-cell lung cancer. J Clin Oncol. 2018;36(28):2872–8.
22. Faje AT, Lawrence D, Flaherty K, Freedman C, Fadden R, Rubin K, et al. High-dose gluco-corticoids for the treatment of ipilimumab-induced hypophysitis is associated with reduced survival in patients with melanoma. Cancer. 2018;124(18):3706–14.
23. Maslov DV, Tawagi K, Kc M, Simenson V, Yuan H, Parent C, et al. Timing of steroid initia-tion and response rates to immune checkpoint inhibitors in metastatic cancer. J Immunother Cancer. 2021;9(7):e002261.
24. Krueger J, Santinon F, Kazanova A, Issa ME, Larrivee B, Kremer R, et al. Hydroxychloroquine (HCQ) decreases the benefit of anti-PD-1 immune checkpoint blockade in tumor immunother-apy. PLoS One. 2021;16(6):e0251731.
25. Verheijden RJ, May AM, Blank CU, Aarts MJB, van den Berkmortel F, van den Eertwegh AJM, et al. Association of anti-TNF with decreased survival in steroid refractory ipilimumab and anti-PD1-treated patients in the Dutch melanoma treatment registry. Clin Cancer Res. 2020;26(9):2268–74.
26. Campochiaro C, Farina N, Tomelleri A, Ferrara R, Lazzari C, De Luca G, et al. Tocilizumab for the treatment of immune-related adverse events: a systematic literature review and a multi-centre case series. Eur J Intern Med. 2021;S0953-6205(21):00266–1.
27. Hailemichael Y, Johnson D, Abdel-Wahab N, Foo WC, Daher M, Haymaker C, et al. Interleukin-6 blockade abrogates immunotherapy toxicity and promotes tumor immunity. Cancer Cell. 2022;9;40(5):509–23.e6. https://doi.org/10.1016/j.ccell.2022.04.004. PMID: 35537412. Epub 2022 May 9.
28. Kim ST, Tayar J, Trinh VA, Suarez-Almazor M, Garcia S, Hwu P, et al. Successful treatment of arthritis induced by checkpoint inhibitors with tocilizumab: a case series. Ann Rheum Dis. 2017;76(12):2061–4.
29. Uemura M, Trinh VA, Haymaker C, Jackson N, Kim DW, Allison JP, et al. Selective inhibi-tion of autoimmune exacerbation while preserving the anti-tumor clinical benefit using IL-6 blockade in a patient with advanced melanoma and Crohn's disease: a case report. J Hematol Oncol. 2016;9(1):81.
30. Murray K, Floudas A, Murray C, Fabre A, Crown J, Fearon U, et al. First use of tofacitinib to treat an immune checkpoint inhibitor-induced arthritis. BMJ Case Rep. 2021;14(2).

Miscellaneous Arthropathies

19

Himanshu Pathak and Karl Gaffney

19.1 Introduction

Adequate knowledge and an index of suspicion are required to diagnose rare musculoskeletal conditions. This chapter discusses certain such arthropathies which when recognized in time and optimally treated, generally have fair outcomes. Amyloidosis is a systemic disorder that may have musculoskeletal manifestations through the accumulation of abnormal proteins in articular and periarticular tissues. Polymerization of abnormal hemoglobin in Sickle cell disease (SCD) leads to sickling of erythrocytes and tissue hypoxia causing painful vaso-occlusive crises, osteonecrosis, dactylitis, and osteomyelitis. Jaccoud's arthropathy (JA) is a reversible deformity of small joints of hands and feet with underlying inflammatory autoimmune disease. Arthritis robustus is a very rare presentation of inflammatory arthritis where the patient has minimal symptoms. In these rare conditions, the pathophysiology of MSK manifestations is not clearly understood, diagnosis is clinical and management of underlying etiology generally improves patient outcomes.

H. Pathak (✉)
Tricolour Hospitals, Vadodara, Gujarat, India

Pramukhswami Medical College, Bhaikaka University, Karamsad, Gujarat, India

K. Gaffney
Norfolk and Norwich University Hospitals NHS Foundation Trust, Norwich, UK

Norwich Medical School, University of East Anglia, Norwich, UK
e-mail: karl.gaffney@nnuh.nhs.uk

19.2   Amyloid Arthropathy

Amyloid arthropathy may be seen in patients with primary amyloidosis (AL type), secondary amyloidosis (AA type), amyloidosis associated with chronic hemodialysis (deposition of beta-2 microglobulins), and transthyretin amyloidosis. AL type amyloidosis is seen with plasma cell dyscrasias while AA type amyloidosis occurs with chronic inflammatory conditions like rheumatoid arthritis, ankylosing spondylitis, Crohn's disease, ulcerative colitis, and chronic infections. The incidence of amyloid arthropathy in plasma cell dyscrasias has been estimated between 3.7 and 9.2% [1, 2].

Amyloidosis is characterized by the deposition of fibrous amyloid fibril proteins in extracellular tissue space. Amyloid fibril proteins are immunoglobulin light chains of either lambda or kappa subtypes. The primary pathogenetic mechanism is considered to be protein misfolding and aggregation of fibril proteins in the extracellular space. On histopathology, amyloid proteins show beta-pleated-sheet-rich configuration and very specific apple-green birefringence with Congo red staining under a polarized light microscope [3]. Immunohistological analysis of synovial membranes in amyloid arthropathy reveals synovitis with inflammatory infiltrates consisting predominantly of macrophages, T cells and absence of B cells and plasma cells [4]. Musculoskeletal manifestations of amyloid arthropathy are characterized by the deposition of amyloid proteins in bones, joints, and extra-articular tissues. The deposition of amyloid can lead to destructive osteoarthropathy at the hips, shoulders, and wrists.

Amyloid arthropathy can have subacute, progressive and rarely a destructive course. It can be bilateral and symmetrical, involving small joints of hands, wrists, knees, and shoulders thereby mimicking rheumatoid arthritis (RA). Infiltration of amyloid proteins into the glenohumeral joint and extra-articular soft tissues can manifest as a shoulder pad sign. Shoulder girdle involvement can result in tendinopathies because of the accumulation of amyloid proteins. In addition to joint swelling, thickening of the palmar and plantar fascia can be seen. Chronic amyloidosis can lead to compressive neuropathies like carpal tunnel syndrome and tarsal tunnel syndrome [2]. Charcot-like arthropathy especially in ankle and knee joints has been reported in amyloidosis patients with underlying polyneuropathy [5]. Deposition of amyloid proteins in the spine can cause compressive myelopathy and nerve root compression. Secondary osteoporosis presenting as osteolytic lesions on long bones and vertebrae can cause pathologic fractures [1–3]. Infiltration of amyloid proteins in muscles can lead to myopathy manifesting as myalgia, pseudo-hypertrophy, and limb weakness. Proximal muscles of the upper and lower limbs are predominantly involved. Serum creatinine kinase levels in the blood can be elevated similar to inflammatory myositis and hereditary myopathies [3]. Macroglossia with teeth indentations is a classical sign of muscle infiltration in amyloidosis.

Radiographs may reveal soft tissue swelling, periarticular osteoporosis, and well-defined subchondral cystic lesions. Thickening of tendons, nodular synovial swelling, effusions, and bursitis are characteristically seen on ultrasound and magnetic resonance imaging ((MRI). Low signal intensity in thickened synovium and periarticular structures on MRI T1 and T2 weighted sequences have also been described in amyloid arthropathy. Similar MRI findings are seen in gout, pigmented villonodular synovitis, and hemophilia. The presence of amyloid protein on histopathology and congo red staining confirms the diagnosis. Biopsies can be taken from the abdominal fat pad, the synovium of the involved joint or muscle [6].

The differential diagnosis of infiltrative amyloid arthropathy includes rheumatoid arthritis, polymyalgia rheumatica, and crystal arthropathies. Soft tissue thickening can also be seen in endocrinopathies like hypothyroidism and acromegaly, which need to be differentiated from amyloidosis in the correct clinical context. Diffuse swelling of fingers and hands can be confused with sclerodactyly seen in scleroderma [7]. Rheumatoid arthritis has multiple similarities to amyloid arthropathy; subacute presentation, and bilateral and symmetrical swelling of metacarpophalangeal and proximal interphalangeal joints. Amyloid-related joint swelling usually lacks clinical features of synovitis (warmth, redness), stiffness after immobility, and significant tenderness. Amyloid arthropathy is very rarely erosive unlike rheumatoid arthritis [2, 3].

The primary management of amyloid arthropathy and myopathy is the treatment of the underlying amyloid subtype disease. Aggressive treatment of multiple myeloma and other monoclonal gammopathies usually improves the underlying MSK manifestations by decreasing abnormal protein production. Pharmacological therapies including non-steroidal anti-inflammatory drugs and low-dose steroids can be used for arthritis, while pregabalin and gabapentin can be used for neuropathic symptoms [7, 8].

19.3 Sickle Cell Disease-Associated Arthropathy

Sickle cell disease is an autosomal recessive hemoglobinopathy that is characterized by a mutation in the beta-globin chain of hemoglobin and subsequent formation of hemoglobin S (HbS). It can be either homozygous (the sickle mutation in the beta-globin chain of hemoglobin (HbSS)) or heterozygous-like sickle beta-thalassemia (sickle beta-globin mutation with another beta-globin mutation) [9].

Sickle cell disease manifests as hemolytic anemia, or tissue ischemia and infarction because of vaso-occlusive crises. The polymerization of hemoglobin S makes sickle-shaped hemoglobin which is more susceptible to degradation in microcirculation. The sickling of red blood cells in bone microcirculation and joint synovium cause thrombosis and infarction. The deformed hemoglobin leads to occlusion of microcirculation and the resultant inflammatory response generated through neutrophils, platelets, and endothelial cells lead to tissue ischemia. Sickling crises may be precipitated by dehydration, hypoxia, sepsis, metabolic acidosis, extremes of temperatures, and certain medications. MSK manifestations of SCD include osteonecrosis, osteomyelitis, osteoporosis, and synovitis [10].

Osteonecrosis usually occurs in the bone marrow of long bones, vertebrae, ribs, and pelvis; however, virtually any part of the skeleton can be involved (Fig. 19.1).

Fig. 19.1 Pelvis MRI
(STIR, coronal) of ilium
bone showing infarct
(yellow arrow) in a
31-year-old patient with
sickle cell disease

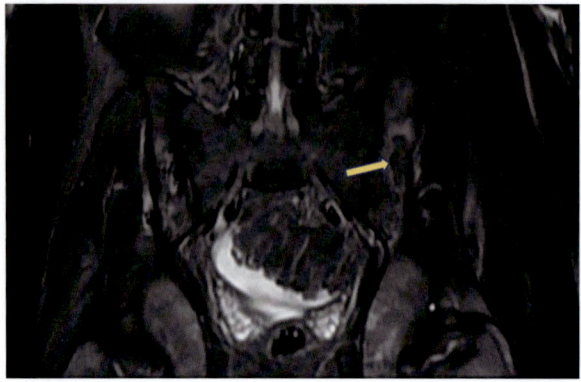

In long bones, osteonecrosis primarily occurs at the femoral head and humeral head which leads to joint destruction. About 50% of HbSS SCD patients will develop osteonecrosis of one or both hips by age of 35 years [9]. In a prospective study of 2590 patients who were followed for an average of 5.6 years, 9.8% had osteonecrosis of one or both femoral heads. The prevalence of osteonecrosis was 21.2% in patients with homozygous HbSS genotype and 11.5% in heterozygous genotype. The incidence of osteonecrosis was highest in patients with hemoglobin SS genotype and alpha-thalassemia (4.5 cases/100 patient-years) [11]. Risk factors for femoral osteonecrosis include older age, male gender, high body mass index, leukopenia, Hb SS with the concurrent α-thalassemia trait (with relatively high Hb), and recurrent vaso-occlusive crisis. Severe pain and restricted movements of the involved site are the main symptoms, however, almost 50% of patients in the early stages of hip osteonecrosis can be pain-free with normal mobility. Pain during deep breathing and spinal movements may suggest rib and vertebral involvement respectively. Pelvic infarctions can produce lower back and buttock pains which worsen during movement [11]. Sickle cell disease is the commonest cause of shoulder osteonecrosis. The risk factors for shoulder osteonecrosis in adults are the presence of hip osteonecrosis and hemoglobin genotype S beta and SC. Like hip osteonecrosis, shoulder osteonecrosis presents with pain and restricted shoulder movements, however, it can be asymptomatic until the later stages of the disease [12].

Sickle cell disease can cause sudden onset joint synovitis and dactylitis. Infiltration of synovium by plasma cells, synovial ischemia, activation of neutrophils, and other inflammatory cytokines in the joint space may all contribute to erosive arthritis. Dactylitis presents as sudden episodes of swelling and tenderness of fingers or toes. Dactylitis associated with SCD may be self-limiting. In SCD gram-positive and gram-negative bacteremia can cause osteomyelitis of hip joints or other large joints. Hyposplenism, complement function dysfunction, and local ischemia have been proposed as possible mechanisms for the increased prevalence of osteomyelitis in SCD. Repeated episodes of bone infarctions in vertebrae and joints can lead to osteoporosis and subsequent increased risk of pathological fractures.

On radiographs of long bones, cystic lesions representing bone infarcts are seen. Radiographs show periarticular osteopenia, erosions, and joint space narrowing which resemble other autoimmune arthritis including rheumatoid arthritis. Early osteonecrosis of hips and shoulder joints can be missed on plain radiographs, thus MRI is the imaging modality of choice for these patients [13].

Hydroxyurea is the initial treatment of choice for SCD. It decreases the polymerization of hemoglobin, increases the level of HbF, and decreases the formation of sickle cells. Adequate management of SCD usually resolves MSK symptoms. Bone marrow transplantation may be required for severe cases of SCD. The management of SCD-associated arthropathies mainly consists of acetaminophen and NSAIDs for pain management. In advanced stages of osteonecrosis of hips and shoulders, hemi or total joint arthroplasty needs to be considered [14].

19.4 Jaccoud's Arthropathy

Jaccoud's arthropathy was first described by a Swiss physician Francois-Sigismond Jaccoud in 1869 among patients with recurrent rheumatic fever. In modern times, JA is seen mainly in patients with systemic lupus erythematosus (SLE); however, rheumatic fever remains a significant etiology. It is characterized by reducible or reversible deformities of the small joints of hands and feet. These deformities include hyperextension at PIP joints and hyperflexion at DIP joints (swan neck), hyperflexion at PIP joints, and hyperextension at DIP joints (Boutonniere deformity), subluxation at MCP joints and thumb, ulnar deviation at wrists and hallux valgus at toes (Fig. 19.2). Few patients can have a severe "mutilans" form of JA with severe synovitis and tenosynovitis [15]. The exact etiology of JA is not known; however, hypermobile joints, chronic mild joint inflammation causing tendon laxity, fibrosis of the joint capsule, and muscular imbalance are proposed as potential mechanisms [16].

Fig. 19.2 Jaccoud's arthropathy in a 32-year-old male with a history of Rheumatic fever in childhood

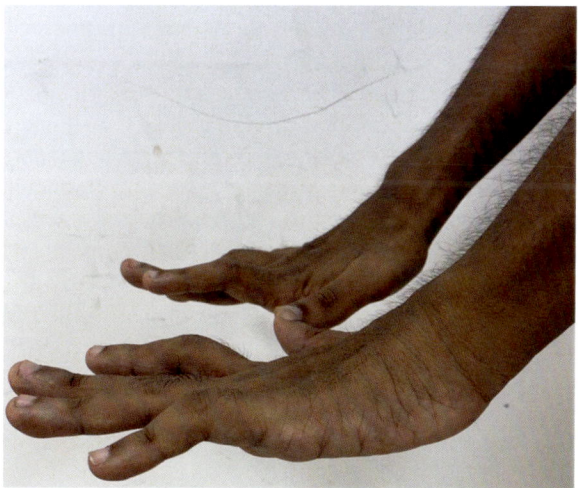

In addition to SLE, JA can be seen in patients with other autoimmune connective tissue diseases including Sjogren's syndrome, dermatomyositis, scleroderma, and sarcoidosis. The prevalence of JA in SLE is between 2 and 5%. A longitudinal cohort study from Latin America showed a higher incidence of renal, hematological and neurological manifestations in patients with SLE who had JA [17].

These deformities can also be found in rheumatoid arthritis, however, in patients with JA, deformities can be corrected and erosive changes are infrequent on plain radiographs. Small joint erosions can be identified on ultrasound and MRI of involved joints.

In chronic forms, reversible deformities of JA can become fixed and difficult to differentiate from rheumatoid arthritis. Factors that are associated with increased risk of erosions in patients with JA are the presence of rheumatoid factor, raised inflammatory markers, and prolonged disease duration. In patients with Rhupus (overlap of SLE and RA), hand deformities can be similar to JA but with erosions. It has been proposed that JA should be diagnosed only in patients with classical deformities, confirmed diagnosis of SLE, and no erosions on radiographs; to prevent confusion with Rhupus [18].

Physical therapy and the use of orthotics for joint protection and strength improvement are key components of the management of chronic JA. The nonerosive form of JA is treated symptomatically with analgesics and treatment of the underlying disease [19]. The presence of clinical synovitis with erosions on imaging requires treatment with disease-modifying anti-rheumatic drugs such as hydroxychloroquine and methotrexate to prevent disease progression [15].

19.5   Arthritis Robustus

About half a century ago when late presentations of arthritis were common and effective treatments options were limited, few reports described a group of patients presenting with proliferative synovitis and deformities in small joints of hands and feet, typical of rheumatoid arthritis but with minimal clinical symptoms. These patients were predominantly male manual workers and the condition was called arthritis robustus (AR) [20]. Similar to typical rheumatoid arthritis, AR patients had bilateral symmetrical joint involvement of carpal and metacarpal joints; however, radiologically subchondral cysts were the predominant findings on x-rays and joint erosions and periarticular osteopenia were less pronounced than typical RA [21]. A lack of recent epidemiological and clinical trial data makes AR more of an observational entity than a specific subtype of inflammatory arthritis. Available medical literature suggests that some patients with AR may progress to typical rheumatoid arthritis and disease-modifying drugs such as methotrexate and leflunomide may be initial treatment options for them [22]. Treatment of AR should be modified according to the patient's clinical phenotype as many patients and clinicians may choose conservative management because of the asymptomatic and slowly progressive nature of the condition. Arthritis robustus may be a rare clinical phenotype of

Table 19.1 Key features of amyloid arthropathy, sickle cell disease-associated arthropathy, Jaccoud's arthropathy, and arthritis robustus

Rare condition	Musculoskeletal manifestations	Management principles
Amyloidosis	• Amyloid arthropathy infiltrative myopathy • Shoulder pad sign, Macroglossia • Compressive neuropathies like carpal tunnel syndrome, tarsal tunnel syndrome, spinal radiculopathies • Osteoporosis of long bones and vertebrae	• Adequate treatment of the underlying cause of amyloidosis • Non-steroidal anti-inflammatory drugs and low dose oral steroids for joint synovitis and tenosynovitis • Gabapentin and pregabalin for symptoms of neuropathy
Sickle cell disease	• Osteonecrosis • Osteomyelitis • Arthritis • Dactylitis	• Treatment of sickle cell disease: Hydroxyurea and bone marrow stem cell transplant • Paracetamol and non-steroidal anti-inflammatory drugs for arthritis and dactylitis • Replacement arthroplasty interventions for osteonecrosis of hips and shoulders
Jaccoud's arthropathy	Reducible deformities of hands: • Swan neck deformity (hyperextension of PIP joint) • Boutonniere deformity (hyperextension at DIP joint) • MCP joints subluxation • Ulnar deviation at wrists	• Physical therapy and orthotics for joint protection and strength improvement • Adequate treatment of underlying connective tissue disease • Non-steroidal anti-inflammatory drugs, low dose steroids, and disease-modifying anti-inflammatory drugs (hydroxychloroquine, methotrexate) for joint synovitis
Arthritis robustus	Involvement of hands and feet in typical rheumatoid arthritis distribution but with minimal symptoms	• Non-steroidal anti-inflammatory drugs, low dose steroids, and disease-modifying anti-rheumatic drugs (such as methotrexate and leflunomide) for joint synovitis and tenosynovitis

rheumatoid arthritis however, this assumption needs further validation from epidemiological studies across the world.

Table 19.1 summarizes key manifestations and management principles of these rare conditions.

19.6 Conclusion

Musculoskeletal manifestations of amyloidosis and SCD indicate poorly controlled and progressive underlying disease whereas arthritis robustus and JA do not necessarily correspond to primary disease activity. An understanding of these conditions in a busy clinic saves precious time for diagnosis and resources which may otherwise generate a long and exhaustive list of investigations. There is a need of increasing awareness about these rare conditions among medical professionals to decrease the chances of incorrect diagnosis. A clear and concise explanation to patients also decreases their anxiety as there is a lack of patient support resources for these uncommon conditions.

References

1. Elsaman AM, Radwan AR, Akmatov MK, Della Beffa C, Walker A, Mayer CT, Dai L, Nativ S, Rygg M, Atsali E, Saijo K, Ogdie AR, Srinivasulu N, Fathi N, Schumacher HR, Pessler F. Amyloid arthropathy associated with multiple myeloma: a systematic analysis of 101 reported cases. Semin Arthritis Rheum. 2013;43(3):405–12.
2. Prokaeva T, Spencer B, Kaut M, et al. Soft tissue, joint, and bone manifestations of AL amyloidosis: clinical presentation, molecular features, and survival. Arthritis Rheum. 2007;56:3858–68.
3. M'Bappé P, Grateau G. Osteo-articular manifestations of amyloidosis. Best Pract Res Clin Rheumatol. 2012;26(4):459–75.
4. Pessler F, Ogdie AR, Mayer CT, et al. Amyloid arthropathy associated with multiple myeloma: polyarthritis without synovial infiltration of CD20+ or CD38+ cells. Amyloid. 2014;21(1):28–34. https://doi.org/10.3109/13506129.2013.862229.
5. Pruzanski W, Baron M, Shupak R. Neuroarthropathy (Charcot joints) in familial amyloid poly-neuropathy. J Rheumatol. 1981;8(3):477–81.
6. Khoo HW, Ding CSL, Tandon AA. Radiologic findings in polyarticular amyloid arthropathy and myopathy in multiple myeloma: a case report. Am J Case Rep. 2018;19:1398–404. Published 2018 Nov 24. https://doi.org/10.12659/AJCR.911212.
7. Garg A, Kumar P, Rao RN, Kashyap R. Myeloma-associated amyloid arthropathy masquerading as seronegative arthritis. South Asian J Cancer. 2020;9(1):37. https://doi.org/10.4103/sajc.sajc_235_19.
8. Patel SN, Koyoda SK, Schwartz D, Ayesha B. Severe hand pain as an extracardiac manifestation of transthyretin amyloidosis. BMJ Case Rep. 2019;12(10):e229677. Published 2019 Oct 23. https://doi.org/10.1136/bcr-2019-229677.
9. Adesina OO, Neumayr LD. Osteonecrosis in sickle cell disease: an update on risk factors, diagnosis, and management. Hematology Am Soc Hematol Educ Program. 2019;6(1):351–8.
10. da Silva Junior GB, Daher Ede F, da Rocha FA. Osteoarticular involvement in sickle cell disease. Rev Bras Hematol Hemoter. 2012;34(2):156–64. https://doi.org/10.5581/1516-8484.20120036.
11. Milner PF, Kraus AP, Sebes JI, Sleeper LA, Dukes KA, Embury SH, Bellevue R, Koshy M, Moohr JW, Smith J. Sickle cell disease as a cause of osteonecrosis of the femoral head. N Engl J Med. 1991;325(21):1476–81.
12. Hernigou P, Hernigou J, Scarlat M. Shoulder osteonecrosis: pathogenesis, causes, clinical evaluation, imaging, and classification. Orthop Surg. 2020;12:1340–9.
13. Ejindu VC, Hine AL, Mashayekhi M, Shorvon PJ, Misra RR. Musculoskeletal manifestations of sickle cell disease. Radiographics. 2007;4:1005–21.
14. Salinas Cisneros G, Thein SL. Recent advances in the treatment of sickle cell disease. Front Physiol. 2020;11:435. Published 2020 May 20. https://doi.org/10.3389/fphys.2020.00435.
15. Santiago MB. Miscellaneous non-inflammatory musculoskeletal conditions. Jaccoud's arthropathy. Best Pract Res Clin Rheumatol. 2011;25(5):715–25.
16. van Vugt RM, Derksen RH, Kater L, Bijlsma JW. Deforming arthropathy or lupus and rhupus hands in systemic lupus erythematosus. Ann Rheum Dis. 1998;57(9):540–4.
17. Quintana R, Pons-Estel G, Roberts K, Sacnún M, Berbotto G, Garcia MA, Saurit V, Barile-Fabris L, Acevedo-Vazquez EM, Tavares Brenol JC, Sato EI, Iglesias A, Uribe O, Alarcon G,

Pons-Estel BA. Jaccoud's arthropathy in SLE: findings from a Latin American multiethnic population. Lupus Sci Med. 2019;6(1):e000343.

18. Santiago M. Jaccoud-type lupus arthropathy: practical classification criteria. Lupus Sci Med. 2020;7(1):e000405. https://doi.org/10.1136/lupus-2020-000405.

19. Santiago M, Machicado V. Images in clinical medicine. Jaccoud's arthropathy. N Engl J Med. 2015;373(1):e1.

20. de Haas WH, de Boer W, Griffioen F, et al. Rheumatoid arthritis, typus robustus. Ann Rheum Dis. 1973;32(1):91–2.

21. Prasad K, Rath D, Kundu BK. Arthritis robustus: review of a case of an "abnormal" rheumatoid. Springerplus. 2014;3:606.

22. Sweeney SE, Harris ED, Firestein GS. Clinical features of rheumatoid arthritis. In: Firestein GS, Budd RC, Gabriel SE, McInnes IB, O'Dell JR, editors. Kelley's textbook of rheumatology, vol. 2. 9th ed. Philadelphia: Elsevier Saunders; 2013. p. 1112.

Index

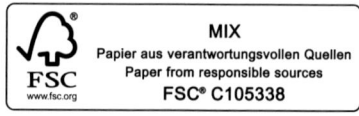